Fundamentals of
Medical Practice
Management

Fundamentals of
Medical Practice
Management

STEPHEN L. WAGNER

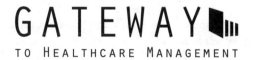

GATEWAY

TO HEALTHCARE MANAGEMENT

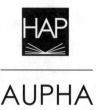

HAP

AUPHA

Health Administration Press, Chicago, Illinois
Association of University Programs in Health Administration, Washington, DC

Library of Congress Cataloging-in-Publication Data

Names: Wagner, Stephen L., 1951– author.
Title: Fundamentals of medical practice management / Stephen L. Wagner,
    Gateway to Healthcare Management.
Description: Chicago, Illinois : Health Administration Press ; Washington, DC
    : Association of University Programs in Health Administration, [2018] |
    Includes bibliographical references.
Identifiers: LCCN 2017026787 (print) | LCCN 2017025405 (ebook) | ISBN
    9781567939316 (ebook) | ISBN 9781567939323 (xml) | ISBN 9781567939330
    (epub) | ISBN 9781567939347 (mobi) | ISBN 9781567939309 (print : alk. paper)
Subjects: LCSH: Medicine—Practice. | Medical offices—Management.
Classification: LCC R728 (print) | LCC R728 .W25 2018 (ebook) | DDC
    610.68—dc23
LC record available at https://lccn.loc.gov/2017026787

The paper used in this publication meets the minimum requirements of American National Standard for Information Sciences—Permanence of Paper for Printed Library Materials, ANSI Z39.48-1984. ⊚ ™

Acquisitions editor: Jennette McClain; Project manager: Joyce Dunne; Cover designer: James Slate; Layout: PerfecType

Found an error or a typo? We want to know! Please e-mail it to hapbooks@ache.org, mentioning the book's title and putting "Book Error" in the subject line.

For photocopying and copyright information, please contact Copyright Clearance Center at www.copyright.com or (978) 750-8400.

Health Administration Press
A division of the Foundation
    of the American College of
    Healthcare Executives
One North Franklin Street
Suite 1700
Chicago, IL 60606-3529
(312) 424-2800

Association of University Programs
    in Health Administration
1730 M Street, NW
Suite 407
Washington, DC 20036
(202) 763-7283

This book is dedicated to my family—Cindy, Matthew, Elizabeth, and Charles.

BRIEF CONTENTS

DETAILED CONTENTS

PREFACE

We are here to make another world.

—W. Edwards Deming

The practice of medicine is one of the oldest and most honorable of professions, but it is facing a revolution that is unprecedented. Navigating this revolution will require skilled and well-prepared practice managers and leaders.

In many ways, the opening quote to this section of the book exemplifies the intention of this text and the current state of medical practice management as a field. Deming, widely considered the father of the quality revolution, often said understanding the "why," not simply the "what," of our work is essential to provide superior services and performance. I had the good fortune to learn from Deming and experience firsthand the foundations of quality management. Through this experience, I gleaned many important insights about the operation of successful practices. Many years have passed since I realized the profound impact of this experience, but Deming's teachings are more relevant today than ever before. Much of his approach has been repackaged for today's industries, but the basis of its truths lies in the tenets Deming demonstrated decades ago.

The true meaning and philosophy of quality and performance excellence get lost in the details of targets, processes, and tools. The details do not replace wisdom or developing an appreciation for what it means to demonstrate excellence and be guided by quality principles. Simply documenting the "right" targets and adopting the right tools is not enough to succeed; process without purpose is pointless. We need to focus less on the completion of discrete functions and more on understanding that function's purpose so that we can know how to improve it. To that end, education for practice managers must incorporate development of deep knowledge of healthcare delivery by the medical practice and its processes. Additionally, today's practice manager must recognize and embrace the need for change in the healthcare industry to provide the care patients need and deserve.

Practice management encompasses a broad range of activities. In large practice organizations, the manager may have responsibility for a narrow range of functions, but many practices are small organizations, in which the management must assume multiple roles. These may include all aspects of operating the enterprise, much like the responsibilities of a small-business owner. So, although practice managers indeed have a lot of "how-to" to learn, this book is more than a how-to text; it is intended to encourage the reader to think about why medical practice managers do what they do and how the roles of other stakeholders interplay with the manager's. How-to textbooks in healthcare become obsolete almost before they are published because the facts are constantly changing. To maintain their relevance, healthcare management texts must also teach when to carry out the tasks and process and why they should be done. Above all else, healthcare education books should emphasize, "First, do the right thing, and then, do it correctly," not unlike the often-repeated words of the Hippocratic Oath, "First, do no harm."

This text focuses on fundamental concepts and knowledge essential to manage, lead, and develop the wisdom to make the changes needed in medical practices to ensure a prosperous and sustainable future. Using strategies that are good for all stakeholders is necessary because healthcare must pose a value proposition for patients and society. This book is ambitious in its coverage of the field and does not assume the reader has prior knowledge of practice management; however, it may not cover particular topics to the depth that some may wish. A book covering every topic applicable to the healthcare administrator would span many volumes.

Although this text discusses many practical topics, from contract law to information technology, its primary focus is on people. We live in a time of diminished emotional, societal, and economic returns from quick-fix accommodations and processes. John Nash recognized this trend in his Nobel Prize–winning research on game theory: Cooperation is often better than competition for all to achieve their objects (Kuhn et al. 1994). This text aims to demonstrate that working together and putting people first is the best way to be successful in healthcare.

As noted in the first chapter, most people agree that the US medical delivery system needs to change, requiring strong, intelligent leaders and managers with a will to see a better future come to fruition. As Ian Malcolm said to John Hammond in the movie *Jurassic Park*, "Your scientists were so preoccupied with whether they could do it that they didn't stop to think if they should" (Spielberg 1993). This dialogue sums up much of what has happened in the practice of medicine over the past several decades. The industry has responded to short-term incentives and fragmented laws, rules, programs, and policies without a clear, unified strategy for the entire healthcare system. Most segments of US healthcare have worked to serve their own interests, so past policies, regulations, advocacy efforts, and so on have made sense from that narrow point of view (Heineman and Froemke 2012). That time has passed.

Due to all the challenges facing the healthcare system, change is essential to the future of the medical practice. Furthermore, practices need to lead that change, not follow the unsatisfactory solutions offered by those who know less about the care of patients than practice managers, staff, and clinicians. The modern practice manager and leader must have courage and the ability to see beyond the immediate and the expedient to do what is necessary for the long-term viability of healthcare practices. Courage is required to face the numerous challenges confronted at every turn without taking the easy route.

To quote one final thought from Deming (2016), "A bad system will beat a good person every time." The objective of this text is to not only provide knowledge but also to change the reader's mind-set about the action, attitude, and fortitude necessary for a new era of practice management to emerge.

REFERENCES

Deming Institute. 2016. "It's Time for a Systems View of Your Organization." Accessed April 13, 2017. https://deming.org/past-events/2016/leading-with-a-systems-view-may.

Heineman, M., and S. Froemke (directors). 2012. *Escape Fire: The Fight to Rescue American Healthcare*. Documentary film. Aisle C Productions and Our Time Projects.

Kuhn, H. W., J. C. Harsanyi, R. Selten, J. W. Weibull, E. van Damme, J. C. Nash Jr., and P. Hammerstein. 1994. "The Work of John C. Nash in Game Theory." Published December 8. www.nobelprize.org/nobel_prizes/economic-sciences/laureates/1994/nash-lecture.pdf.

Spielberg, S. (director). 1993. *Jurassic Park*. Motion picture. Universal Pictures and Amblin Entertainment.

ACKNOWLEDGMENTS

I would like to acknowledge the help of Elizabeth A. Wagner, PhD. As a professional writer and educator, she proofread the early draft of the text and gave valuable suggestions and insights.

CHAPTER 1

THE ORIGINS AND HISTORY OF MEDICINE AND MEDICAL PRACTICE

Not everything that counts can be counted, and not everything that can be counted counts.

—William Bruce Cameron

LEARNING OBJECTIVES

➤ Appreciate the history of medical practice.

➤ Explore the eight domains of medical practice management.

➤ Understand the forces of change affecting medical practice.

➤ Develop a perspective on the changes affecting medical practice.

➤ Understand the importance of the medical practitioner.

INTRODUCTION

Healthcare tends to be an accurate barometer of US society. Consider that virtually every aspect of social dysfunction, or of the human enterprise in general, becomes intertwined with the healthcare system. Most of the US population is born in a hospital, and many die there. The healthcare system is a place of joy and sorrow, hope and despair. The importance of the health system is hard to overstate, and the role that the medical providers play is a key factor in how the future system of care will take shape. This near-universal involvement with the healthcare system of virtually every person makes healthcare an accurate barometer of our society.

Often, the physician practice is the first line of care delivery, and for many patients, the physician provides the longitudinal care that sustains health and well-being (DiMatteo 1998). Therefore, the medical practice is a fundamental component of the healthcare delivery system, making the management and leadership of the medical practice a key to reforming that system. Because the physician practice is often the entry point for most patients into the healthcare system, in many ways it embodies the challenges of practice management, and the choices made to overcome these challenges may be endless and require achieving a careful balance of the art and the science of management.

This balance requires what W. Edwards Deming, the father of modern quality management, referred to as "profound knowledge," as well as the expertise to know when and how to use it (Deming Institute 2016). Deming's concept of profound knowledge is based in systems theory. It holds that every organization is composed of four main interrelated components, people, and processes, which depend on management to carefully orchestrate this interaction:

- ◆ Appreciation of a system
- ◆ Theory of knowledge
- ◆ Psychology of change
- ◆ Knowledge about variation

How do we keep up with the rapidly changing environment of healthcare in this new era? What metrics do we use, and what do we ignore? This journey demands that we answer these and more questions to bring about change in our healthcare system. It requires the full engagement of the provider community if meaningful and lasting change is to occur. Once change is effected, a new paradigm of care delivery will require a new mind-set that moves the industry from healthcare as the goal of the US healthcare system to well-being (Gawande 2014, 2016). Although health is critical to overall well-being, it is not the only issue. This text provides technical information on the management of the medical practice, but it also offers insight into necessary new skill sets providers and other healthcare leaders must have and roles they must play to create a paradigm of sustainable care for the future to optimize well-being as well as health.

LIFELONG LEARNING

Practice management is changing rapidly in response to the ever-changing landscape of healthcare and the medical practice. Practice managers need to be committed to lifelong learning and be active in our professional organizations to ensure they are up-to-date on current knowledge.

The Medical Group Management Association (MGMA), with its academic arm, the American College of Medical Practice Executives (ACMPE), is the premier practice management education and networking group for practice managers. The organization dates back to 1926 and represents more than 33,000 administrators and executives in 18,000 healthcare organizations in which 385,000 physicians practice. MGMA (2016a) has been instrumental in advancing the knowledge of practice management, and ACMPE offers a rigorous **certification** program in practice management that is widely recognized in the industry.

ACMPE has identified eight areas that are essential for the practice manager to understand (exhibit 1.1).

This text examines each of these domains of the practice management body of knowledge to provide a sound, fundamental base for practice managers and practice leaders. It includes a comprehensive overview that does not assume a great deal of prior education in the field of practice management. Furthermore, it seeks to provide not only specific information about the management of the medical practice but also context in the larger US healthcare system. Too often, different segments of the healthcare system see themselves as operating in isolation. This point of view must change if medical practices are to transform and if managers are to lead successful practices in the future, whether a small, free-standing practice or a large practice integrated with a major healthcare system.

Another prominent organization for the education and advancement of practice management is the American College of Healthcare Executives (ACHE). ACHE is a professional organization of more than 40,000 US and international healthcare executives who

Certification
A voluntary system of standards that practitioners meet to demonstrate accomplishment or ability in their profession. Certification standards are generally set by nongovernmental agencies or associations.

Business operations	Financial management
Human resource management	Information management
Organizational governance	Patient care systems
Quality management	Risk management

Source: MGMA (2016b).

EXHIBIT 1.1
The Eight Domains of the Body of Knowledge for Practice Managers

lead healthcare systems, hospitals, and other healthcare organizations. Currently with 78 chapters, ACHE offers board certification in healthcare management as a Fellow of ACHE, a highly regarded designation for healthcare management professionals (ACHE 2016).

THE AMERICAN HEALTHCARE SYSTEM

The practice of medicine drives the US healthcare system and its components, and medicine is heavily influenced by the system as well. Medical practice and the healthcare system both are built on the foundation of the physician–patient relationship. Although the percentage of total healthcare costs attributed to physicians and other clinical practitioners was 20 percent in 2015, the so-called clinician's pen, representing the prescribing and referral power of medical practice clinicians, indirectly accounts for most healthcare system costs. Administrators do not prescribe medication, admit patients, or order tests and services. This fact is just one illustration of a fragmented system whose segments can act independently. This fragmentation must be addressed if medical practices are to provide high-quality healthcare to patients at the lowest cost possible.

To begin our study of practice management, the book first offers some perspective of medical practices in terms of the overall US healthcare system. A complete history of the practice of medicine is beyond the scope of this text, but the lengthy and enduring nature of medical practice is important to recognize. The first known mention of the practice of medicine is from the Old Kingdom of Ancient Egypt, dating back to about 2600 BC. Later, the first known code of conduct, the Code of Hammurabi, dealt with many aspects of human **behavior** and, most importantly for our study, established laws governing the practice of medicine. The first medical text was written about 250 years later (Nunn 2002).

Exhibit 1.2 provides a sample of some significant points in the development of the physician medical practice from ancient times to the present. The reader may wonder why such a diverse series of events is listed, ranging from the recognition of the first physician to the occurrence of natural disasters and terrorist acts. Medicine, whether directly or indirectly, influences virtually every aspect of human life. Events such as Hurricane Katrina, the 9/11 terrorist attacks, the emergence of the human immunodeficiency virus (HIV), and the Ebola virus outbreak have had major impacts on the healthcare system and physician practice. Before 9/11, medical practices thought little about emergency preparedness and management; such activities were seen as under the purview of government agencies. Until HIV was identified in 1983 as the cause of acquired immunodeficiency syndrome (AIDS), and reinforced by the Ebola crisis of 2014, medical practices spent few resources and little time thinking about deadly infectious disease and the potential for it to arrive from distant locales. A traveler can reach virtually any destination in the world within a 24-hour period, which is well within the incubation period of most infectious agents. Modern air travel has made the world of disease a single place, so practices must be mindful of patients' origins and travels.

Behavior
How an individual acts, especially toward others.

2600 BC	Imhotep, a famous doctor, is the first physician mentioned in recorded history. After his death he is worshiped as a god. (Hurry 1978)	**EXHIBIT 1.2** Selected Major Events in the History of Medicine and Medical Practice
1792–1750 BC	The Code of Hammurabi is written, establishing laws governing the practice of medicine. (Johns 2000)	
1500 BC	The Ebers Papyrus is the first known medical book. (Hinrichs'sche, Wreszinski, and Umschrift 1913)	
500 BC	Alcamaeon of Croton in Italy says that a body is healthy as long as it has the right balance of hot and cold, wet and dry. If the balance is upset, the body falls ill. (Jones 1979)	
460–370 BC	Hippocrates lives. He stresses careful observation and the importance of nutrition. (Jones 1868)	
384–322 BC	Aristotle lives. He says the body is made up of 4 humors or liquids: phlegm, blood, yellow bile, and black bile. (Greek Medicine.net 2016)	
130–200 AD	Roman doctor Galen lives. Over following centuries, his writings become very influential. (Sarton 1951)	
1100–1300 AD	Schools of medicine are founded in Europe. In the 13th century, barber-surgeons begin to work in towns. The church runs the only hospitals. (Cobban 1999; Rashdall 1895)	
1543	Andreas Vesalius publishes *The Fabric of the Human Body*. (Garrison and Hast 2014)	
1628	William Harvey publishes his discovery of how the blood circulates in the body. (Harvey 1993)	
1796	Edward Jenner invents vaccination against smallpox. (Winkelstein 1992)	
1816	Rene Laennec invents the stethoscope. (Roguin 2006)	
1847	Chloroform is used as an anesthetic by James Simpson. (Ball 1996)	
1865	Joseph Lister develops antiseptic surgery. (Bankston 2004)	
1870	The Medical Practice Act is passed. Licensure of physicians becomes a state function. (Stevens 1971)	
1876	The American Association of Medical Colleges is founded. (Coggeshall 1965)	
1880	Louis Pasteur invents a vaccine for chicken cholera. (Debré 2000)	

(continued on next page)

EXHIBIT 1.2
Selected Major
Events in the
History of
Medicine and
Medical Practice
(continued)

1895	Wilhelm Conrad Röntgen discovers X-rays. (Glasser 1933)
1910	The Abraham Flexner report on medical education is published. (Flexner 1910)
1928	Penicillin is discovered by Scottish scientist Alexander Fleming, and it is established that the drug can be used in medicine. (Ligon 2004)
1929	The first employer-sponsored health insurance is created at Baylor Teachers College as Blue Cross. (Buchmueller and Monheit 2009)
1931	The electron microscope is invented. (Palucka 2002)
1943	Willem Johan Kolff invents the first artificial kidney (dialysis) machine. (Heiney 2003)
1951	Epidemiology studies identify cigarette smoking as a cause of lung cancer. Sir Richard Doll is the first to make this link. (Keating 2009)
1953	Jonas Salk announces he has developed a vaccine for polio. (Koprowski 1960)
1953	The structure of DNA is determined. (Dahm 2008)
1965	Medicare and Medicaid are passed into Law. (Social Security Administration 2016)
1967	The first heart transplant is performed by Christiaan Barnard. (Barnard 2011)
1971	MRI scanning is invented. (Lauterbur 1973)
1973	The HMO Act is passed. (Dorsey 1975)
1989	President George W. Bush signs the Omnibus Budget Reconciliation Act of 1989, enacting a physician payment schedule based on a resource-based relative value scale. (AMA 2017)
1996	The Health Insurance Portability and Accountability Act is passed as an amendment to the HMO Act. (Atchinson and Fox 1997)
2001	The 9/11 terrorist attacks occur. (Bernstein 2003)
2003	The human genome is sequenced. (National Human Genome Research Institute 2010)
2005	Hurricane Katrina devastates the Gulf Coast, including New Orleans. (Knabb, Rhome, and Brown 2005)
2008	The Triple Aim for healthcare delivery is proposed by the Institute for Healthcare Improvement. (Berwick, Nolan, and Whittington 2008)

2008	Medicare Part D is enacted. (Hargrave et al. 2007)
2010	The Affordable Care Act is passed. (HHS 2010)
2012	High-deductible health plans become more common. (Bundorf 2012)
2014	The Ebola crisis emerges in West Africa. (CDC 2016b)
2016	Zika virus becomes a serious health threat. (CDC 2016c; Wang and Barry 2016)

EXHIBIT 1.2
Selected Major Events in the History of Medicine and Medical Practice *(continued)*

The evolution of medical practices has coincided with and been driven in part by the development of medical technology and the scientific revolution. Medicine was limited in scope and primitive until the middle of the nineteenth century. Theories of disease were arcane, and diagnostic tools were largely absent (Rosenberg and Vogel 1979). Prior to 1850, medical education constituted an apprenticeship that was inconsistent and poorly preceptored, with no standard curriculum (Rothstein 1972). Procedures focused on expelling the disease with bleedings and emetics. Surgery was limited because of the lack of anesthesia, and as a result, being fast was better than being good. Patients often directed the physician as to the care they should receive. One might say early medical practice was the first iteration of patient-centered care (Burke 1985).

PRACTICE MANAGEMENT RESOURCES

Now, however, the amount of information available about medicine and medical practice management is virtually endless, representing many points of view; ideas; political world views; notions about funding and access; and the numerous disciplines in the broader management field, such as **accounting**, finance, human resources management, organization development, and logistics. With the vast expanse of knowledge available, students of healthcare and practice management are encouraged to develop lifelong learning skills. The field is changing so rapidly that the need for continuous updating of knowledge and skills is essential.

Accounting
A system for keeping score in business, using dollars.

For example, practice managers need to build a virtual library of accurate and reliable sources. The list that follows comprises the foundation of that library, which should be referred to frequently (see the appendix to this text for each resource's website):

◆ Centers for Medicare & Medicaid Services (CMS)

◆ Advisory Board

◆ Dartmouth Atlas

◆ National Committee for Quality Assurance

◆ Institute for Healthcare Improvement

◆ Institute of Medicine

◆ Institute for Health Policy and Innovation

◆ Kaiser Family Foundation

◆ Robert Wood Johnson Foundation

◆ Annenberg Foundation

◆ Commonwealth Fund

◆ Centers for Disease Control and Prevention

◆ Agency for Healthcare Research and Quality

THE DIMENSIONS OF MEDICAL PRACTICE

Medical practices can take many forms, ranging from small sole proprietorships to large multispecialty medical practices. Recent years have seen more medical practices embedded in large healthcare organizations, which also may be solo practices or large multispecialty entities (see exhibit 1.3).

    A group practice is defined as a medical practice consisting of two or more practitioners working in a common management and administrative structure. Single-specialty groups are those that focus on one aspect of medicine, such as general surgery, family practice, orthopedics, cardiology, or internal medicine. Multispecialty medical groups contain more than one medical specialty in the organization. Multispecialty practices are highly integrated, with a common **governance** leadership and common management structure, and they have a highly developed corporate system for managing finances and dealing with regulatory agencies. Their operation and function are much more complex than those of solo or small practices.

    Integrated delivery systems (IDSs) are networks of healthcare organizations under a single holding company or parent organization that contain multiple components of healthcare delivery. An IDS often includes hospitals, physicians and other clinicians, and payment organizations, often referred to as third-party payer organizations. The **goal** is to provide as complete a continuum of care as possible.

Governance
A system of policies and procedures designed to facilitate oversight of the management of the enterprise. Serves as the foundation of how the practice will behave, compete, and document its actions.

Goal
A specific target that an individual or a company tries to achieve.

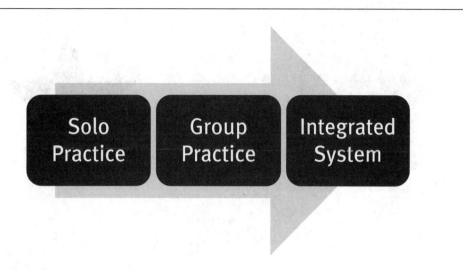

EXHIBIT 1.3
Practice
Structures—Simple
to Complex

TYPES OF PRACTITIONERS

Physicians have, of course, played a pivotal role in the US healthcare system since its inception. Physicians—and now, other nonphysician providers such as nurse practitioners (discussed later)—care for patients by

◆ assessing the patient's health status,

◆ diagnosing the patient's condition, and

◆ prescribing and performing treatment.

It has been said that the most expensive instrument in the healthcare industry is the provider's pen. An amusing statement, it also carries a lot of truth because all diagnostic and surgical procedures as well as office-based and hospital-based assessments—in fact, all care in general—is either performed or ordered by a provider.

Furthermore, the medical practice is unlike any other organization in the medical field because the nature and identity of the practice is closely linked to the individual providers in the practice. The providers are the primary producers and the primary governance body, and they are held accountable for the performance of the practice in a personal way. Their income is directly tied to the practice's performance, more closely than for other medical field workers. Exhibit 1.4 shows the fundamental components of a medical practice.

Often, the challenge in practice management is to serve the interests of the providers while maintaining a focus on the patient, with patient focus being the True North of the practice.

Exhibit 1.4
The Practice
Management
Model

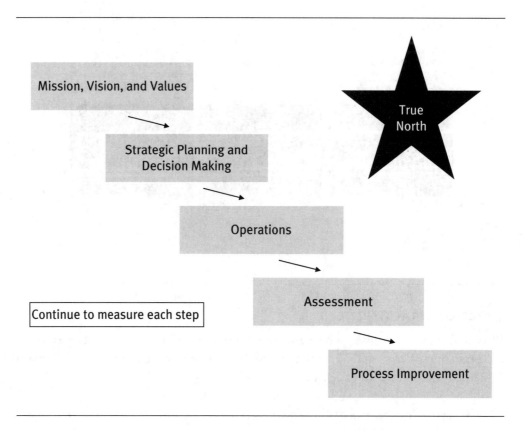

"True North" is a concept taken from Lean management that embodies the ideal state of a practice, its providers' vision of perfection, and the type and quality of practice it should strive to achieve every day. True North should transcend the individual and his or her personal goals or actions. Achieving personal objectives is not mutually exclusive but coincidental with True North.

Exhibit 1.5 shows the number of physicians practicing in the United States. This number can be further broken down into the number of practices by size and multispecialty versus single specialty, as shown in exhibit 1.6. Note the increasing size of practices over time, a trend that is expected to continue.

Exhibit 1.5
Total Active
Physicians in the
United States,
April 2017

Primary Care Physicians	Specialist Physicians	Total
443,962	479,346	923,308

Source: Kaiser Family Foundation (2017).

Number of Physicians in Practice	Single-Specialty Practice	Multispecialty Practice
1	1.5%	0.3%
2 to 4	42.0%	13.8%
5 to 10	31.7%	20.8%
11 to 24	13.7%	17.2%
25 to 49	6.7%	11.1%
50+	4.5%	36.9%
Total	100%	100%
N	1,452	836

EXHIBIT 1.6
Distribution of Single- and Multispecialty Physicians by Practice Size, 2014

Source: Kane (2014).

A primary care physician (PCP) is often the first contact for a patient with an undiagnosed health concern. In addition, PCPs frequently provide continuing care for many medical conditions that are not limited by cause, organ system, or diagnosis. This purview of practice differs from that of a medical specialist, who has completed advanced education and clinical training in a specific area of medicine and typically focuses on the diagnosis and treatment of one organ system of the body and its diseases.

Nurse practitioners and physician assistants are a growing segment of medical service provider, as seen in exhibit 1.7. A physician assistant (PA) is a nationally certified and state-licensed medical professional. PAs practice medicine with physicians and other providers and are allowed to prescribe medication in all 50 states, the District of Columbia, the majority of US territories, and the uniformed services. A nurse practitioner (NP) is a registered nurse qualified, through advanced training, to assume some of the duties and responsibilities of a physician.

PAs and NPs are sometimes referred to as advanced practice professionals or mid-level providers; however, the term *mid-level provider* is considered obsolete.

State laws vary as to the specific duties PAs and NPs are allowed to perform, so the practice manager must be fully informed on these regulations.

Advanced practice professionals are becoming increasingly important to medical practices because they can replace physicians in care delivery for many services, reserving the physician for more complex care requiring their expertise. For example, PAs and NPs often work as part of a care team with physicians. They may examine the patient first; collect facts and findings; and then, in collaboration with the physician, make a diagnosis

Provider Type	Total	Percent Primary Care	Practicing Primary Care
Nurse practitioners	106,073	52.0%	55,625
Physician assistants	70,383	43.4%	30,402

Source: AHRQ (2011).

and develop a treatment plan. The physician supervises the process and conducts his or her own examination of the patients to ensure that the proper care is delivered. The physician often checks critical elements of the exam and establishes a relationship with the patient. The PA or NP typically follows up with the patient once the treatment plan is established.

PRACTICE OWNERSHIP

In addition to the area of medicine practiced, physician practices can be classified by type of ownership. Exhibit 1.8 shows the distribution of medical practices by ownership. Note the trend—also expected to continue—toward practice ownership by hospitals and healthcare systems.

LICENSING PHYSICIANS

All 50 states require physicians and medical providers to hold a license. The licensing of medical providers is performed under the auspices of a medical examining board. These boards have the right to grant a license to practice medicine and the responsibility to investigate and discipline providers in cases of inappropriate conduct.

These licenses provide the practitioner a general right and privilege to practice medicine, but they usually do not grant specific privileges to practice a particular medical specialty. This activity is beyond the scope of **licensure** and typically is conducted by the hospital or hospitals at which the physician or advanced practice provider delivers care.

Licensure
A mandatory system of state-imposed standards that practitioners must meet to practice a given profession.

The licensing process includes a thorough, painstaking review and verification of the training and experience the physician or provider has received. Criminal background checks and reviews of the National Practitioner Data Bank (NPDB) are conducted in this process. The NPDB contains documentation of any disciplinary acts leveled against the physician, malpractice settlements, and other practice restrictions the physician may have received.

Reciprocity, or the reciprocal granting of a medical license by states based on licensing of the provider in another state, has become a thing of the past because of concerns

	2012	2014
At least some hospital ownership	23.4%	25.6%
Wholly owned by hospital	14.7%	15.6%
Jointly owned, physicians and hospital	6.0%	7.3%
Unknown whether wholly or jointly owned	2.6%	2.7%
Direct hospital employee	5.6%	7.2%
Not-for-profit	6.5%	6.4%
Other	4.4%	4.0%
Total	100%	100%
N	3,466	3,500

EXHIBIT 1.8
Distribution of Physicians by Practice Ownership Structure, 2012 and 2014

Source: Kane (2014).

that practitioners with a poor record or history of committing fraud can simply cross state lines and begin anew.

Licensure should not be confused with certification. Many medical specialties offer special recognition through board certification, which indicates the practitioner has acquired additional, specific training and testing in an area of medicine (see exhibit 1.9). Contrary to licensure, the absence of board certification by itself does not prohibit a physician from practicing in a medical specialty in most states.

MEDICAL TRAINING

According to the American Association of Medical Colleges (AAMC 2016), 145 accredited US and 17 accredited Canadian medical schools; nearly 400 major teaching hospitals and health systems, including 51 US Department of Veterans Affairs medical centers; and more than 80 academic societies offer medical education. In addition, the American Association of Colleges of Osteopathic Medicine (AACOM 2016) reports that 31 colleges of osteopathic medicine are in operation. Although both are fully licensed physicians in the United States and very similar in many respects, doctors of osteopathy (DOs), or osteopaths, differ from medical doctors (MDs) in the educational path they take for their medical education. DOs

Exhibit 1.9

Partial List of
Medical Specialties

Allergies and immunology	Anesthesiology	Cardiology
Dermatology	Emergency medicine	Genetics
Gerontology	Gynecology	Hematology
Internal medicine	Neurology	Obstetrics
Oncology	Otolaryngology	Palliative care and hospice
Pathology	Pediatrics and related subspecialties	Preventive medicine
Primary care practice	Psychiatry	Radiation oncology
Radiology	Surgery and related subspecialties	Urology

attend osteopathic medical schools, and MDs attend allopathic medical schools. Each type of school teaches the diagnosis and treatment of disease, but the disciplines vary somewhat in philosophy, with the osteopathic approach focusing more on a holistic view of human disease and treatment. Also worth noting is that DOs often complete their postgraduate training in allopathic residencies and fellowships, which further reduces the distinction between the two types of physician.

Among them, these organizations employ more than 128,000 faculty members, educate 83,000 medical students, and host 110,000 resident physicians (AAMC 2016).

What Is Changing?

The Conundrum

Three fundamental aspects of practice management and care delivery are important to focus on in any discussion of medical practice: high quality, high access, and low cost.

Economists may argue that a practice can succeed as a business with any two of those three components, for instance, high quality and a high level of access, where cost is not low. Indeed, economic theory holds that a business cannot achieve all three simultaneously. However, medical practices must achieve each to be an effective and high-quality practice.

Consider that in some countries, to limit healthcare costs, a concern around the world, their healthcare systems limit access. For example, delays are seen with hip replacements, knee replacements, and even some essential surgeries. In the United States, these procedures can be undertaken almost immediately. But healthcare costs for care and treatment are much higher than in other countries. Thus, one job of the practice manager and leader is to maximize or optimize the relationship between cost, access, and quality (see exhibit 1.10).

SOCIAL CHANGE

As US society has changed, so has the practice of medicine. In social terms, the country has moved from a time when information about health and our healthcare was the sole purview of the medical professional to a time when individuals have access to an enormous amount of information. The Internet has had a profound impact on healthcare. Patients are now able to read about virtually any condition, diagnosis, or treatment, and in many cases, they make judgments about what option is in their best interest.

Patients also have demonstrated new, or renewed, interest in alternative forms of healthcare. A variety of terms are associated with alternative medicine, including *complementary medicine* and *integrative medicine*. Complementary and alternative medicine (CAM) modalities include acupuncture, energy therapies, magnetic field therapies, therapeutic touch, Reiki, Ayurvedic medicine, herbal medicine, and Chinese medicine, to name a few.

The effectiveness of these therapies has been demonstrated to varying degrees, but Americans spent more than $33.9 billion in 2007 on CAM products and services, according to a National Institutes of Health survey conducted by the National Center for

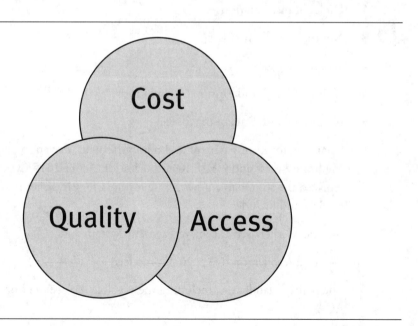

EXHIBIT 1.10
The Practice
Conundrum

Complementary and Integrative Health (2009). These findings indicate that patients are seeking solutions that suit their healthcare needs better than traditional medicine does.

What Are Some of Today's Challenges?

To develop an appreciation for some of the important changes and challenges facing medical practice, this section touches on a few important issues, including the following:

◆ The cost of care

◆ The Patient Protection and Affordable Care Act of 2010 (ACA)

◆ Health policy issues, such as changes to Medicare and Medicaid

◆ Changing disease burden and rise of chronic disease

◆ Lack of a coordinated system of care

◆ Rising consumerism and patient-centered care

◆ Patient safety and quality concerns

◆ Demographic changes in the population

◆ Rapidly changing technologies and treatments

◆ Digital transformation

◆ Nontraditional providers

◆ Workforce issues

◆ Uninsured and underinsured populations

◆ Financial constraints of practices

◆ Changing forms of payment and reimbursement, driven in part by the Medicare Access and CHIP Reauthorization Act of 2015 (MACRA), which replaced the sustainable growth rate formula for physician reimbursement for services and includes

— the Merit-Based Incentive Payment System and

— advanced alternative payment models

◆ The political landscape, including the possible replacement or repeal of the ACA

THE PERFECT STORM

The "perfect storm" metaphor describes the coalescing of multiple events to create dramatic and unique consequences. Similar to the scenario depicted in a novel with this title by Sebastian Junger (2009), in which he describes a catastrophic storm off the coast of New Bedford, Massachusetts, some US healthcare observers would describe what is happening today in healthcare as a perfect storm. Elements of the perfect storm in the practice of medicine are shown in exhibit 1.11.

THE COST OF CARE

No factor has affected the sense of urgency to reform the US system of healthcare more than the cost. According to CMS (2015), US healthcare spending increased 5.3 percent to $3.0 trillion in 2014, or $9,523 per person. This growth was primarily the result of the coverage expansions under the ACA, particularly for Medicaid and private health insurance. Of course, the trend of rapidly increasing healthcare costs was seen long before the passage and enactment of the ACA: The share of the US economy devoted to healthcare spending was 17.5 percent, up from 17.3 percent in 2013 and almost 2.5 times that of other Western countries.

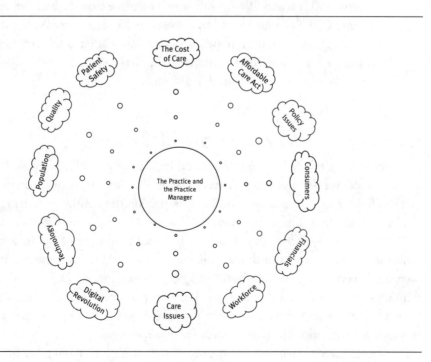

EXHIBIT 1.11
The Forces of Change Acting on Medical Practices: "The Perfect Storm"

The Institute of Medicine, a prestigious federal research and policy organization established in 1970 as part of the National Academy of Sciences, estimates that roughly a third of US healthcare dollars is wasted, amounting to between $700 and $800 billion. This enormous amount of waste is a result of unnecessary services, insufficient care that leads to readmissions and other repeat care, excess administrative costs, and increasing prices (IOM 2001). As one might expect, waste and the resulting excess expenditure in the US healthcare system is one area of tremendous criticism from many observers.

According to the Organisation for Economic Co-operation and Development (OECD 2015), an international economic group composed of 34 member nations based in Paris, the important factors that differentiate the US healthcare system from that of other countries are as follows:

◆ The United States has fewer physicians per capita than many other OECD countries have, at 2.4 practicing physicians per 1,000 people in 2010, below the OECD average of 3.1 practicing physicians per 1,000 people.

◆ The number of hospital beds in the United States was 2.6 per 1,000 people in 2009, whereas the OECD average was 3.4 beds.

◆ In the United States, life expectancy at birth increased by nearly nine years between 1960 and 2010, while it rose by more than 11 years on average in other OECD countries and by more than 15 years in Japan. In 2010, the average American lived to be 78.7 years—more than a full year below the average for other OECD countries. Cultural factors, lifestyle issues, and health habits play a role in this difference.

THE AFFORDABLE CARE ACT AND OTHER LEGISLATION

Since the passage of Medicare and Medicaid legislation in 1965, no other law has had a greater impact on the healthcare delivery system than the ACA. We discuss the ACA in detail in later chapters; here, we consider its impact on the healthcare system as well as the challenges and opportunities it brings.

The timeline shown in exhibit 1.2 includes a number of significant changes to healthcare regulations. As healthcare moved from a trade to a profession, its regulation increased. Every state now licenses the practice of medicine and enforces educational and training standards toward that end. Medical practices must comply with all regulations related to corporations and businesses in the state in which they operate and are subject to employment regulations by state and federal government.

Major pieces of legislation have been instrumental in shaping the direction of the practice of medicine in some important ways; they include the following:

◆   Corporate Practices Act

◆   Medicare and Medicaid legislation

◆   Balanced Budget Act of 1997, which created the resource-based relative value scale

◆   ACA

◆   MACRA

THE CHANGING DISEASE BURDEN AND THE RISE OF CHRONIC DISEASE

Disease Burden

Another significant issue facing the modern healthcare practice is how the burden of disease, or the impact of a health problem as measured by financial cost, mortality, morbidity, or other indicators, has changed and whether providers can keep up with these changes. In 1900, gastrointestinal infections, tuberculosis, pneumonia, and influenza were significant potential detriments to Americans' health and longevity. By 2010, however, cancer and heart disease became the major causes of mortality in the United States (Jones, Podolsky, and Greene 2012). Add to these conditions emerging diseases such as fibromyalgia and infections from the Zika virus—some of which may not have become known until recently—and the enormity of disease states medical practices must be equipped to treat is daunting.

The number of services provided in practice offices is substantial. Most individuals receive most of their care in a medical practice; the following statistics are just a sampling of the scale (NCHS 2015a):

◆   Number of drugs ordered or provided—2.6 billion

◆   Percentage of visits involving drug therapy—75.1 percent

◆   Most frequently prescribed therapeutic classes

   — Analgesics

   — Antihyperlipidemic agents

   — Antidepressants

◆   Percentage of persons using at least one prescription drug in the past 30 days—48.7 percent (2009–2012)

◆   Percentage of persons using three or more prescription drugs in the past 30 days—21.8 percent (2009–2012)

◆ Percentage of persons using five or more prescription drugs in the past 30 days—10.7 percent (2009–2012)

Chronic Disease

Almost half of US residents have at least one chronic condition, and more than 85 percent of those older than 65 have a chronic disease. As defined by the Centers for Disease Control and Prevention (CDC 2016a), chronic diseases are those that persist for three months or more. They generally cannot be prevented by vaccines or cured by medication, and they do not disappear spontaneously. Chronic disease is a major driver of cost because approximately 80 percent of healthcare resources expended are used by people with chronic conditions. Importantly, most of the treatment of these diseases occurs in the medical office setting.

According to the CDC (2016a), chronic diseases are responsible for seven out of ten deaths in the United States. Common chronic diseases include the following:

◆ Diabetes

◆ Heart disease

◆ Arthritis

◆ Kidney disease

◆ HIV/AIDS

◆ Lupus

◆ Multiple sclerosis

Because chronic disease cannot be cured, prevention is the key to reversing the cost, morbidity, and mortality trends currently seen in the healthcare system. Prevention is viewed as taking place in one of three levels:

1. Primary prevention seeks to avoid the onset of a disease using risk-reduction strategies such as altering behaviors or eliminating exposures that can lead to disease, or by enhancing resistance to the effects of exposure to a disease agent. An example of primary prevention is vaccination against flu.

2. Secondary prevention includes procedures that detect and treat so-called preclinical health status changes and controlling disease progression. An example of secondary prevention is mammography to detect early breast cancer.

3. Tertiary prevention reduces the impact of disease on the patient's functioning, longevity, and quality of life. An example of tertiary prevention is cardiac rehabilitation following a heart attack.

A Large and Growing Problem: The Number of People with Chronic Conditions

Boyle and colleagues (2001) projected a 165 percent increase in diabetes by 2050 to a prevalence of 7.2 percent of the population, affecting 29 million US residents. More recent evidence suggests those figures might be underestimations (CDC 2012). Unless that incidence curve is changed, US society will continue to see the devastating complications of this disease, including neuropathy (nerve damage), blindness, kidney failure, and heart disease.

Type 2 diabetes and many other chronic diseases are classified as "lifestyle diseases" because they are preventable and closely related to diet, exercise, and other lifestyle behaviors (Al-Maskari 2010).

In addition to causes such as obesity, observers expect to see a steady increase in the number of people with chronic conditions, in part because the US population is aging, and older people tend to have more chronic disease than younger people have.

Health-conscious behavior, including a focus on eating natural and chemical-free foods, has become a more popular way to combat chronic disease. Medicine has come a long way from the time of Hippocrates, but we are wise to remember what he said: "Let medicine be thy food and let food be thy medicine" (Lloyd 1950). That old wisdom must be reinserted into medical practice, at least to some degree.

LACK OF A COORDINATED SYSTEM OF CARE

The US healthcare system currently does not pay adequate attention to the continuum of health services and the continuum of care. As human beings, we have healthcare concerns starting before we are born and present or emerging all the way until the end of our lives. An effective system of care needs to reflect all the stages of one's life.

In particular, end-of-life care is an issue that lacks a coordinated model in the United States. Many observers consider that the US healthcare delivery system does not deal with end-of-life care well. For example, a significant amount of money is spent at the end of life for care that, in many cases, is at best futile and at worst harmful to the patient and his or her family.

A coordinated system of care also should be concerned with the determinants of health. Exhibit 1.12 shows some major factors that determine health status. Healthcare is a component, but many others are present. The increased focus on the determinants of health points to the need for medical practices to be aware of and attend to the other

EXHIBIT 1.12
Determinants of
Health

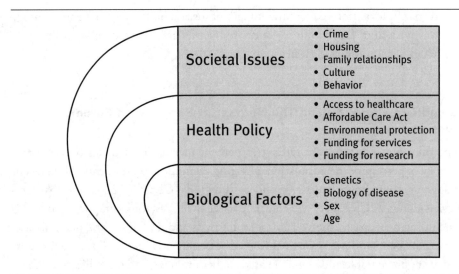

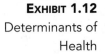

factors. Practices can do more in this area than they are currently; we discuss those ideas in later chapters.

RISING CONSUMERISM

An area of medical practice and healthcare in general that also has received regular attention recently is the experience of the patient and his or her family. In considering this issue, one must first distinguish between two primary modes of practice as they relate to patient care.

Provider-Directed Care

The first is provider-directed patient care. In this model, which has been practiced for decades in the United States, the provider makes the vast majority of decisions and determines the type and extent of care the patient receives.

One concern related to provider-directed care is that the patient may have little understanding about the treatment being received and, therefore, be less committed to complying with instructions. For provider-directed healthcare to result in satisfactory outcomes, a patient must have both the desire and the ability to comply with treatment recommendations; thus, his or her individual circumstances are very much a part of the treatment equation.

Patient-Centered Care

The second model is patient-centric healthcare. In this model, the patient and his or her family play a central role in conjunction with the provider (Jones 2014). The provider offers multiple options to the patient, all of which are medically acceptable, and the patient assumes greater decision-making responsibility regarding the approach to treatment.

Patient-centered care can be seen in decisions related to treating prostate cancer. Prostate cancer is often a slow-growing tumor. In fact, more than 80 percent of men older than age 80 have prostate cancer, but the disease has limited medical consequences in many of these cases. Due to the slow-advancing nature of prostate cancer, two viable approaches are considered for its treatment. One approach, known as watchful waiting, involves careful monitoring of the patient's condition whereby aggressive intervention is not undertaken until definitive signs indicate the cancer is growing. The second option is aggressive therapy. This approach may involve surgery, chemotherapy, or other forms of treatment.

The question is, which to choose? According to a study published in the *New England Journal of Medicine* (Bill-Axelson et al. 2014), the benefits of aggressive therapy were found to be highly dependent on the age of the patient and the type of prostate cancer. This finding gives enhanced credence to the notion of watchful waiting, which may also reduce unnecessary surgery, side effects, and cost.

One major initiative in population health management related to patient-centric care that involves the medical practice is the patient-centered medical home (PCMH).

The PCMH provides a starting place for the patient to receive all his or her nonemergency medical care. The model is characterized by 24/7 access to tightly coordinated care by a team of providers. Primary care is offered at the PCMH location, and other medical services are referred to specialists as appropriate (NCQA 2014).

Today, physicians are becoming increasingly patient centered. In addition to bringing the patient to the decision-making table, they are accommodating him or her in other ways, such as adopting alternate forms of communication, such as e-mail (Dalal et al. 2016).

PATIENT SAFETY AND QUALITY CONCERNS

In terms of patient safety and quality, the medical practice must ensure that it provides healthcare that meets the following standards (IOM 2001; AHRQ 2016):

◆ *Safe*—Protecting patients from being harmed by the care that is intended to help them. This goal includes the prevention of nosocomial infections, which are infections acquired in the hospital or healthcare setting; wrong-site surgery; medication errors; falls; and other harmful events.

◆ *Effective*—Providing services on the basis of scientific knowledge to all who can benefit and refraining from providing services to those not likely to benefit (i.e., avoiding underuse and misuse, respectively).

◆ *Patient centered*—Providing care that is respectful of and responsive to individual patient preferences, needs, and **values** and ensuring that patient values guide all clinical decisions.

◆ *Timely*—Reducing wait times for and eliminating harmful delays in care.

◆ *Efficient*—Avoiding waste, including waste of equipment, supplies, ideas, and energy.

◆ *Equitable*—Providing care that does not vary in quality because of personal patient characteristics such as race, gender, ethnicity, geographic location, and socioeconomic status.

Values
The beliefs and guidelines an individual uses to make choices when confronted with a situation.

DEMOGRAPHIC CHANGES

The Graying of America

The baby boom generation is retiring at the rate of about 10,000 people per day. In fact, the most rapidly growing segment of the US population is people older than age 85. US residents are living much longer than in the past, and as people age, they tend to need more healthcare. Although healthcare is a major contributor to longevity, it is not the only important contributor; other factors may have an even more significant impact on length of life (Nelson 2016). Only in the past 100 years has longevity been linked to healthcare. Before that time, life expectancy was largely determined by uncontrollable risk, such as infections, accidents, childbirth, starvation, and other similar events. For example, George Washington died from acute laryngitis, a condition that is easily treated today with an antibiotic (Knox 1933).

The graying of America will continue to be a significant issue for medical practices, as from age 65, on average, men and women will live almost 20 additional years (NCHS 2015b):

◆ Both sexes at 65 years—19.3 years of average additional life expectancy

◆ Men at 65 years—17.9 years of average additional life expectancy

◆ Women at 65 years—20.5 years of average additional life expectancy

CHANGES IN THE US POPULATION

The increase in immigration to the United States and the diversity of the population are major new considerations for medical practices. US providers encounter more languages, customs, and beliefs than in the past, making service to patients an increasing challenge. Mastering the nuances of diversity is essential for a modern practice to be successful.

RAPIDLY CHANGING TECHNOLOGIES AND RELATED TREATMENTS

The healthcare industry has seen a dramatic shift in the types and complexity of medical technology and the available treatments for patients. This unrelenting trend has led to commensurate complexity of care and increased cost, as well as the need for greater specialization in the delivery of services.

Digital Transformation and Nontraditional Providers

Not only have the science and technology of treatment changed, but the way healthcare is delivered is rapidly changing as well. A major transformational force in the medical practice has been the rise of digital media tools and the nontraditional provider who has been enabled by digital innovations.

Transformation often does not occur from within the industry being transformed, and healthcare is no exception. In 2015, more than 165,000 healthcare apps were available for smartphones and tablet computers, many of them targeted to the **ambulatory care** environment and most developed outside the healthcare industry (Terry 2015).

The medical practice must compete with entrants from the information technology industry, the retail pharmaceutical industry, the insurance industry, medical device companies, and Internet-based providers from around the world. The emergence of web-based providers has created a whole new mobile health industry known as mHealth.

The digital transformation of healthcare is not limited to the alternative delivery modes; it also has revolutionized the availability of information. One may consider this development to have a democratizing effect on healthcare, as information about virtually any condition, treatment, or procedure is available on the Internet. Like most innovations, it can carry both positive and negative consequences. Although a tremendous amount of information is available, this information is often of limited value unless it can be properly interpreted by a professional. A patient may be aware of information, but he or she may not understand it and certainly will not be able to apply it to the situation at hand.

Another major issue regarding Internet-based information is its accuracy. Physicians are often concerned that patients access information that is either misunderstood or, in some cases, blatantly inaccurate, which can cause difficulties in the physician–patient

Ambulatory care
Healthcare services provided to patients on an outpatient basis, rather than by admission to a hospital or another healthcare facility.

relationship. The patient may be skeptical of information provided by the physician because it conflicts with inaccurate information the patient obtained from another source and believes to be true. One solution to this problem is to provide patients with high-quality sources for Internet-based information about their condition and encourage them to obtain more detailed information. Therefore, the Internet can be an educational resource for the physician practice when proactively embraced and used properly.

WORKFORCE ISSUES

For the first time in US history, four generations of employees are in the workforce, and that workforce is becoming increasingly diverse in many other areas as well. These factors present unprecedented challenges, as each generation and ethnic group brings its own temperament; belief system; and preferences for structure, authority, and workplace inter-action (Knight 2014).

One issue that arises from intergenerational and ethnic diversity is that people tend to focus on differences instead of looking for similarities to forge collaborations and embrace new ideas. This is a key consideration, as the process of collaboration allows people to produce the best outcome possible.

How do we get multiple generations to work effectively in a collaborative fashion? Everyone has much to contribute and share, and practice managers must devise ways for the organizations to tap the power of diversity. One means to do so is to focus on the shared objective in light of the value each generation and group brings to the work environment. By making the most of our diverse workforce, practice managers and leaders can combine new concepts and innovations to solve problems together.

FINANCIAL CONSTRAINTS

By definition, constraints limit the scope, the time, or the quality of the product or service being provided. As resources are limited, decisions must be made in an effort to optimize the constraint relationship and thereby deliver optimum outcomes. Of course, financial resources are no different. Financial constraints limit the freedom to act and provide support for people and projects in the organization (Travis et al. 2004).

In a later chapter, we delve into the issues related to fighting financial constraints in more detail. Here, we consider the unique nature of healthcare financing as a source of concern for the practice manager. Although practices set their own fees, in most cases healthcare is paid for by so-called third-party payers, such as Medicare. Medicare establishes reimbursement limits for services, effectively setting the fees for the practice. Similarly, in the case of nongovernmental payers, such as insurance companies, fees may be negotiated, but negotiation is often limited by the size and market power of the practice. Small practices may be dealt with on a take-it-or-leave-it basis. Most enterprises have their actual payment rate or price established by external **stakeholders**; these represent a unique and challenging aspect of medical practice management.

> **Stakeholder**
> Individual or group that has a vested interest in the practice.

As in a society, practice managers and leaders must balance the ideal outcome with what is possible given that all resources are limited to some extent. Doing so requires a combination of personal responsibility and practice accountability.

LEADERSHIP CHALLENGES

The list of challenges discussed to this point is significant. To address them, medical practice leaders and managers must be adept at guiding change in their practice.

THE REIMBURSEMENT PARADIGM SHIFT

The paradigm of medical practice is currently experiencing a seismic shift. Most businesses and industries undergo transitions of their business and operational models over time as the environment of the industry changes. However, the current **paradigm shift** means medical practices will be paid differently than in the past, placing a lot of pressure on how practices adapt to other changes occurring in the healthcare system, such as the way medical care is delivered.

> **Paradigm shift**
> A change in the way a practice views its business.

What Happens to Organizations When a Paradigm Shift Occurs in an Industry?

A paradigm is the way stakeholders think an industry should behave—the model they hold in their mind. This model has a strong hold, like a set of strong beliefs; thus, changing a paradigm is difficult.

A paradigm shift is a major change in the way the world thinks about something. One example of a paradigm shift occurred in the photography industry when cameras became digital. Kodak, a company with a history spanning more than a hundred years, was fixated on film and slides, and the cameras that used these photographic modes. As digital photography became widely adopted, Kodak refused to act on the paradigm shift and continued to focus on film and cameras and more film. Essentially, Kodak's leaders forgot that the business they were in was not about photography but about people. And people—consumers—had become less interested in film cameras; they were more interested in recording their lives and preserving memories. The modality mattered less to them than the activity. The irony is that Kodak invented digital photography but chose not to pursue the technology for the commercial market (Lucas and Goh 2009). Steve Jobs of Apple Computer saw the potential of making the digital camera part of the popular iPhone, providing an effortless way to take pictures that met the needs of most photography consumers.

This is an example of the *second curve*. This concept was introduced by healthcare futurist Ian Morrison in 1996. He posits that service and product innovation go through a series of curves. Each curve represents a product or service that matures over time and is then replaced by either a new or improved service or product. Entities that operate in an industry undergoing a paradigm shift must move past the first curve or be doomed to failure. In healthcare, the second curve is represented by **telemedicine**, web-based medical services, on-demand medical services, and new information technologies used to analyze and understand patient populations and their needs. Those practices that fail to enter the second curve will become obsolete as well. An important aspect of paradigm shifts is that they cause participants' knowledge base to shrink; every player starts over to build a new model of care.

The transition point from the first curve to the second curve is called the strain. Here, the demand for and provision of healthcare shift from being experienced predominantly the old way to predominantly the new way, for example, from office visits to virtual visits. The strain is a difficult point in a practice's operational life, and many businesses fail during this period. The organization must function in both paradigms simultaneously, aiming to move safely from the first curve to the second curve. Because the US healthcare system is changing incrementally from volume-based reimbursement (the old paradigm) to value-based reimbursement or **pay for performance** (the new paradigm), the second curve challenge for medical practices is that they must continue to operate in a volume-based system while slowly transitioning to the value paradigm. At the time of this writing, the majority of **revenue** for medical practices remains volume based (Center for Healthcare Quality and Payment Reform 2013).

What Is Value?

Value is a function of cost and quality, as demonstrated by the following equation:

$$Value = f(Cost/Quality)$$

In practical terms, value is what we are willing to pay for: what we see as a fair exchange of our resources (money) for something we receive (healthcare). Cost comprises all the economic and noneconomic input needed to receive the service. It includes money, of course, but also such factors as waiting time, access issues, perception of caring, and many others that may be particular to the individual expending the cost.

Quality is a measure of how good the service is. In healthcare, it can be determined by many factors. Some questions that may help ascertain quality include the following:

◆ Did I get well?

◆ Was the service timely?

Telemedicine
Involves the use of electronic communication and information technologies to provide or support clinical care at a distance.

Pay for performance (P4P)
Mechanism whereby providers are reimbursed on the basis of their level of success in meeting specific performance measures.

Revenue
The amounts received by or due to a practice for goods or services it provides to customers. Receipts are cash revenues; revenues may also be represented by accounts receivable.

◆ Were the staff and physicians friendly?

◆ Do I understand what the follow-up treatment entails?

Medical practices often quantify quality by metrics such as the following:

◆ Time to third available appointment (a measure of appointment availability)

◆ Number of calls that go unanswered (a measure of access)

◆ Waiting time (a measure of timeliness)

◆ Whether follow-up on lab and imaging services took place as needed, and length of time to follow-up (a measure of thoroughness)

◆ Patient satisfaction scores (a measure of the patient's perception of overall quality)

DETERMINANTS OF HEALTH

Another important issue in practice management, and healthcare administration in general, is understanding the determinants of health. (Review the select factors listed in exhibit 1.12 that go into determining health.) Many determinants are outside of individuals' control, such as in what generation or era one is born and one's biological sex, race, and other genetic and biological factors. Others, including individual behaviors; family and community networks; living and working conditions; and broad social, economic, cultural, health, and environmental conditions, are controllable to greater or lesser degrees. All these determinants can have a tremendous impact on overall health.

Every practice must consider its role in mitigating these issues, which go beyond what are traditionally considered to be "healthcare issues." Practices should engage patients in improving self-care and self-management, and they must be leaders and advocates for change in the lifestyle behaviors that have led to increases in the disease burden.

Furthermore, public policy plays a major role in health determinants, such as equity of care, and healthcare professionals should advocate for improvements to health policy that influences these issues.

CHANGES IN HEALTH COVERAGE

Since health insurance became commonplace after World War II, numerous changes have occurred in how healthcare is paid for. Originally, health insurance was primary indemnity coverage. This coverage provided payment to physicians or repaid the patient for the out-of-pocket costs incurred by the patient in seeking medical treatment as set forth in the policy.

Managed care became common in the 1980s and has gone through a number of transitions over the years. A relatively recent invention in health insurance, the consumer-directed health plan (CDHP), is having a profound impact on the medical environment. CDHPs provide coverage for medical services, but only after a substantial out-of-pocket deductible has been met by the patient. This requirement has led some patients to delay care or fail to pay the provider for care received because they do not have sufficient funds to cover the deductible. The latter results in the provider or medical practice encountering increasing amounts of **bad debt**.

Healthcare finance is covered in detail in a later chapter.

Bad debt
Amount owed to a practice that will not be paid.

CHANGES IN ORGANIZATIONAL STRUCTURE

In modern times, the predominant form of medical practice has been solo practice or small practice groups and partnerships. However, as the US healthcare system has evolved in response to value-based reimbursement and other **environmental factors**, consolidation of medical practices is occurring. Much more about this topic is covered throughout the remainder of the book.

Environmental factors
Forces that influence the business but are external to the business itself, such as public policy, regulations, and economic conditions.

THE COMPLEXITY OF THE HEALTHCARE ENVIRONMENT

The healthcare environment has become highly complex and will only continue to increase in complexity. Numerous new technologies and services as well as increasing volumes of information lead to new management challenges. For example, as discussed in depth in chapters 6 and 7, the move from using the International Classification of Diseases, Ninth Edition, Clinical Modification (ICD-9-CM) to ICD 10 for documenting diagnostic codes for reimbursement increased the number of codes from approximately 14,000 to more than 69,000. In addition, an entirely different set of codes, Current Procedural Terminology codes, recently increased to more than 71,000 codes from the previous set of 3,824 codes (CDC 2015).

SCIENTIFIC AND TECHNOLOGICAL CHANGE

The technological achievements in healthcare have been nothing short of remarkable. Consider that just a few years ago major surgery was a common treatment option for a person suffering from stomach ulcers, requiring a hospital stay and posing surgical risk. Today, many people with stomach ulcers can be treated with a simple over-the-counter medicine known as a proton pump inhibitor.

Another example of technological advances is related to diagnostic imaging. Until the introduction of advanced imaging technology such as computed tomography, ultrasound, and magnetic resonance imaging, exploratory surgery was often necessary to determine the patient's ailment.

THE CLOUD OF ANXIETY

All this change and attendant pressure on the modern medical practice has created a "cloud of anxiety," as illustrated in exhibit 1.13. With so many variables to address and the prospects of disruption to deal with on a daily basis, the seemingly constant uncertainty requires a new type of leader for this new era, one who can accurately interpret reality, explain the present, paint a compelling vision of the future, and lead the necessary change (exhibit 1.14). To ensure the success of the future medical practice, the practice manager must be this kind of leader.

EXHIBIT 1.13
The Cloud of Anxiety

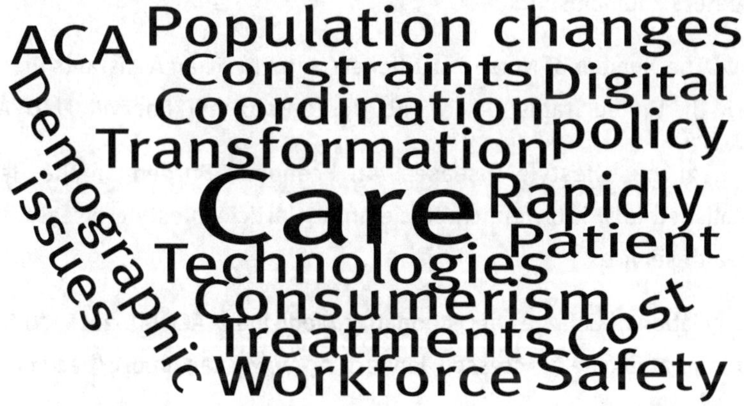

Interpret reality in an understandable way.

Explain the present in clear and factual terms.

Paint a compelling picture of the future.

Develop followers, and help them become problem solvers.

Lead change, and move toward the vision of the future.

EXHIBIT 1.14
What Leaders Must Do

DISCUSSION QUESTIONS

1. Discuss the importance of the medical practitioner to the healthcare system.

2. Describe several of the forces of change affecting the medical practice.

3. What are some challenges faced by the medical practice manager?

4. The metaphor "the perfect storm" has been used to describe the changes in healthcare. What does it mean in the healthcare context?

5. Describe and discuss several of the models of medical practice.

REFERENCES

Agency for Healthcare Research and Quality (AHRQ). 2016. "The Six Domains of Health Care Quality." Accessed February 24. https://cahps.ahrq.gov/consumer-reporting/talking quality/create/sixdomains.html.

————. 2011. "The Number of Nurse Practitioners and Physician Assistants Practicing Primary Care in the United States." AHRQ Pub. No. 12-P001-3-EF. Rockville, MD: AHRQ.

Al-Maskari, F. 2010. "Lifestyle Diseases: An Economic Burden on the Health Services." Published July. http://unchronicle.un.org/article/lifestyle-diseases-economic-burden-health-services.

American Association of Colleges of Osteopathic Medicine (AACOM). 2016. "U.S. Colleges of Osteopathic Medicine." Accessed January 29. www.aacom.org/become-a-doctor/us-coms.

American Association of Medical Colleges (AAMC). 2016. "Medical Schools." Accessed January 29. www.aamc.org/about/membership/378788/medicalschools.html.

American College of Healthcare Executives (ACHE). 2016. "About ACHE." Accessed January 31. www.ache.org/aboutache.cfm.

American Medical Association (AMA). 2017. "RBRVS Overview." Accessed April 20. www.ama-assn.org/rbrvs-overview.

Atchinson, B. K., and D. M. Fox. 1997. "The Politics of the Health Insurance Portability and Accountability Act." *Health Affairs* 16 (3): 146–50.

Ball, C. 1996. "James Young Simpson, 1811–1870." *Anaesthesia and Intensive Care* 24 (6): 639.

Bankston, J. 2004. *Joseph Lister and the Story of Antiseptics (Uncharted, Unexplored, and Unexplained)*. Bear, DE: Mitchell Lane.

Barnard, M. 2011. *Defining Moments*. Cape Town, South Africa: Random House Struik.

Bernstein, R. B. 2003. *Out of the Blue: A Narrative of September 11, 2001*. New York: Times Books.

Berwick, D. M., T. W. Nolan, and J. Whittington. 2008. "The Triple Aim: Care, Cost, and Quality." *Health Affairs* 27 (3): 759–69.

Bill-Axelson, A., L. Holmberg, H. Garmo, J. R. Rider, K. Taari, C. Busch, S. Nordling, M. Häggman, S.-O. Andersson, A. Spångberg, O. Andrén, J. Palmgren, G. Steineck, H.-O. Adami, and J.-E. Johansson. 2014. "Radical Prostatectomy or Watchful Waiting in Early Prostate Cancer." *New England Journal of Medicine* 370: 932–42.

Boyle, J. P., A. A. Honeycutt, K. M. Narayan, T. J. Hoerger, L. S. Geiss, H. Chen, and T. J. Thompson. 2001. "Projection of Diabetes Burden Through 2050: Impact of Changing Demography and Disease Prevalence in the U.S." *Diabetes Care* 24 (11): 1936–40.

Buchmueller, T. C., and A. C. Monheit. 2009. "Employer-Sponsored Health Insurance and the Promise of Health Insurance Reform." NBER Working Paper Number 14839. Cambridge, MA: National Bureau of Economic Research.

Bundorf, M. K. 2012. "Consumer-Directed Health Plans: Do They Deliver?" Published October. www.rwjf.org/en/library/research/2012/10/consumer-directed-health-plans.html.

Burke, J. 1985. *The Day the Universe Changed*. London: London Writers.

Center for Healthcare Quality and Payment Reform. 2013. "Payment Reform Barrier #3: Physician Compensation Based on Volume, Not Value." Published February 28. http://chqpr.org/blog/index.php/2013/02/payment-reform-barrier-3-physician-compensation-based-on-volume-not-value.

Centers for Disease Control and Prevention (CDC). 2016a. "Chronic Disease." Updated May 24. www.cdc.gov/chronicdisease.

———. 2016b. "2014–2016 Ebola Outbreak in West Africa." Accessed January 22, 2016. www.cdc.gov/vhf/ebola/outbreaks/2014-west-africa.

———. 2016c. "Zika Virus." Updated January 29. www.cdc.gov/zika/index.html.

———. 2015. "International Classification of Diseases, (ICD-10-CM/PCS) Transition— Background." Updated October 1. www.cdc.gov/nchs/icd/icd10cm_pcs_background.htm.

———. 2012. "Increasing Prevalence of Diagnosed Diabetes—United States and Puerto Rico, 1995–2010." *Morbidity and Mortality Weekly Report*. Published November 16. www.cdc.gov/mmwr/preview/mmwrhtml/mm6145a4.htm.

Centers for Medicare & Medicaid Services (CMS). 2015. "National Health Expenditures 2014 Highlights." Accessed April 20, 2017. www.cms.gov/Research-Statistics-Data-and-Systems/Statistics-Trends-and-Reports/NationalHealthExpendData/Downloads/highlights.pdf.

Cobban, A. B. 1999. *English University Life in the Middle Ages*. Columbus: Ohio State University Press.

Coggeshall, L. T. 1965. *Planning for Medical Progress Through Education*. Evanston, IL: Association of American Medical Colleges.

Dahm, R. 2008. "Discovering DNA: Friedrich Miescher and the Early Years of Nucleic Acid Research." *Human Genetics* 122 (6): 565–81.

Dalal, A. K., P. C. Dykes, S. Collins, L. S. Lehmann, K. Ohashi, R. Rozenblum, D. Stade, K. McNally, C. R. C. Morrison, S. Ravindran, E. Mlaver, J. Hanna, F. Chang, R. Kandala, G. Getty, and D. W. Bates. 2016. "A Web-Based, Patient-Centered Toolkit to Engage Patients and Caregivers in the Acute Care Setting: A Preliminary Evaluation." *Journal of the American Medical Informatics Association* 23 (1): 80–87.

Debré, P. 2000. *Louis Pasteur*. Baltimore, MD: Johns Hopkins University Press.

Deming Institute. 2016. "The Deming System of Profound Knowledge® (SoPK)." Accessed January 1. https://deming.org/theman/theories/profoundknowledge.

DiMatteo, M. R. 1998. "The Role of the Physician in the Emerging Health Care Environment." *Western Journal of Medicine* 168 (5): 328–33.

Dorsey, J. L. 1975. "The Health Maintenance Organization Act of 1973 (P.L. 93-222) and Prepaid Groups." *Medical Care* 13 (1): 1–9.

Flexner, A. 1910. *Medical Education in the United States and Canada*. New York: Carnegie Foundation for the Advancement of Teaching.

Garrison, D. H., and M. H. Hast (trans.). 2014. *The Fabric of the Human Body*. Basel, Switzerland: Karger.

Gawande, A. 2016. "An Evening with Dr. Atul Gawande." Live performance. Charlotte, NC, February 25.

———. 2014. *Being Mortal*. New York: Metropolitan.

Glasser, O. 1933. *Wilhelm Conrad Röntgen and the Early History of the Roentgen Rays*. London: John Bale, Sons and Danielsson.

GreekMedicine.net. 2016. "Aristotle." Accessed January 31. www.greekmedicine.net/whos_who/Aristotle.html.

Hargrave, E., J. Hoadley, K. Merrelli, and J. Cubansk. 2007. "Medicare Part D 2008 Data Spotlight: Specialty Tiers." Menlo Park, CA: Kaiser Family Foundation.

Harvey, W. 1993. *The Circulation of the Blood and Other Writings*. Translated by K. J. Franklin. London: Orion.

Heiney, P. 2003. *The Nuts and Bolts of Life: Willem Kolff and the Invention of the Kidney Machine*. Charleston, SC: History Press.

Hinrichs'sche, W., I. Wreszinski, and J. C. Umschrift. 1913. *Der Papyrus Ebers*. Leipzig, Germany: Buchhandlung.

Hurry, J. B. 1978. *Imhotep*, 2nd ed. New York: AMS Press.

Institute of Medicine (IOM). 2001. *Crossing the Quality Chasm: A New Health System for the 21st Century*. Washington, DC: National Academies Press.

Johns, C. H. W. (trans.). 2000. *Hammurabi, King; The Oldest Code of Laws in the World*. Clark, NJ: Lawbook Exchange.

Jones, D. S., S. H. Podolsky, and J. A. Greene. 2012. "The Burden of Disease and the Changing Task of Medicine." *New England Journal of Medicine* 366: 2333–38.

Jones, K. B. 2014. "Patient-Centered Care Versus Patient-Directed Care." Published December 12. www.physicianspractice.com/blog/patient-centered-care-versus-patient-directed-care.

Jones, W. 1979. *Philosophy and Medicine in Ancient Greece*. New York: Arno Press.

Jones, W. H. S. 1868. *Hippocrates Collected Works I*. Cambridge, MA: Harvard University Press.

Junger, S. 2009. *The Perfect Storm: A True Story of Men Against the Sea*. New York: W. W. Norton.

Kaiser Family Foundation. 2017. "Total Professionally Active Physicians." Published April. http://kff.org/other/state-indicator/total-active-physicians.

Kane, C. 2014. "AMA Policy Research Perspectives, Updated Data on Physicians Practice Arrangement: Inching Toward Hospital Ownership." Chicago: American Medical Association.

Keating, C. 2009. *Smoking Kills: The Revolutionary Life of Richard Doll*. Oxford, UK: Signal.

Knabb, R. D., J. R. Rhome, and D. P. Brown. 2005. *Hurricane Katrina*. Miami, FL: National Hurricane Center.

Knight, R. 2014. "Managing People from 5 Generations." Published September 25. https://hbr.org/2014/09/managing-people-from-5-generations.

Knox, J. H. M., Jr. 1933. "The Medical History of George Washington, His Physicians, Friends and Advisers." *Bulletin of the Institute of the History of Medicine* 174–91.

Koprowski, H. 1960. "Historical Aspects of the Development of Live Virus Vaccine in Polio-myelitis." *British Medical Journal* 2 (5192): 85–91.

Lauterbur, P. C. 1973. "Image Formation by Induced Local Interactions: Examples of Employing Nuclear Magnetic Resonance." *Nature* 242: 190–91.

Ligon, B. L. 2004. "Penicillin: Its Discovery and Early Development." *Seminars in Pediatric Infectious Diseases* 15 (1): 52–57.

Lloyd, G. E. R. (ed.). 1950. *Hippocratic Writings*. Translated by J. Chadwick. London: Penguin.

Lucas, H. C., and J. M. Goh. 2009. "Disruptive Technology: How Kodak Missed the Digital Photography Revolution." *Journal of Strategic Information Systems* 18: 46–55.

Medical Group Management Association (MGMA). 2016a. "About MGMA." Accessed February 16. www.mgma.com/about/overview.

———. 2016b. "Body of Knowledge for Medical Practice Management." Accessed February 16. www.mgma.com/education-certification/certification/body-of-knowledge/medical-practice-management-body-of-knowledge.

Morrison, I. 1996. *The Second Curve: Managing the Velocity of Change*. New York: Ballantine.

National Center for Complementary and Integrative Health. 2009. "Americans Spent $33.9 Billion Out-of-Pocket on Complementary and Alternative Medicine." Published July 30. https://nccih.nih.gov/news/2009/073009.htm.

National Center for Health Statistics (NCHS). 2015a. "International Classification of Diseases, (ICD-10-CM/PCS) Transition - Background." Accessed February 4, 2016. www.cdc.gov/nchs/icd/icd10cm_pcs_background.htm.

———. 2015b. "Older Persons' Health." Accessed March 1, 2016. www.cdc.gov/nchs/fastats/older-american-health.htm.

National Committee for Quality Assurance (NCQA). 2014. *Standards and Guidelines for NCQA Patient Centered Medical Homes 2014*. Washington, DC: NCQA.

National Human Genome Research Institute. 2010. "The Human Genome Project Completion: Frequently Asked Questions." Updated October 30. www.genome.gov/11006943.

Nelson, T. D. 2016. "The Age of Ageism." *Journal of Social Issues* 72: 191–98.

Nunn, J. F. 2002. *Ancient Egyptian Medicine*. Norman: University of Oklahoma Press.

Organisation for Economic Co-operation and Development (OECD). 2015. "Focus on Health Spending OECD Health Statistics 2015." White paper. Paris: OECD.

Palucka, T. 2002. "Overview of Electron Microscopy." Updated December 10. http://authors.library.caltech.edu/5456/1/hrst.mit.edu/hrs/materials/public/Electron Microscope/EM_HistOverview.htm.

Rashdall, H. 1895. *The Universities of Europe in the Middle Ages*, 3 vols., revised by F. M. Powicke and A. B. Emden. Oxford, UK: Clarendon.

Roguin, A. 2006. "Rene Theophile Laennec (1781–1826): The Man Behind the Stethoscope." *Clinical Medicine and Research* 4 (3): 230–35.

Rosenberg, C. E., and M. J. Vogel (eds.). 1979. "The Therapeutic Revolution: Medicine, Meaning, and Social Change in Nineteenth-Century America." *Perspectives in Biology and Medicine* 20 (4): 485–506.

Rothstein, W. G. 1972. *American Physicians in the Nineteenth Century: From Sect to Science*. Baltimore, MD: Johns Hopkins Press.

Sarton, G. 1951. *Galen of Pergamon*. Lawrence: University of Kansas Press.

Social Security Administration. 2016. "Vote Tallies for Passage of Medicare in 1965." Accessed February 1. www.ssa.gov/history/tally65.html.

Stevens, R. 1971. *American Medicine and the Public Interest*. New Haven, CT: Yale University Press.

Terry, K. 2015. "Number of Health Apps Soars, but Use Does Not Always Follow." Published September 18. www.medscape.com/viewarticle/851226.

Travis, P., S. Bennett, A. Haines, T. Pang, Z. Bhutta, A. A. Hyder, N. R. Pielemeier, A. Mills, and T. Evans. 2004. "Overcoming Health-Systems Constraints to Achieve the Millennium Development Goals." *Lancet* 364 (9437): 900–906.

US Department of Health & Human Services (HHS). 2010. "About the Affordable Care Act." Accessed January 18, 2016. www.hhs.gov/healthcare/about-the-law/index.html.

Wang, Y. A., and M. Barry. 2016. "Zika Outbreak Bears an Eerie Resemblance to the Spread of Ebola." Published February 9. www.latimes.com/opinion/op-ed/la-oe-0209-wang-barry-zika-ebola-20160209-story.html.

Winkelstein, W., Jr. 1992. "Not Just a Country Doctor: Edward Jenner, Scientist." *Epidemiology Review* 14 (1): 1–15.

CHAPTER 2

PRACTICE MODELS AND LEGAL ORGANIZATION

Culture eats strategy for breakfast.

—Peter Drucker

➤ Describe the wide range of medical practice models.

➤ Characterize the relationships between physicians and healthcare institutions.

➤ Understand the duties and responsibilities of the practice manager.

➤ Appreciate the importance of the mission, vision, and values of the practice.

STRUCTURES AND ORGANIZATION

The healthcare portion of the US economy continues to increase due to population growth, the aging population, and other factors, all of which are discussed later in the text. This continued growth is one reason the US healthcare system needs transformation and reform.

Medical practices play an increasingly important role in this transformation as practices become integrated into the overall delivery system. As such, reform cannot occur without physician involvement. One change already taking place is a trend toward large, integrated practices (Adamopoulos 2014). Integrated practices are those that are part of other organizations. In 2013, 26 percent of physicians identified themselves as employed by a healthcare organization (Jackson Healthcare 2013). Adamopoulos (2014) also noted a trend toward larger and more complex organizational practice structures. Multispecialty practices are growing, with the share of physicians in multispecialty practices having increased to 25 percent in 2014 from 22.1 percent in 2012.

These shifts bring new challenges for practice management professionals related to competitive pressures and the complexity of managing a large medical practice.

THE HEALTHCARE SYSTEM HIERARCHY

Before one can begin to address these challenges, one must understand the medical practice in the context of the overall healthcare system. As shown in exhibit 2.1, the medical practice plays a pivotal role in the US healthcare system because it provides continuity in the delivery of healthcare. Many, if not most, patients enter the healthcare system and are cared for at the individual provider level—often the medical practice—and are followed over time by the same practice. All aspects of the healthcare system rely on the direction of the physician to function and to trigger the use of resources.

MISSION, VISION, AND VALUES

A fundamental aspect of any organization, including the medical practice, is its governance framework, which includes the board of directors or trustees and senior management. As

EXHIBIT 2.1
The Healthcare
System Hierarchy

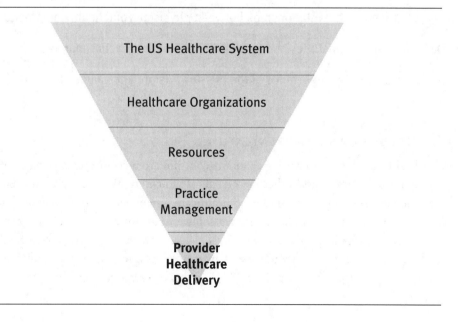

The US Healthcare System

Healthcare Organizations

Resources

Practice Management

Provider Healthcare Delivery

illustrated in exhibit 2.2, governance is guided by a mission, a vision, and values for the organization. This philosophical foundation provides a basis for strategic planning, which is a means of creating the goals and operational objectives of the medical practice. All aspects of decision making by the practice manager should be guided by the mission, vision, and values of the practice.

The mission of the organization is the reason it exists. The mission statement describes the overall purpose and intent of the organization. The vision of the organization describes the future state of the organization if it is successful in achieving its mission. The values of an organization indicate those beliefs the organization holds most dear and how it behaves as an entity in adhering to those values.

RELATIONSHIP OF THE PRACTICE TO ITS STAKEHOLDERS

Medical practices have many stakeholders—both internal and external to the organization. The effective medical practice is conscious of all of these relationships and carefully engages with them to carry out its mission. The practice manager and other practice leaders must understand the needs and concerns of all these constituencies and are critical conduits who

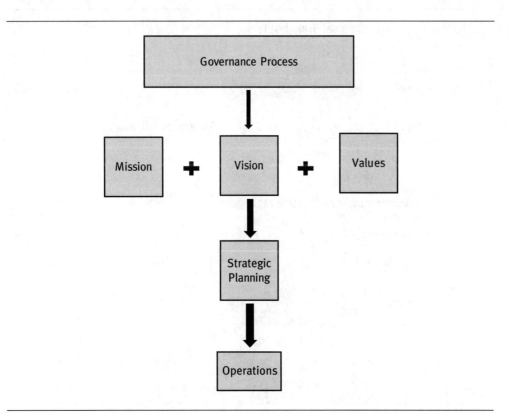

EXHIBIT 2.2
Mission, Vision, and Values

must translate the input of the governing body and external stakeholders to the operational units of the practice. Exhibit 2.3 illustrates the interrelationships of different stakeholders in a medical practice.

GENERAL STRUCTURE OF THE MEDICAL PRACTICE

Exhibit 2.4 illustrates a functional structure for the medical practice. It demonstrates the relationship between the operational aspects of the practice, where care is provided to patients, and the internal and external functions that support practice operations and engage with the external environment.

TAXONOMY OF PRACTICE MODELS AND LEGAL ORGANIZATION

Practices are organized in a wide range of forms, from a small, individual or solo practice to a large, highly organized practice with hundreds or even thousands of providers (exhibit 2.5). In general, the larger the organization, the more structured, complex, and integrated it will be (Galbraith 2014).

EXHIBIT 2.3
Stakeholder
Relationships
of the Medical
Practice

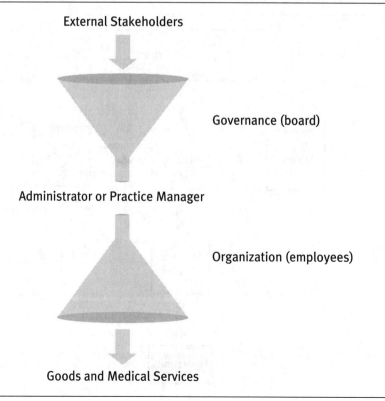

External Stakeholders

Governance (board)

Administrator or Practice Manager

Organization (employees)

Goods and Medical Services

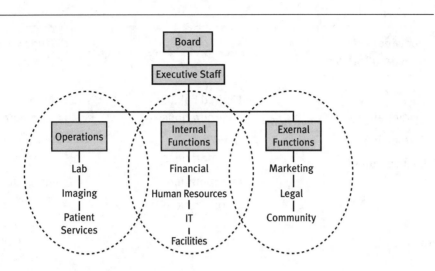

EXHIBIT 2.4
Operational
Structure of the
Medical Practice

The degree to which a practice is integrated ranges from virtually no integration, as with the solo practice, to moderate integration, such as a group practice, which may include many providers and numerous specialties, to a fully integrated practice that is a wholly owned subsidiary of a healthcare delivery system or an accountable care organization (ACO). Integration of medical practices is discussed in terms of two dimensions. First is the issue of integrating business and administrative services, such as billing and marketing. Second is the issue of clinical services integration.

Two key characteristics of multispecialty group practices include that they are highly integrated, with a common governance and leadership or management structure, and they have a highly developed corporate system for managing finances and ensuring compliance with regulatory agencies. They differ greatly in operation and governance from solo practices, which are largely overseen by the practitioner who owns the practice. The specific differences are discussed in detail later in the book.

Practices may choose to integrate for any number of reasons. The most prevalent is the economies of scale achieved by pooling resources to carry out the necessary functions of the medical practice. One of the most important economies of scale to medical practices is the ability to manage the complex aspects of today's practice, including finances, the regulatory environment, and the increasing need for the practice to respond to the changing healthcare environment.

CHARACTERISTICS OF PRACTICE ORGANIZATIONS

Many important organizational elements must be considered when planning the form the medical practice will take. These factors include taxation, liability, the number of members,

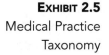

EXHIBIT 2.5
Medical Practice
Taxonomy

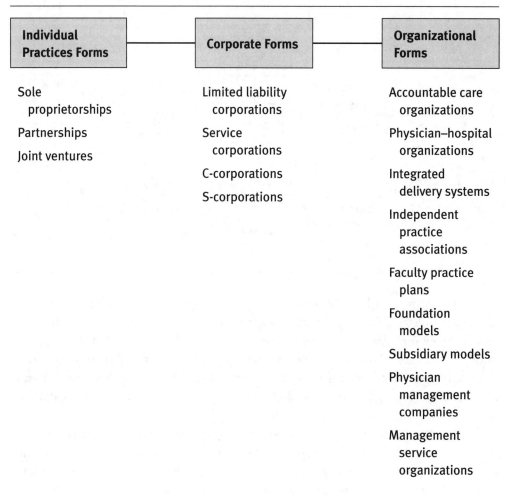

Individual Practices Forms	Corporate Forms	Organizational Forms
Sole proprietorships	Limited liability corporations	Accountable care organizations
Partnerships	Service corporations	Physician–hospital organizations
Joint ventures	C-corporations	Integrated delivery systems
	S-corporations	Independent practice associations
		Faculty practice plans
		Foundation models
		Subsidiary models
		Physician management companies
		Management service organizations

Capital
Resources, usually cash, available to invest or use for operations.

ownership, extent of personal flexibility and autonomy allowed, transferability of ownership, **capital** formation, and vision (Wagner 2013).

Practices that are sole proprietorships place individual responsibility on the individual practitioner to fulfill the financial, service, and other obligations of the organization. This form of ownership offers the advantage of control but holds the practitioner accountable for the entire operation.

Practices also may be formed as corporations, which, in the eyes of the law, are discrete entities (Showalter 2017). This status means that a corporation may enter into legally binding contracts, including debt obligations. In addition, because a corporation is seen by the law as an artificial person, it can be prosecuted for a variety of criminal behavior, such as fraud, wrongful death, and other criminal acts. It can be sued for negligence or liability, can be licensed, and must pay income taxes. These features provide part of the appeal for a medical practice forming as a corporation because it may act as a single entity even though it may include many individual practitioners and areas of the organization that may carry out separate functions. Corporations generally shelter the individuals in the organization from its liabilities. The major exception to this protection in a medical practice is that the corporation cannot shield the individual practitioner from medical negligence and liability.

Corporations can be for-profit or not-for-profit. For-profit organizations have shareholders and pay taxes. Some advantages of the taxable corporate form over the not-for-profit include the following:

◆ Easier to set up

◆ More flexible in terms of governance

◆ Less regulation

◆ Can legally manage taxable income

◆ Less restriction on compensation arrangements

Two disadvantages of a for-profit entity are that they

◆ must pay income taxes to both the state and federal treasury when profitable and

◆ cannot seek tax-deductible donations for nonprofitable services.

Not-for-profit, or tax-exempt, organizations are established under section 501(c)3 of the Internal Revenue Code. They, too, carry distinct advantages and disadvantages (IRS 2017). Some advantages of not-for-profit over for-profit organizations include the following:

◆ They are allowed to solicit tax-deductible donations.

◆ They may enjoy a more positive public image.

◆ They do not pay taxes to the state or federal treasury as long as the organization operates within the tax-exempt guidelines.

Disadvantages of not-for-profit status include the following:

◆ Additional paperwork is required to apply for tax-exempt status.

◆ Not-for-profit organizations are required to follow Internal Revenue Service regulations regarding tax-exempt organizations.

◆ They are required to have a board of directors that has community representation.

◆ All of their financial transactions must be performed at arm's length, meaning insider dealing is prohibited.

◆ Compensation arrangements may be restricted.

A common scenario in today's healthcare environment is one in which practices are owned by large healthcare entities such as a hospital or healthcare system. These larger entities may be for-profit or not-for-profit. In the case of for-profit hospitals or healthcare systems, they may be privately held or publicly traded organizations; the latter form means that the shareholders may be any individuals or entities that wish to buy shares in the organization.

AFFILIATION VERSUS EMPLOYMENT MODELS AND THE CORPORATE PRACTICE OF MEDICINE

The extent to which medicine may be practiced is dictated by each state, either by statute or by other means such as licensure. These rules are generally codified in state regulations known as corporate practice of medicine doctrines. These doctrines prohibit a corporate entity from owning practices and directing medical practitioners to eliminate the control of medical care by those not trained or motivated to provide care in the best interest of patients. Many states prohibit any ownership of a medical practice by nonproviders for the same reason. At one time, these rules placed limits on physicians being employed by corporations or selling their practices to hospitals and other healthcare entities. In roughly the past decade, these laws have been clarified to lift many restrictions on the employment of providers (Michal, Pekarske, and McManus 2006).

The employment of physicians or affiliation of physician practices with other healthcare entities takes different forms, as described in the paragraphs that follow.

THE EMPLOYMENT ARRANGEMENT

The most straightforward is the employment arrangement. In this arrangement, the physician or provider becomes an employee of the organization, and often the working arrangement is detailed in an employment agreement. Exhibit 2.6 lists some features of an employment agreement.

Benefits and Compensation

Benefits and compensation provisions specified in the employment contract include the salary the provider is to receive and how that salary is calculated; many practices use formulas

		EXHIBIT 2.6
Benefits and Compensation	Restrictive Covenants	Key Features of
Salary	Perfect Performance	an Employment
Nonsalary Terms	Contract Terms	Agreement
Ownership/Partnership	Termination Provisions	
Outside Activities	Tail Insurance	
Job Requirements	Nonassignability	

to determine compensation (discussed in more detail in a later chapter.) The contract also includes important nonsalary benefits, such as the following:

♦ Vacation pay

♦ Health insurance

♦ Disability insurance

♦ Pension or retirement savings **account**

♦ Allowances for meetings and entertainment **expenses**

♦ Car allowances

♦ Continuing education benefits

In addition, the contract often specifies practice accoutrements that the provider receives, such as cell phones, office furnishings, and other equipment or accessories.

Ownership

Some private practices offer physicians the opportunity to purchase an ownership stake or to become a partner in the practice. Such terms are typically detailed in the contract or included by reference in a separate agreement that specifies how the provider becomes an owner. Inclusion by reference is an important concept in contract law. Contracts that reference a document, such as a policy, essentially make the referenced document part of the terms of the contract. All the parties to the contract must be clear on what terms from the document are incorporated into the contract to avoid future disputes and misunderstandings.

Many practitioners engage in entrepreneurial activities such as book writing, software development, and other types of medical enterprise. The employment contract should specify the terms and conditions under which these activities are permissible and to what extent, if any, the benefits from these activities belong to the contract holder. Such provisions are

Account
A record of financial transactions; usually refers to a specific category or type.

Expense
An expenditure that is chargeable against revenue during an accounting period resulting in the reduction of an asset.

often overlooked in contracts and can lead to misunderstanding and difficulties when the issue arises post facto (after the contract has been signed).

The job requirements may also be delineated in the contract. These may entail working hours, the location at which the practitioner is expected to work, the number of days per week that the provider will be available to practice, the amount of call coverage to be taken, and the method for distributing call coverage among the practitioners.

Restrictive Covenants

A controversial area of contracts is the restrictive covenant. This provision sets certain parameters usually related to future working restrictions if the provider leaves the practice. Simply put, it restricts the practitioner from engaging in the practice of medicine for a certain period of time in a certain specified distance from the previous practice. In some states, such provisions are prohibited; in other states, they are discouraged but legal. In states where the restrictive covenant is permissible, the covenant is almost always bound by certain reasonableness standards. The first standard is the length of time that the restrictive covenant may be in place: The shorter the time, the more enforceable the covenant may be. The second standard considers how far the practitioner must move to be compliant with the covenant. Obviously, a restrictive covenant that prohibits practice in an entire region or state is unreasonable and would be found unenforceable by a court of law.

In many cases, the restrictive covenant calls for "perfect performance," meaning the provision can only be satisfied by doing what is specifically stated in the contract. In other cases, the restrictive covenant may offer a buyout provision, allowing the practitioner leaving the practice to pay a certain sum to negate the restrictive covenant. Regardless of the provisions, the practitioner must understand the nature of the restrictive covenant and be willing to abide by its terms.

Terms of the Contract

Contract terms are always stated in the contract. They include length of the contract, under what state laws the contract is governed, whether arbitration will be used as a method for settling disputes, and any other conditions related to how the contract is administered.

Effective contracts also include a termination process or termination provisions. These clauses specify how the parties to the contract will conduct themselves once the contract has expired and how the contract can be otherwise terminated. Contracts can typically be terminated for failure to perform by either party. For example, if the practice refuses to pay the provider, the provider has a claim of nonperformance under the contract. Conversely, if the provider fails to provide medical care as specified under the contract, the practice has cause to terminate the contract. Some contracts simply expire. In this case, decisions must be made to determine how medical records are handled and any continuation of benefits or access to practice resources. Any restrictive convent usually survives the expiration of the contract, meaning it is enforceable after the contract has ended.

Tail Coverage or Extended Reporting Endorsement

One aspect of ending the practice relationship involves the provision of tail coverage for malpractice insurance. This coverage extends insurance protection to the provider for all prior occurrences of alleged or actual malpractice that occurred while employed by the practice. These policies can be expensive; therefore, the contract should specify who is responsible for purchasing tail coverage. The practice almost always requires that malpractice tail coverage be purchased by the practitioner (see also chapter 4).

Nonassignability Clause

Most provider employment agreements contain a nonassignability clause. This provision simply states that the contract may not be assigned to another individual, in essence allowing someone else to take the provider's place in the practice. Although this limitation may seem obvious, the clause is an important part of the employment agreement.

Some Final Details About Employment Contracts

For a contract to be enforceable and considered legally binding, it must contain these five elements (McKendrick 2012):

- ◆ An intent to enter into an agreement.

- ◆ An offer.

- ◆ Acceptance of the offer.

- ◆ Consideration, which means, in the case of an employment agreement, economic benefits, such as a salary, in exchange for services rendered to the practice.

- ◆ A legal capacity to enter into the agreement. Although unlikely in the case of a provider service agreement, a minor cannot enter into a legally binding agreement.

In addition to these five elements, the subject matter of the contract must be of a legal nature. This component is particularly important in the area of medical services because of the many private inurement rules and anti-kickback provisions that exist in the regulatory environment of the medical practice (see chapter 4 for details). If the contract contains requirements to break the law, it cannot be enforced. Notably, although contracts are usually enforced and governed by specific state laws, federal issues arise related to Medicare, Medicaid, and regulations that govern the practice of medicine.

Severability clauses may be important elements as well. In some states, if any provision of the contract is held to be unenforceable, the entire agreement is unenforceable. In other jurisdictions, only the offending clause is voided. Contracts may also contain language that requires the parties to negotiate a resolution to any clause of the contract that is found unenforceable or illegal to bring the contract into compliance. This is an important consideration in today's healthcare environment, as laws and regulations change so quickly that an acceptable activity may become illegal due to policy changes, requiring those aspects of the contract to be changed or eliminated.

The development and execution of an employment agreement in the medical practice require expertise in state and federal law. Often, this is an area for which the practice seeks outside counsel to be certain these important documents are handled correctly.

AFFILIATION AGREEMENTS WITH OTHER ORGANIZATIONS

In an affiliation agreement, the practice signs a contract with another party, typically a healthcare entity, to provide certain specific services under a contractual arrangement. A major difference between an affiliation agreement and an employment contract is that under an affiliation agreement the provider remains an independent contractor and continues to own and manage his or her practice. Any restrictions on the practice are enumerated in the affiliation agreement.

Affiliation agreements vary widely and may involve the provision of specific medical services, educational affiliations, and management services. Such agreements are often entered into because one or both parties do not wish to become fully integrated but see a need for specific services to be delivered and some level of cooperation to do so (see, e.g., Blum 2013).

CULTURE AND ORGANIZATION

Strategy
The science of business planning whereby an organization plans its approach to achieving its goals.

Culture is defined as the beliefs, customs, practices, and behaviors of a particular group (*Merriam-Webster* 2016). Simply put, culture dictates how an organization conducts business, what it values, how it gets things done, and how it views itself. The culture of an organization defines how it treats its members and what behaviors it expects from them. Culture is a powerful force; as Peter Drucker is widely said to have stated, "Culture eats **strategy** for breakfast."

The relationships between practitioners and institutional providers, such as hospitals and healthcare systems, have often been strained because of the significant cultural differences between the parties. Almost by definition, medical practices have been less formal and are what Robbins (1990) refers to as professional collegial organizations. In these organizations, the primary producer is also the owner and governs the organization. Often the cultures of the two healthcare segments clash and create management problems that must be addressed by the medical practice (Schein 2016).

Part of the problem centers on expectations of each party being established prior to the acquisition or affiliation. A cultural fit survey is essential to determining compatibility, as is having a clear understanding of what each party wishes to accomplish as a result of the combination of the organizations. As exhibit 2.7 shows, culture dictates virtually every aspect of the organization by influencing

- ◆ organizational structure and governance;

- ◆ mission, vision, and values;

- ◆ goals, tasks, and incentives;

- ◆ performance and the expectations of people in the organization; and

- ◆ information systems and other operational infrastructure.

Culture is both codified by formal policy and procedure and imbued by informal means through the behavior of its members. The more the culture is aligned with positive

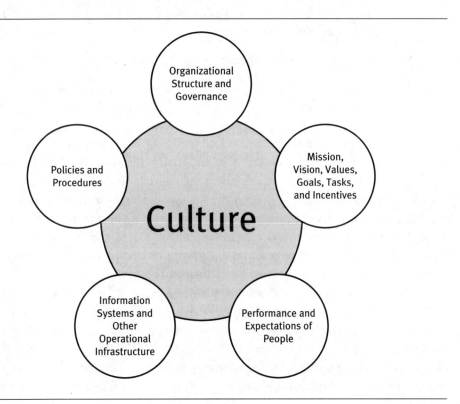

EXHIBIT 2.7
Culture Affects All Aspects of the Practice

behavior, the more effective the organization is. For example, if organizational leaders say they value and expect courteous treatment of others but allow disrespectful behavior to go unchallenged, they degrade the culture (Drucker 2006).

ACADEMIC MEDICAL CENTERS AND PHYSICIAN PRACTICE MANAGEMENT

About 400 of the more than 5,500 hospitals in the United States carry the special designation of academic medical center (AMC) (AHA 2017). AMCs are typically members of the Association of American Medical Colleges (AAMC) and its subsidiary, the Council of Teaching Hospitals (AAMC 2016). As are other hospitals, they also are often members of the American Hospital Association (AHA). An AMC has an organizational structure that is different from other for-profit or not-for-profit solo or multispecialty practices.

The number of AMCs and their associated medical practices, as with most healthcare organizations, grew rapidly after World War II when federal funding for medicine was greatly increased. Specific factors in this growth include the following:

◆ The advent of the third-party payer following World War II

◆ The introduction of Medicare and Medicaid in 1965, which stimulated research and allowed for the application of the resulting technologies in the treatment of many more patients

◆ A great increase in the expectations of the US healthcare system by patients

◆ The creation of many new medical specialties that focused on the treatment of complex illnesses

Physician practices often are involved with AMCs, so practice managers must be knowledgeable of several elements of this important healthcare organizational structure. AMCs are typically integrated in the teaching and research functions of the medical schools at major research universities. They often offer unique and highly specialized medical services requiring the availability of physicians with specific training in complex areas of medicine. Examples are Level I trauma services, transplantation services, and the use of sophisticated diagnostic technology such as positron emission tomography scanners. Physicians who practice in AMCs are often involved in teaching and research functions.

Making generalizations about how physician practices associate with AMCs is difficult. The physicians in the practice may be employed as faculty to provide clinical services; the practice may be affiliated by contract as previously discussed, fulfilling specific needs of the AMC; or the practice may be wholly owned by the AMC. One important distinguishing characteristic related to the medical practice in an AMC is that it is often mission based, and as a result, less emphasis is placed on productivity as a function of patients seen, or relative value units produced. Productivity may include such aspects of medical activity as research, time devoted to teaching, presenting at conferences, and other scholarly endeavors.

ACCOUNTABLE CARE ORGANIZATIONS

One of the most influential developments in determining the structure and organization of medical practices is the ACO. These healthcare delivery constructs are a central feature of the Affordable Care Act (ACA) of 2010 (McCanne 2010) and, in many ways, are defined more by what they do than by their structure. In general, an ACO is a group of providers who share responsibility for a population of patients regarding the quality, cost, and coordination of their care. Two notable features of ACOs are that they can

◆ be any a combination of group practices, practice networks, hospitals, or hospital-employed physicians and providers and

◆ be joint ventures, with the proviso that they must be able to receive and distribute payments.

All members of the ACO do not have to belong to a single entity; they can be bound by a contract. However, an ACO must include physicians in its membership (AAFP 2016).

The ACO works with insurers, the largest being Medicare, to achieve improved health outcomes. Specifically, they seek to accomplish the following goals, referred to as the Triple Aim (IHI 2017; see chapter 10):

◆ Improve population health

◆ Improve the patient experience

◆ Reduce total cost of care

Most of the arrangements between the payers and the ACO involve incentives for reducing cost such that the ACO receives payments if agreed-on targets are met. A central aspect of the ACO is to provide enhanced preventive care; therefore, the care delivered by ACO primary care providers is central to the success of the ACO.

Although more sophisticated in some respects, the ACO is reminiscent of the health maintenance organization (HMO) because it places a heavy emphasis on wellness and prevention as a health and economic strategy and focuses on primary care. HMOs are prepaid or capitated health insurance plans for which the patient (or his or her employer) pays a fixed fee each month instead of paying for the cost of each service received. These are delivered by providers who are under contract with (or are employees of) the HMO. ACOs provide incentives for shared savings, making prevention a hallmark of the concept. Patients and providers both benefit, in theory, through attentive patient management, improved outcomes, and reduced cost. In addition, economic opportunity accrues for the physicians, hospitals, and other provider organizations that are part of the ACO.

The ACA established an ACO for Medicare providers called the Medicare Shared Savings Program (MSSP) as part of reforms to the Medicare delivery system. The MSSP is intended to improve outcomes and increase the value of care by rewarding ACOs that "lower their growth in health care costs while meeting performance standards on quality of care and putting patients first" (CMS 2017). Additional ACOs are being developed with commercial insurance carriers, and as of January 2015, the total number of ACOs was 744 (Muhlestein 2015). All 50 US states now have at least one ACO.

CLINICAL INTEGRATION

Clinical integration is receiving much more attention than in the past as an alternative care delivery model concept. More than a type of organizational structure, integrated delivery systems (IDSs) seek to provide integrated clinical services. Specifically, the clinical integration model aims to provide care to the patient in a longitudinal (or long-term and coordinated) manner without necessarily having all of the providers of care reside in a single entity.

Joining or developing an IDS requires the following elements to be in place:

- Collaborative leadership
- Involved governing body
- Compliant legal structure
- Effective payer strategy
- Culture change
- Aligned incentives for physicians
- Value-based compensation
- Program infrastructure
- High performance
- Network physician leadership and support
- Clinical programs
- Disease programs
- Care protocols
- Clinical metrics
- Population health management

◆ Technology infrastructure

◆ Health information exchange

◆ Disease registries

◆ Patient longitudinal record

◆ Patient portal to enable engagement

Considering the longitudinal nature of clinical integration, the model focuses much more on developing procedures geared toward achieving excellent outcomes than relying on organizational structure to maximize the benefits. The clinical integration model is an approach to solving the problem of fragmented care. The essential features of clinical integration are as follows (Strandberg-Larsen et al. 2010):

◆ Providing care across the continuum of services

◆ Improving individual care outcomes

◆ Improving the health of all of the patients served by the organization (population health)

Clinical integration can be accomplished by contracting with other providers; merging with other practices or being acquired by a health system; or having all the clinical care providers agree to established protocols of care, which provides for a more seamless continuum of care for the patient and greater economic synergy.

PATIENT-CENTERED MEDICAL HOMES

The patient-centered medical home (PCMH) is a concept introduced by E. H. Wagner in 1998. Unlike many of the approaches pervasive in the healthcare field today, such as more efficient treatment, better drugs, and new care modalities to care for the sick, the PCMH is focused on prevention and early intervention for patient care. This focus is especially appropriate for the chronically ill, as early intervention can delay a worsening condition and prevent the emergence of further complications and other consequences of the **chronic illness**, such as kidney failure in diabetic patients. The PCMH helps ensure continuity of care and offers expert guidance in navigating the healthcare delivery system by serving as the starting point for all of a patient's medical concerns. Any physician practice can become a PCMH by adhering to the following six principles and standards, which form the basis for certification by the National Committee for Quality Assurance (NCQA 2016, 2017):

◆ Patient-centered access: The practice must be able to provide needed care 24 hours a day.

Chronic illness
Diseases characterized by one or more of the following criteria: they are permanent; leave residual disability; are caused by nonreversible pathological alteration; require special training of the patient for rehabilitation; or require a long period of supervision, observation, or care.

◆ Team-based care: All members of the practice must be engaged in providing the patient with needed information and meeting the cultural and linguistic needs of the patient.

◆ Population health management: The practice must collect data for population health management purposes.

◆ Care management and support: The practice must support evidence-based guidelines for prevention and for acute and chronic care management.

◆ Care coordination and care transitions: The practice must track and coordinate tests, referrals, and care transitions.

◆ Performance measurement and quality improvement: The practice must use data and experience for purposes of continuous improvement.

Physician practices that are interested in becoming a PCMH should reflect on the following questions before beginning the process:

1. Does the practice value the patient as an active participant in his or her own healthcare?

2. Is the practice able to develop and maintain an ongoing personal relationship with the patient for achieving continuity of care?

3. Can the practice lead a team of professionals, inspiring and empowering them to fulfill the mission of the medical home concept?

4. Is the practice able to establish solid professional relationships with other physicians, particularly those who specialize in different fields, to secure specialized care for patients?

5. Does the practice believe in the concept of prevention of disease and illness and a holistic approach to medicine?

6. Is the practice able to help the patient navigate the complex field of healthcare?

7. Is the practice open to patient feedback and to seeking quality improvement based on that feedback to ensure that patient expectations are met (and in some cases exceeded)?

8. Does the practice embrace technology to support patient communication, care, and education?

9. Is the practice prepared to adopt the needed workflow and process modifications? Does the practice have adequate staff (in both number and skill) to manage the increased accessibility to its patients (increased volume

of e-mails and after-hours phone calls)? Does the practice have adequate information technology (IT) staff to manage video chat capabilities and mobile health applications?

10. Does the practice have the IT infrastructure to support the services offered by a PCMH? Does it have an electronic health record system (EHR) in place? Is the EHR interoperable with the rest of the community healthcare providers, such as hospitals, rehabilitation centers, and other medical practices?

11. Does the practice staff have adequate training to provide health coaching? For example, are they experienced with techniques such as motivational interviewing? Does the practice have the capacity to organize disease-specific support groups? What behavioral or mental health services will it offer its patients?

12. What kind of care teams will the practice provide its patients? What specialists and care providers will make up these care teams? Do they have adequate relationships with other providers who are willing to join the PCMH?

13. Is the practice prepared to assess process and outcome improvements? What performance measures will it use to track its progress?

14. Does the practice wish to become a certified PCMH? If so, has it chosen a national accrediting body through which to apply for certification?

15. Is the practice currently financially stable enough to take on the **risk** of shifting to the value-based purchasing model of the PCMH?

> **Risk**
> The possibility of loss, inherent in all business activities. High risk requires high return. All business decisions must consider the amount of risk involved.

Not enough practices ask these important questions as they begin to develop a PCMH. As with so many decisions in the healthcare world, mind-set is everything. Practice leaders must have a deep understanding of what the practice wishes to accomplish and how best to implement the effort.

Additional Considerations Related to Medical Homes

The overall promise of the PCMH is that it helps frame a medical practice's approach to offering value-based care. One way it does so is by allowing the practice to seek simplification for a complex environment. The payment system that drives practice management encourages incremental improvement efforts, bolting on process after process, procedure upon procedure, making systems difficult to work with, rather than taking the time to think through the value that each process adds and how it operates.

Consider waiting time. The scheduling structure in medical practices is largely dictated by the reimbursement system. Practices have determined that they need to see a certain number of patients in a given amount of time to break even or be profitable as a business. Regardless of the individual patient's needs, the practice may schedule an elderly or disabled person for the same 15-minute appointment length given any other patient when, realistically, the elderly or disabled individual requires more time and attention.

With modern data analytics processes, however, medical practices could match appointment times with the specified needs of the patient, including his or her demographic characteristics, giving older patients or those with complex medical issues more time than patients with relatively straightforward and simple problems. The PCMH is often a prominent feature of the ACO because it aligns well with the goals and strategies of reduced cost through better, more coordinated care.

INTEGRATED DELIVERY SYSTEMS

Although a detailed discussion of IDSs is beyond the scope of this text, a brief discussion is relevant to the physician practice because practices are often part of an IDS. Essentially, the IDS can be either a horizontally or a vertically integrated healthcare organization. Vertically integrated organizations increase their reach by adding similar service lines, such as hospitals, whereas a horizontally integrated organization increases in reach by adding related but different service lines; for example, a hospital organization might add physician practices. IDSs are generally characterized as being a large organization capable of providing a variety of services to their patients. An IDS may include any or all of the following services or entities:

- ◆ Hospital services
- ◆ Physician services
- ◆ Ambulatory care services
- ◆ Surgical centers
- ◆ Urgent care centers
- ◆ Nursing homes
- ◆ Palliative and hospice care facilities
- ◆ Home health care services
- ◆ Pharmacy services
- ◆ Telemedicine services
- ◆ Telehealth services

Some IDSs also include an insurance arm, thereby providing the financing of care as well as the provision of services. Although IDSs have similarities to ACOs, they are not the same model. In essence, all ACOs are likely IDSs, but not all IDSs are ACOs.

PROS AND CONS OF INTEGRATION

All structural forms have pros and cons, and this maxim is true of integration. Some advantages of participation in an IDS are as follows:

◆ Economies of scale can be leveraged.

◆ Patient care decisions can be improved through the coordination of care across affiliated providers.

◆ Cost-effectiveness is more likely to be achieved.

◆ Patients may be better served with an increased scope of service.

◆ A larger financial base may afford a practice more access to capital.

◆ More specialty staff with greater expertise may be hired.

◆ Competition erodes, as little antitrust activity in healthcare has been seen in the past two or three decades.

Disadvantages of integration are the following:

◆ Friction among physicians may emerge because, as a function of their training, many tend to work better independently than they do as part of a team in large, integrated organizations (Groopman 2008).

◆ Decisions are made differently in larger integrated practices than members are typically accustomed to, requiring an adjustment for some providers.

◆ Seamless integration of information systems is needed and often difficult to achieve.

◆ Standardizing processes and workflows to reduce variation is often resisted by practice physicians and can be difficult to achieve.

◆ Changes in policies must be reconciled. This can be a difficult process, and it may be costly because government regulations may require enhancement of the benefits package of the acquiring organization to comply with nondiscrimination rules, such as pension and health benefits (IRS 2016).

Increased complexity is another issue that often arises with increasing organization size and scope. By definition, medical care is complex, and it is often delivered on an individualized basis. This factor makes streamlining processes and organizational structures difficult, and streamlining also tends to reduce innovative activities due to environmental uncertainty. This uncertainty leads to unintended consequences, unpredictability, indecision, and lack of clarity of goals (Star 2013).

MERGERS AND ACQUISITIONS

Tremendous growth has been seen in recent years in the size and scope of medical practices, as noted earlier in the chapter. This growth is usually accomplished in one of two ways: by "organic growth," which constitutes additions to an existing practice by recruiting new members, or through mergers and acquisitions. A merger is a transaction that creates a new, single entity from combining two or more previously single organizations. An acquisition occurs when one organization purchases the **assets** of another entity. In the case of an acquisition, the acquiring organization usually remains intact.

One danger that can arise from a merger or an acquisition is illustrated in exhibit 2.8: the creation of too many silos for patients to navigate. Healthcare professionals often see their work as a series of discrete activities, each under separate control. The patient or the patient's family view healthcare activities differently; they see their encounter with the practice as a single event and part of an overall experience. When mergers or acquisitions take place, the practices involved need to fully integrate all parts of the new practice to avoid silos. Keeping the patient experience in mind helps practice leaders improve the functioning of their medical practices.

While drawbacks to mergers and acquisitions are evident, especially in terms of culture issues, they allow a practice to grow quickly and may also allow it to acquire new services and prevent the duplication of services that can lead to an oversupply and potential overutilization.

These activities require great care and expertise. As shown in exhibit 2.9, numerous details must be resolved to ensure a successful transaction.

Asset
Item of value owned by a business. May be a physical property, such as a building; a physical object, such as a stock certificate; or a right, such as the right to use a patented process.

EXHIBIT 2.8
Rearranging How We Think About Care

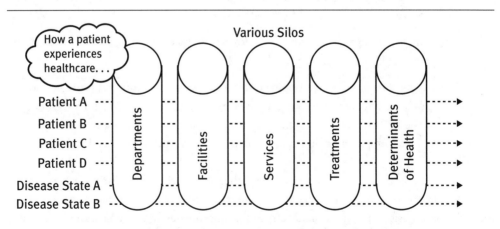

PREMERGER ASSESSMENT
- Review each practice's finances.
- Review employee payroll and benefits for each practice.
- Review coding practices.
- Review fee schedules.

NEW PRACTICE ENTITY
- Partnership or corporation?
- Professional association?
- Effective date of merged operations?

ASSETS THAT WILL BE CONTRIBUTED TO NEW ENTITY BY EACH PRACTICE
- Hard assets (will be leased from existing and new entities).

Accounts Receivable (A/R):
- What amount will be contributed?
- How will remainder of physician A/R be accounted for?

Inventory and Other Assets

NEW PRACTICE'S ASSUMPTION OF DEBT OF EACH PRACTICE
Review physician's existing debts:
- Accounts payable.
- Notes and other payables.
- Lease obligations.
- Defined benefit plan.

FORMULA FOR COMPENSATION OF THE DOCTORS (USUALLY BASED ON PREASSESSMENT)
- Physician collections and shared and allocated overhead.
- Fixed compensation plus bonus.
- Bonus based on percentage of collections.
- Bonus based on percentage of net production.
- Equal compensation for all physicians.
- Fixed compensation plus percentage of net production.
- Percentage of net production.
- Compensation formula for nonowner physicians.

OPERATIONAL ISSUES
- Call schedule.
- Billing/collection policies.

Exhibit 2.9
Merger Checklist

(continued on next page)

EXHIBIT 2.9
Merger Checklist
(continued)

- Computer system (hardware and software to use).
- Appointment scheduling, including systems to schedule.
- Office forms.
- Medical charts.
- Superbill.
- Fee schedule.
- Notification of insurance carriers of new entity, if applicable.
- New group provider number.
- Banking (and banking contact).
  Insurance:
  - Group health, life, and disability.
  - Malpractice.
  - Office contents.
  - Other.
- Office hours, all locations.
- Telephone numbers, all locations.
- Purchasing function, establish controls and systems.
- Professional assistance.
- Choose practice's accountant.
- Choose practice's attorney.
- Establish and wire for computer networking.
- Other operational issues.

ASSESS HIDDEN COSTS TO MERGE
- Nonproductive time (lost patient billing).
- Marketing costs.
- Professional fees to merge.
- Moving costs, if applicable (schedule moving assistance).
- Malpractice tail premium.
- Cost to equalize fringe benefits.
- Cost to develop common operational policies.
- Possible facility costs.
- Buyout of existing leases.
- Additional leasehold improvements.
- Write-off of unproductive or abandoned assets.
- Other hidden costs.

PERSONNEL
- Determine practice's administrator and related employment contract.
- Review current compensation of employees and existing benefit plans.
- Decide which employees stay and which may have to leave.
- Write or update employee manual.

- Establish new fringe benefits.
- Establish job duties for each employee.
- Technicians to be assigned or pooled?
- Identify potential employee conflicts.
- Establish annual office and clinical personnel job assessment and evaluation program.

FACILITIES
Review current lease obligations of each practice:
  - Office leases.
  - Equipment leases.
- Determine if offices will consolidate into one location.
- Decide how specific equipment will be used in the practice.
- Review issues related to physician ownership of office building, if applicable.
- Establish lease formula for existing equipment and equipment to be acquired.

MANAGING PHYSICIAN
- Who will be managing physician? (or)
- Establish "office of managing physician."
  Decide on duties of managing physician vs. administrator:
  - Manage day-to-day operations.
  - Supervise employees.
  - Supervise billing/collection activities.
  - Ensure that all insurance as required by the group is paid and maintained.
  - Acquire fixed assets for less than $[dollar amount].
  - Authorize contracts on behalf of the group not in excess of $[dollar amount].
  - Maintain bank accounts.
  - Make sure all tax returns are prepared and filed on time.
  - Make sure all licenses are renewed.
  - Supervise payment of accounts payable.
  - Implement business decisions of the group practice.
  - Call to order regular meeting of the physicians.
  - Serve as liaison with community hospitals, referral networks, other medical practices.
  - Other duties.
- Will managing physician be compensated? If so, how much?
  How will managing physician be elected each year?
  - Vote of the physicians.
  - Annual rotation.

PRACTICE'S RETIREMENT PLAN
- Will there be a new plan? What features will it include?
- Decide what to do with current plan(s).

Exhibit 2.9
Merger Checklist
(continued)

(continued on next page)

EXHIBIT 2.9
Merger Checklist
(continued)

- Choose retirement plan administrator.
- Choose investment counselor.

NEW NAME OF THE GROUP PRACTICE
- Adopt name of one of the practices or decide on name of the new practice.

SPECIFIC PHYSICIAN CONTRACT ISSUES
Voluntary withdrawal by owner:
- Required notice [number of days or months].

Involuntary termination of an owner:
- Death.
- Owner's right to practice medicine in the state is suspended, revoked, or canceled.
- Owner loses privileges to any hospital at which the practice regularly maintains admission privileges.
- Owner fails to follow reasonable policies or directives established by the practice.
- Owner commits acts amounting to gross negligence or willful misconduct to the detriment of the practice or its patients.
- Owner is convicted of a crime.
- Owner breaches the terms of his or her employment agreement.
- Physician becomes uninsurable for medical malpractice coverage.
- Disability of an owner:
  - Owner becomes and remains disabled for [number] months (six months?).
  - Continued compensation to a disabled owner:
  - How long?
  - How much? (Based on a percentage of receivables collected over [number] months.)
  - Permanent vs. temporary disability.

Physician fringe benefits:
- Vacation.
- Sick leave.
- Effect on compensation if physician chooses to take extra time off for vacation, continuing medical education (CME) study, etc.
- Expenses (CME, etc.)—dollar allowance.
- Time off (regular afternoon) during week.

Malpractice tail-end premium:
- Who pays in event of owner's withdrawal?

Exhibit 2.9
Merger Checklist
(continued)

BUYOUT OF AN OWNER
Address these events requiring a buyout:
- Death.
- Disability.
- Retirement.
- Withdrawal from the practice.

How will ownership interest be valued?
- Appraisal.
- Fixed formula.
- Deferred compensation (payout a percentage of patient receivables).
- Will a goodwill calculation be required?

Payout of ownership interest:
- Death:
  - Insurance proceeds.
  - How much insurance to obtain.
  - Proper structure for "key man" insurance.
- Disability, retirement, withdrawal:
  - Installment payments or lump sum.
  - Interest rate for installment payments.
  - When will installment payments begin?

Admission of a new owner:
- Required vote.
- Required net production dollar volume.
  How to value buy-in amount:
  - Appraisal.
  - Fixed formula.
- Installment payments, interest rate.

DISSOLUTION OF THE GROUP PRACTICE
- Required vote of the current owners.
- Method of dissolution.

MAJOR DECISIONS BY THE GROUP
- Majority or unanimous approval?
- Hiring and firing of personnel.
- Amending practice fee schedule.

(continued on next page)

Exhibit 2.9
Merger Checklist
(continued)

- Purchase of fixed assets in excess of $[dollar amount].
- Adopting or amending retirement plan.
- Any expenditure in excess of $[dollar amount].
- Designating of changing signatories on group bank accounts.
- Borrowing money.
- Entering into lease contracts.
- Offering ownership to a physician (probation or trial period).
- Terminating a physician's ownership.
- Withdrawals from group bank accounts.
- Negotiating and settling claims against the group practice.
- Determining which expenses of the individual physicians should be paid for by the group practice.
- Dissolution of the group practice.
- Purchase of insurance.
- Sale of group practice assets.
- Time intervals to reevaluate owner physician compensation formula; management group assignments; nonowner physician compensation formula.
- Other.

PROMOTION OF THE NEW GROUP PRACTICE
- Develop marketing strategy.
- Budget costs for marketing implementation.

The "Great Double Cross"

Psychologist and author Wayne Sotile discusses one of the most compelling issues weighing on the minds of medical group practice members. That issue is the "great double cross." Sotile asserts that the physician has always enjoyed the admiration of society and the promise of a comfortable living in return for providing care to patients—and that status is changing. Now-perpetual reductions in reimbursement are leading to ever-declining financial rewards, and lawsuits and the increasing scrutiny of physicians' practice of medicine have eroded the esteem many physicians feel. In addition, they are required to devote more time than in the past to charting in the EHR and performing other non-patient-care duties, further separating patients from physicians. The result has been a continued decrease in satisfaction with the practice of medicine (Sotile and Sotile 2002). Of those physicians currently in practice, 36 percent plan to retire in the next ten years, and only 58 percent of physicians are satisfied or very satisfied with their practice. They are also less likely to recommend medical practice as a profession (Jackson Healthcare 2013).

One important function of a practice's governance structure is to help restore and maintain practice satisfaction and address issues of burnout (see chapter 8). In addition, practice leaders must deal with a whole host of other issues in today's modern healthcare era, including the following:

◆ Decisions about the ownership structure

◆ New providers and their contractual relationship with the practice

◆ Practice relationships with outside entities

◆ Duties and contributions of the practice manager

◆ Physician involvement in practice management

◆ Provider relations

◆ Emerging model of healthcare delivery

Part of the practice leader's job is to manage the important relationships among physician practice stakeholders. We return to these and other issues in the chapters ahead.

DISCUSSION QUESTIONS

1. What is the purpose of the mission, vision, and values of the medical practice?

2. Who are some of the stakeholders of the medical practice?

3. What are some of the operational, internal, and external functions of the practice?

4. What are the components of organizational culture that affect the medical practice?

5. Describe some of the key organizational forms that include medical practices.

REFERENCES

Adamopoulos, H. 2014. "10 Key Healthcare Transaction Trends." Published February 7. www.beckershospitalreview.com/hospital-transactions-and-valuation/10-key-health care-transaction-trends.html.

American Academy of Family Physicians (AAFP). 2016. "Accountable Care Organizations." Accessed May 31. www.aafp.org/practice-management/payment/acos/sell.html.

American Hospital Association (AHA). 2017. "Fast Facts on US Hospitals." Updated January. www.aha.org/research/rc/stat-studies/fast-facts.shtml.

Association of American Medical Colleges (AAMC). 2016. "Council of Teaching Hospitals and Health Systems (COTH)." Accessed June 1. www.aamc.org/members/coth.

Blum, B. A. 2013. *Examples & Explanations: Contracts*, 6th ed. Alphen aan den Rijn, Netherlands: Aspen.

Centers for Medicare & Medicaid Services (CMS). 2017. "Shared Savings Program." Modified January 18. www.cms.gov/Medicare/Medicare-Fee-for-Service-Payment/shared savingsprogram/index.html?redirect=/sharedsavingsprogram.

Drucker, P. F. 2006. *Classic Drucker: Wisdom from Peter Drucker from the Pages of Harvard Business Review*. Boston: Harvard Business Review Press.

Galbraith, J. 2014. *Designing Organizations: Strategy, Structure, and Process at the Business Unit and Enterprise Levels*, 3rd ed. San Francisco: Jossey-Bass.

Groopman, J. 2008. *How Doctors Think*. New York: Houghton-Mifflin.

Institute for Healthcare Improvement (IHI). 2017. "The IHI Triple Aim." Accessed April 24. www.ihi.org/engage/initiatives/TripleAim/Pages/default.aspx.

Internal Revenue Service (IRS). 2017. "Exemption Requirements - 501(c)(3) Organizations." Updated January 26. www.irs.gov/charities-non-profits/charitable-organizations/exemption-requirements-section-501-c-3-organizations.

———. 2016. "A Guide to Common Qualified Plan Requirements." Updated October 28. www.irs.gov/retirement-plans/a-guide-to-common-qualified-plan-requirements.

Jackson Healthcare. 2013. "Filling the Void: 2013 Physician Outlook & Practice Trends." Accessed April 22, 2017. www.jacksonhealthcare.com/media/191888/2013 physiciantrends-void_ebk0513.pdf.

McCanne, D. 2010. "How Does the Affordable Care Act Define ACOs?" Published October 28. http://pnhp.org/blog/2010/10/28/how-does-the-affordable-care-act-define-acos.

McKendrick, E. 2012. *Contract Law: Text, Cases, and Materials*, 5th ed. Oxford, UK: Oxford University Press.

Merriam-Webster Collegiate Dictionary. 2016. "Culture." Accessed March 2. www.merriam-webster.com/dictionary/culture.

Michal, M. H., M. S. L. Pekarske, and M. K. McManus. 2006. "Corporate Practice of Medicine Doctrine 50 State Summary." New York: Center for Advanced Palliative Care.

Muhlestein, D. 2015. "Growth and Dispersion of Accountable Care Organizations in 2015." Published March 31. http://healthaffairs.org/blog/2015/03/31/growth-and-dispersion-of-accountable-care-organizations-in-2015-2.

National Committee for Quality Assurance (NCQA). 2017. "NCQA Patient-Centered Medical Home: Improving Experiences for Patients, Providers and Practice Staff." Accessed April 22. www.ncqa.org/Portals/0/PCMH%20brochure-web.pdf.

———. 2016. "Patient-Centered Medical Home (PCMH) Recognition." Accessed March 5. www.ncqa.org/Programs/Recognition/Practices/PatientCenteredMedicalHomePCMH.aspx.

Robbins, S. P. 1990. *Organizational Theory: Structure, Design, and Applications*, 3rd ed. Upper Saddle River, NJ: Prentice-Hall.

Schein, E. 2016. *Organizational Culture and Leadership*, 4th ed. San Francisco: Jossey-Bass.

Showalter, J. S. 2017. *The Law of Healthcare Administration*, 8th ed. Chicago: Health Administration Press.

Sotile, W., and M. Sotile. 2002. *The Resilient Physician: Effective Emotional Management for Doctors & Their Medical Organizations*. Chicago: American Medical Association Press.

Star, P. 2013. "Law and the Fog of Healthcare: Complexity and Uncertainty in the Struggle over Health Policy." *Saint Louis University Journal of Health Law and Policy* 6: 213–28.

Strandberg-Larsen, M., M. Schiøtz, J. Silver, A. Frølich, J. Andersen, I. Graetz, M. Reed, J. Bellows, A. Krasnik, T. Rundall, and J. Hsu. 2010. "Is the Kaiser Permanente Model Superior in Terms of Clinical Integration? A Comparative Study of Kaiser Permanente, Northern California and the Danish Healthcare System." *BMC Health Services Research* 10 (91): 1–13.

Wagner, E. H. 1998. "Chronic Disease Management: What Will It Take to Improve Care for Chronic Illness?" *Effective Clinical Practice* 1 (1): 2–4.

Wagner, S. L. 2013. "Organization and Operation of Medical Group Practice." In *Physician Practice Management: Essential Operational and Financial Knowledge*, 2nd ed., by Lawrence Wolper, 45–83. Burlington, MA: Jones & Bartlett Learning.

CHAPTER 3

INFORMATION TECHNOLOGY AND MANAGEMENT

Knowledge is power.

—Iman Ali Talib

LEARNING OBJECTIVES

➤ Assess the information technology needs of the medical practice.

➤ Consider the challenges of applying information technology in the medical practice.

➤ Recognize when to receive outside help on information technology issues.

➤ Articulate meaningful use and other regulatory requirements.

INTRODUCTION

We have all experienced the advantages of the digital world. It influences how we listen to music, how we pay our bills, how we conduct commerce, and how we learn and collect information. The information technology (IT) system is the backbone of the modern medical practice and is essential to supporting its operations and clinical functions. Virtually every aspect of the practice is potentially enhanced by the use of IT. Knowledge and information are power, and that power allows the practice to serve its patients as well as the community in a more precise and effective way than it could without IT capabilities.

Information technology in medical practices varies widely, from simple practice management systems (PMSs) to sophisticated longitudinal healthcare enterprise information systems, which may integrate a number of entities and functions (Nelson and Staggers 2018). Some electronic systems serve as health information exchanges (HIE), which connect organizations in a region or healthcare system (discussed in more depth later in the chapter).

For our purposes, the terms *digital* and *electronic* are used interchangeably, as are *information technology* and *electronic records*. Exhibit 3.1 illustrates the purpose and characteristics of an electronic system in the medical practice. Notice that the modern system is intended to service multiple stakeholders, so its design must be usable for a variety of purposes to enhance all stakeholders' performance. A system that does not fulfill these expectations will not be used, a situation that has plagued the digital transformation of medical practices.

PERFORMANCE

One of the biggest barriers to the acceptance of IT systems in medical practices is the performance of the system. How reliable is the system? How much of the time is it up and running? Unreliable systems encourage practices to maintain parallel paper systems "just in case," which is ultimately a waste of time and resources and should be avoided by implementing the most reliable IT systems available.

EXHIBIT 3.1
What IT Systems Should Do

For Whom?	Patients
	Providers
	Support Staff
For What Purpose?	Patient Care
	Documentation
	Research
	Picture Archiving and Capture
	Other Ancillaries
	Communication
	Decision Support
What Characteristics Should They Have?	Usable
	Specific
	Secure
	Smooth Flow
	Implementable
	Scalable

A related issue is whether use of the system adds steps to a process previously performed manually. The practice needs to determine if these additional steps are worth the value added by the system. Additional tasks can increase the time needed to perform the functions of the practice and may increase employee frustration and reduce acceptance of the IT system if they do not add clear value.

To paraphrase a theme from the 1951 movie *The Day the Earth Stood Still*, it is easy to be impressed with the technology. The practice manager and governing body need to analyze the performance of the IT systems with great care and attention before making purchasing decisions. The focus should be on bringing value to the practice and its patients, which in turn depends on the selection and proper implementation of the right system for the practice (Cryts 2016).

INTERFACE

Simply put, the IT user interface is how individuals interact with the information technology systems. It is the connection between the human beings and the technology, and it is critical to the successful implementation of any information system.

The easier the IT system is to use, the more likely it will be accepted by the stakeholders. Providers often complain that the old paper way was faster. What this sentiment does not take into account is that more people than just the provider were involved in completing the old process, and the total effort expended may have been greater than the provider realized. With that said, protecting and supporting the productive capacity of the clinicians is essential because they are the primary limiting factor for the productivity of any medical practice.

The interface with other systems inside and outside of the practice is an important consideration as well, with interoperability, or the ability to communicate with the other systems, being a critical element. Does the practice intend to connect with hospital systems, payer systems, regional health information networks, or other vendors and service providers? The answer to this question greatly influences the IT system the practice should choose.

EDUCATION AND TRAINING

Education and training are essential to the proper implementation and use of the IT system; however, the value of these activities is often underappreciated by medical practices. As a result, inadequate resources are devoted to having all members of the practice properly educated on the use of the system. This lack of training leads to frustration and, of course, the inefficient implementation of the IT system.

A carefully devised plan for the education and training of practice members is essential to the successful implementation of any IT system. Developing such a plan is often difficult, however, because devoting time to education and training takes away from the time available for clinical activities. As illustrated in exhibit 3.2, the initial loss of productivity that inevitably occurs with new systems may be regained, and productivity improved, as the use of the system becomes routine.

Protecting the physicians' time has always been an important issue for the medical practice. Although no concrete evidence has emerged at this point indicating that electronic records improve clinical productivity, they are essential to the administrative and operational side of the practice. One way to maximize the time of physicians and improve their productivity is to employ scribes. Scribes are individuals who help collect information for the physician by attending patient visits and taking notes from the history and physical and any other discussion that takes place. They then enter the data into the patient's electronic record, eliminating that step for the physician. The scribe has become a familiar member of the care team.

MEANINGFUL USE

Health Insurance Portability and Accountability Act (HIPAA)
Legislation covering many aspects of patient privacy and the sharing of private health information.

The Health Information Technology for Economic and Clinical Health Act (HITECH) was passed as part of the American Recovery and Reinvestment Act of 2009. HITECH provides significant provisions for medical practices intended to encourage a more rapid adoption of electronic health information systems than was occurring prior to the act's passage. It also includes provisions to enhance enforcement of the **Health Insurance Portability and Accountability Act (HIPAA)** and requires practices to engage in the meaningful use of electronic health information systems in a series of three stages (GPO 2009).

EXHIBIT 3.2
The IT Learning
Curve

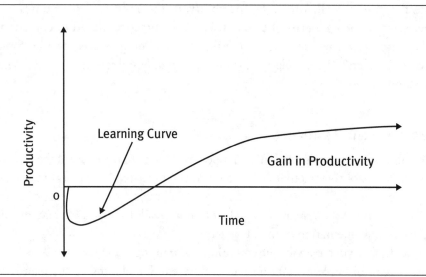

The term *meaningful use* refers to the IT capabilities practices adopt for providing care and engaging patients. The three stages of meaningful use are as follows (HealthIT. gov 2013):

1. Patient access

2. Patient–provider messaging; educational resources; and information gathering, such as the ability of the system to upload data from home monitoring devices

3. Self-management tools and electronic reporting on the patient care experience

As can be seen in exhibit 3.3, stage 1 begins the electronic records implementation effort with a focus on capturing and sharing data. Stage 2 focuses on establishing criteria for advanced clinical processes, and stage 3 looks at improving outcomes. Stage 3 is of

EXHIBIT 3.3
Meaningful Use Initiative

Stage 1: Meaningful Use Criteria Focus on Data Capture and Sharing	Stage 2: Meaningful Use Criteria Focus on Advanced Clinical Processes	Stage 3: Meaningful Use Criteria Focus on Improved Outcomes
Electronically capturing health information in a standardized format	More rigorous health information exchange (HIE)	Improving quality, safety, and efficiency, leading to improved health outcomes
Using that information to track key clinical conditions	Increased requirements for e-prescribing and incorporating lab results	Decision support for national high-priority conditions
Communicating that information for care coordination processes	Electronic transmission of patient care summaries across multiple settings	Patient access to self-management tools
Initiating the reporting of clinical quality measures and public health information	More patient-controlled data	Access to comprehensive patient data through patient-centered HIE
Using information to engage patients and their families in their care		Improving population health
Timeline: 2011–2012	Timeline: 2014	Timeline: 2016

Source: Adapted from HealthIT.gov (2013).

particular significance because it requires the meaningful interaction of patients with the provider using electronic means and encourages the practice to focus on improving the population's health.

Practices were expected to have achieved stage 3 by 2016.

HITECH has indeed provided the needed impetus for accelerating the use of electronic health information systems in medical practices and moving practices from stand-alone IT systems to fully integrated systems, as shown in exhibit 3.4.

A general mental model of the information management process is illustrated in exhibit 3.5 in terms of the policies, processes, and goals of the organization. It shows the continuum of information to knowledge as data are collected and processed to create a knowledge base that can be used for decision making and operations.

EXHIBIT 3.4
Continuum of IT
System Integration

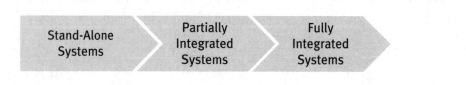

EXHIBIT 3.5
Data Collection,
Processing, and
Reporting

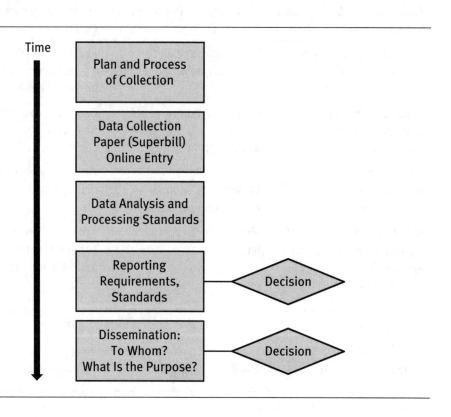

PRACTICE MANAGEMENT SYSTEMS

An important part of the overall IT system for medical practices is the PMS. PMSs perform the following functions (AMA 2016):

◆ Capture patient demographics

◆ Schedule appointments

◆ Preregister patients for upcoming procedures (including insurance eligibility and benefits confirmation)

◆ Determine the patient's financial responsibility to facilitate payment collection at the point of care

◆ Maintain lists of insurance payers

◆ Perform billing tasks

◆ Generate administrative reports

PMSs also can perform the aggregation of large data sets over time, which allows the practice to take a broad view of important management and healthcare issues. This process is difficult, if not impossible, using paper record systems.

Because data management is an important component of effective medical practice operations, practice managers require some knowledge about what it is, when it is used, and for what purpose it is used. Data management is a vast field, a thorough understanding of which may be beyond the scope of most practice management generalists. Suffice to say here that data management focuses on ensuring that the practice properly maintains and makes available the data needed to operate the practice effectively and efficiently. It is a database management function, sometimes referred to as a data warehouse, that allows the practice to store vital information in an interactive and retrievable format, thus facilitating the creation of custom reports.

Some important functions of data management include the following:

◆ *Decision support*—This function assists practices in justifying the business case for actions. For example, a multispecialty practice may consult a report generated by the data management system to determine whether to hire a geriatrician on the basis of the number of patients older than age 65 seen in the practice. Similarly, a practice manager may notice a trend in the data showing the increased ordering of a particular procedure and decide to purchase a new piece of equipment to accommodate the increase in demand.

◆ *Business intelligence*—This attribute of data management takes the data available in the practice from its information and data systems and converts it into information that can be used in developing strategic plans or to provide better service to patients. For example, a practice may glean an opportunity from the business intelligence gathered on the zip codes of the patient base for a possible location of a new practice satellite office.

◆ *Creation of metrics for improvement and **dashboards** for tracking progress*—By analyzing the raw data of the practice, data management tools can compile a relevant series of metrics and create dashboards that help practice leaders evaluate the performance of the practice.

Modern PMSs should include **analytical** tools that assist with these and more processes. Exhibit 3.6 illustrates a typical data collection, processing, and reporting structure. In developing these systems, practices must be sure to consider how the system will function and what it is expected to produce before purchasing the system.

OTHER IMPORTANT SYSTEMS IN THE MEDICAL PRACTICE

Some additional electronic systems in the medical practice that comprise IT and management functions are the following:

◆ Medical records

◆ Laboratory testing and results

◆ Imaging, sometimes referred to as picture archiving and communication systems

◆ Human resources

◆ Accounting

◆ Financial management

One could argue with great success that the patient medical record is the most valuable and important document in the medical practice. With that in mind, we focus on describing the medical records system in this section.

MEDICAL RECORDS

The maintenance and safekeeping of a patient's medical record is the principal function of the medical records unit. The records contain the proof of what activities were undertaken,

Dashboard
Similar to a car's dashboard, provides a medical practice integrated and consistently presented operational data for decision making.

Analytical
Decision-making style in which the decision maker gives careful consideration to the uniqueness of situations. This style is typically used when tolerance for ambiguity is high and decision makers are rational in their thinking.

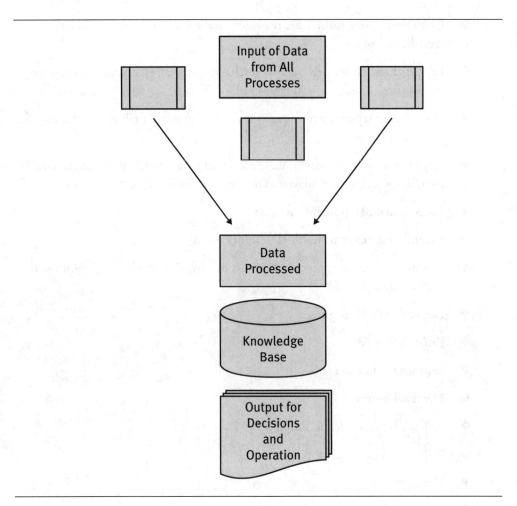

EXHIBIT 3.6
Information
Management
Model

by whom, how they were done, why they were necessary or appropriate, and where they were performed. In addition, medical records capture a plan for future care.

Most medical practice records contain the following information:

◆ Physician notes, including a treatment plan and treatments provided

◆ Operative notes related to surgical procedures

◆ Laboratory test orders and results

◆ X-ray test orders and results

◆ Documentation of any **ancillary services** provided or indicated, such as laboratory or audiology services

Ancillary services
Range of services
provided to support
the work of a primary
physician, classified
into three categories:
diagnostic, therapeu-
tic, and custodial.

◆ Communications from other providers in the form of letters, copies of records, and so on

◆ Patient's hospital records, such as discharge summaries, operative notes, and copies of test results from the hospital

◆ Consultative reports, which describe the background, evaluation, and plan for the care of the patient

◆ Any treatment plans other than those documented in the physician notes, including goals to be achieved as through a rehabilitation plan

◆ Patient's demographic information

◆ Patient's insurance or health plan information

◆ Patient's upcoming appointments with the practice or related appointments with another provider

◆ Past and current diagnoses

◆ Patient's allergies

◆ Patient's medication list

◆ Physician orders

◆ Patient's home health or hospice care information

◆ Follow-up indicated for the patient

◆ Nurse's notes

◆ Patient's self-care status

◆ Patient's disabilities and impairments

◆ Patient's equipment requirements

◆ Patient's nutrition details

◆ Therapist notes

◆ Social service agency notes

Patient Records Completed Through Clinical Content Integration

One of the great challenges of medical records management is completeness because patient records come from so many sources. Practices should consider opportunities to join local, regional, and national HIEs to gain access to more complete and accurate information from other participating practices, thereby helping to ensure that patients receive improved service and care.

HIEs are just part of the movement toward increasing the completeness of patient records through clinical content integration. Healthcare systems are integrating practices that are not owned but are affiliated, providing them access to critical patient clinical information.

The term *health information exchange* refers to an organization of reliable and interoperable electronic health-related information sharing conducted in a manner that protects the confidentiality, privacy, and security of the information. Currently, regional health information organizations (RHIOs) are the most common form of HIE organization. A RHIO governs the exchange of health information between so-called healthcare stakeholders within a defined geographic area. The goal of this exchange is to improve healthcare for people in the community (Jones and Groom 2017).

RHIOs typically include a range of participating healthcare provider entities as well as other health stakeholders, such as payers, laboratories, and public health departments. They are often managed by a board of directors composed of representatives from each participating organization. For a RHIO to be established, stakeholders in the proposed RHIO must reach consensus on what information can be shared among different participating entities. In addition, prior to exchanging information, the entities need to sign data use agreements. Because the capacity to effectively store and manage clinical data electronically is a prerequisite for participating in an HIE, RHIOs often offer programs to assist affiliated providers with health IT adoption at the institutional level (AHRQ 2017).

These exchanges employ nationally recognized standards for interoperability and security (HealthIT.gov 2014a, 2014b). Medical practices that participate in these exchanges have wider access to not only patient data but population health information as well.

Population health management is a healthcare approach that focuses on improving healthcare outcomes for an entire group or population. The concept of population health takes a broad view of patient care by emphasizing engagement of physicians, other providers, and the patient. The idea is not to reduce the quality of care for the individual but rather to broaden the scope of care to consider the larger group as well as the individual.

Data are essential for population health management, as they inform the medical practice about the health status of the community. If a practice does not understand the status of its patient group, it will fail to know whether its health improvement efforts work. Take, for example, the A1c levels of a group of diabetic patients. The A1c level is a measure of how well the patient's diabetes is controlled. To measure the effectiveness of a care strategy for diabetic patients, the practice must be able to compile an aggregate measure of the A1c level for the entire group of patients under its care or in the population.

HIEs allow a medical practice to integrate patient information from multiple provider sources, as illustrated in exhibit 3.7.

EXHIBIT 3.7
Health Information
Exchange

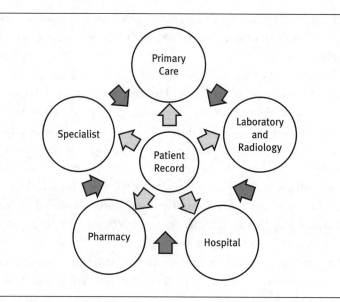

The Wisconsin Health Information Exchange, known as WISHIN, provides a good example of how an HIE can be organized and work for the benefit of medical practices and their patients. The exchange connects more than 1,000 providers and, in addition to health data sharing, offers a platform for practices to conduct research and focus on health issues that are of particular interest to the region (WISHIN 2013).

THE PATIENT FLOW PROCESS AND IT'S ROLE

The effective practice carefully considers process flow issues. Many processes can be improved using digital technology: Consider the example in exhibit 3.8, which illustrates a simple process flowchart for a patient visit. Each of these processes can be enhanced with digital technology, and each step may provide opportunities for improvement, as discussed in chapter 10. In this case, reminders, decision points, and standardization of procedures are enhanced with the digital technology.

THE NEED TO STANDARDIZE PROCESSES IN A PRACTICE

As illustrated by the flowchart in exhibit 3.8, applying digital technology to procedures requires careful attention to process standardization for each activity to function effectively. This requirement has been a barrier to technology adoption by the healthcare industry because it can only be effective if the practice standardizes its processes. That standardization involves a learning curve that, in the short run, will reduce the efficiency of the operation

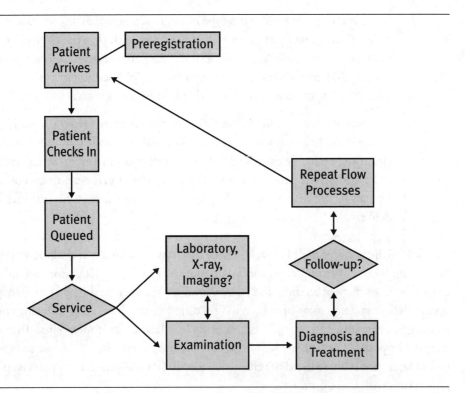

EXHIBIT 3.8
Patient Flow
Process

and therefore its productivity. Practices often find this side effect untenable and are unwilling to invest the time and financial resources needed to make the conversion. However, the short-term disadvantages of adoption are often outweighed by the long-term gains. Exhibit 3.2 earlier in the chapter illustrates this phenomenon.

INTEROPERABILITY

As defined by the Healthcare Information and Management Systems Society (HIMSS 2016), "Interoperability means the ability of health information systems to work together within and across organizational boundaries in order to advance the effective delivery of healthcare for individuals and communities. There are three levels of health information technology interoperability: 1) Foundational; 2) Structural; and 3) Semantic." The following explanation of each level is adapted from HIMSS (2016):

1. *Foundational* means there is the ability for data exchange to occur between one information technology system and another without data interpretation. Albeit an oversimplification, data interpretation is a term that describes the conversion of data from one computer language to another.

2. *Structural* interoperability is a type of data exchange that allows movement of healthcare data from one system to another such that the clinical or operational purpose and meaning of the data are preserved and unaltered. It ensures that data exchanges between information technology systems can be interpreted at the data field level. This is known as syntax.

3. *Semantic* interoperability is the ability of two or more systems to exchange information in a usable way. This level of interoperability supports the electronic exchange of patient summary information among caregivers and other authorized parties via potentially disparate EHR systems and other systems to improve quality, safety, efficiency, and efficacy of healthcare delivery.

Initially, most of the IT systems in medical practices were stand-alone systems with little integration. For example, practices used separate systems for laboratory activities, radiology functions, patient records, and administrative processes via the practice management system. These systems were often created by different vendors using different computer languages, protocols, and procedures, resulting in a lack of interoperability. That made it virtually impossible or, at best, very expensive for the systems to talk to one another. This lack of interoperability reduced the effectiveness of EHRs and thus further reduced practices' satisfaction with these products.

More modern systems tend to use common computer languages and standardized interfaces, which allow for greater interoperability.

VALUE-BASED CARE AND IT

A modern IT system is essential if a practice wishes to participate in value-based care (CMS 2017). The ability to provide value-based care depends on a practice having contemporaneous (real-time) data for its patient base on the care provided, the outcomes achieved, and the costs incurred from practice operations. This level of data acquisition simply is not realistic with a manual system; manual data capture is difficult, inaccurate, time-consuming, and costly.

POPULATION HEALTH

For most of the US healthcare system's history, the provision of care has focused on the individual patient. Although this aim is clearly a very important and necessary goal that still needs to be pursued, it is insufficient for healthcare in the new era. Taking good care of individual patients must be accompanied by a focus on the care of an entire population of patients. Population health management reflects second-curve medicine (HRET 2013; see also chapter 1).

Population health management is a process by which patient data are collected from multiple sources, compiled into the patient record, and accessed by providers to inform them of the population's health status. Metrics are such an important aspect of population health management that practices may be putting their business at risk in terms of reimbursement if they ignore value-based measures. And of primary importance, a practice that cannot measure the outcomes it seeks to achieve will not be able to measure the improvements its innovations are creating.

In short, having well-developed IT systems in place is essential to effective population health management.

PRACTICAL ASPECTS OF MEDICAL PRACTICE INFORMATION SYSTEMS

In this section, we discuss several practical issues surrounding IT in medical practices, including system selection, installation failure, the cloud, governance, and privacy and security.

SELECTING A SYSTEM FOR THE PRACTICE

When considering electronic systems for the medical practice, whether purchasing cloud services (discussed later in the section) or hosting servers on site at the practice, practice leadership must address the following questions for successful implementation:

◆   How usable is the system? A major complaint of clinicians about electronic systems is that they are not user-friendly or intuitive and therefore are disruptive to workflow. The practice leader must be sure to ascertain the ability of the system to adapt to the unique needs of the users.

◆   How customized is the system to the practice? The capabilities of the system should closely match the needs and expectations of the practice, and the system should fit seamlessly into the practice structure. Achieving such compatibility may require the development of special templates for different specialties by a consultant or vendor.

◆   How compatible is the system's operation with the natural workflow of the practice? Disruption of workflows can be a major impediment to implementation and may decrease practice efficiency if attention is not paid to this detail early on.

◆   How deployable is the system? System launch requires careful planning to be sure that the system can be integrated into the practice with minimal disruption to its operations. Another important consideration is the amount of training needed for staff to properly use the system. Most medical practices are busy environments, and large blocks of time to devote to training can be difficult to schedule.

◆   Is the system scalable? In other words, can it grow and adapt with the practice to keep up with the demands of an increasing workload? Determining scalability at the beginning of the selection process helps prevent the need to find new systems in the future as a practice grows.

STEPS IN THE SYSTEM SELECTION PROCESS

The selection of an IT system for the medical practice demands a disciplined project management approach. Exhibit 3.9 illustrates the constrained relationships among scope, time, cost, and quality that typically develop when any project is undertaken. All projects require an optimization of their scope, the time required to complete them, and the quality (value or cost could be substituted here) of the desired outcome. The larger the scope, the more the project will cost or the quality will be reduced, and the longer it will take to implement. Similarly, as scope decreases, cost is reduced, and quality increases, and the time to implement may decrease. These rules may be simple, but they are critical to consider in the planning of a project such as information systems implementation. Many IT projects undertaken in medical practices have failed because practice leaders failed to account for the relationships among scope, quality, cost, and time to implement. For example, medical practices often fall victim to the fierce urgency of now and rush to complete a project, risking the long-range goals of the project.

Exhibit 3.9
The Constrained
Relationship
in Project
Management

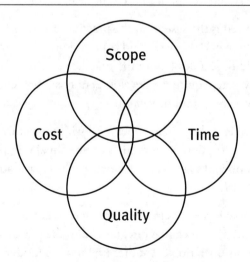

The system selection process, whether for a practice management system, an EHR, or another IT system, requires the completion of several important steps.

Step 1.   Consider the need for outside independent expertise. IT is a rapidly changing field and requires a level of expertise that may not be available in the practice. The leadership should consider obtaining outside independent expertise before undertaking a major selection process for an IT product. In this process, however, it should emphasize the importance of independence to prevent conflicts of interest that may be present if the outside expert is affiliated with the vendor of the IT system being implemented.

Step 2.   Conduct a needs assessment. This step should involve members from every department and service area of the practice. Focus on the outcomes desired and the problems the practice is attempting to address by implementing an IT solution.

Step 3.   Develop a list of must-have criteria. Be sure the practice has a way to measure the success of the project prior to system selection; developing a list of criteria will help make that a reality.

Step 4.   Find appropriate comparables. Medical practices vary widely in the services they offer, their size, and many other characteristics. Seek advice from practices that are similar to yours to help establish criteria that may be useful in the selection process. This step offers the practice manager and other leaders an opportunity to discuss the project with individuals in similar circumstances who have previously gone through the process.

Step 5.   Develop a list of potential vendors. Checking with industry contacts, leaders at the comparable practices, and professional organizations may be useful for creating this list. Consider attending information system trade shows as an effective way to gain firsthand knowledge of the marketplace.

Step 6.   Develop a request for proposal (RFP). The RFP helps standardize the responses from the vendors, making comparisons straightforward. In addition, requesting specific information contained in the RFP will ensure that the vendors respond to the needs of the practice and that the must-haves are being addressed.

Step 7.   List the top vendors who seem to offer the best solutions for the practice.

Step 8.   Interview each vendor on the list of top candidates. This step provides practice leadership the opportunity to receive clarification on any questions that arise from responses on the RFP and can offer a sense about the vendor's reliability and expertise.

Step 9. Negotiate a contract with the vendor of choice. This contract should pay careful attention to the scope of the project, including the following elements:

◆ Specific features that are included in the products and services to be provided

◆ The price to be paid and the terms of payment

◆ The timeline for delivery of the agreed-on products and services

◆ Any penalties for failure to deliver as scheduled

◆ Guarantees and other warranties for the products and services

◆ Any future promise of services and support

Information system contracts should be as specific as possible to prevent misunderstandings related to the installation of the system and any follow-up service. IT projects in medical practices are notorious for going over budget, falling behind schedule, and in general being frustrating to execute.

Step 10. Prepare for implementation. This is a critical step in the process because time must be set aside for training staff and testing the system. Alternative operating scenarios will need to be used during the implementation process. Preparation for implementation also includes thorough discussions with all members and stakeholders in the practice to be sure they understand the implications of the implementation process. IT projects tend to be very disruptive, so a comprehensive, understandable, and convincing presentation about the nature of the implementation and potential consequences is essential.

Step 11. Implement the new system. Following the plan that has been constructed for implementation is a key to success in this step, as is frequent communications with all stakeholders as implementation proceeds.

Step 12. Reflect on the project. Projects rarely go completely according to plan, and important lessons always come from reflecting on the ways the project rollout varied from expectations. One way to conduct a meaningful reflection on the project is to gather all the key players in the implementation of the project in a structured meeting that adheres to the following guidelines:

◆ Establish the purpose and background of the meeting so participants understand it is not intended to assign blame but to share lessons that can be applied to future projects.

◆ Establish ground rules and guidelines for the meeting process. These guidelines include asking attendees to be open and honest, encouraging everyone in the meeting to participate, reducing external distractions by turning off cell phones and other devices, maintaining an atmosphere of confidentiality, and keeping the discussion on target. If unrelated issues arise during the discussion, defer them to another forum (and be sure to follow up as promised).

◆ Ask the following questions:

— What went well with the implementation?

— What would we do again for future projects?

— What did not go well, and what did we learn that we can improve on?

— Specifically, what would we do differently for future projects?

◆ Summarize the discussion and any follow-up measures that arose.

◆ Thank the participants for their involvement, and let them know how future information regarding the meeting will be communicated.

COMMON REASONS FOR INSTALLATION FAILURES

Much of the success of an installation of a new electronic system depends on the attentive leadership and governance of the project. Leadership typically takes the form of a steering committee that includes the practice leadership and physician representation. The committee determines measurable goals and the best means for system testing, including pre- and post-live measurements to assess success.

Leadership is responsible for establishing reasonable expectations of what will likely occur in the process as well as what the result of the implementation will be. One good way to develop these expectations is to ask the stakeholders what success will look like to them once the system is implemented. If the expectations of the stakeholders seem unrealistic or beyond the scope of the project, these discrepancies should be resolved before the project proceeds.

Complicated and intricate interfaces can be difficult to implement and manage. However, such innovations as voice recognition technology have improved greatly, providing convenient and efficient interfacing with the IT system, especially the EHR. Thus, advanced technology should not be dismissed merely because it is complicated and difficult to implement.

CLOUD COMPUTING AND THE MEDICAL PRACTICE

The impact that the Internet has had on the medical practice would have been difficult to imagine 30 years ago. And it will continue to have a major, largely unforeseen, influence in the future. One such impact that has emerged is the use of cloud computing, sometimes called software as a service (SaaS).

Cloud computing allows virtually every aspect of medical practice IT services to be performed "on the cloud." *The cloud* is a generic term that refers to the ability to access services and computing power through a service provider via the Internet without maintaining the hardware and software on-site at the practice. The practice must still maintain equipment by which to access the Internet and to input to or download information from the cloud, but the amount of equipment needed is greatly reduced from that needed for a stand-alone system, or a system that is primarily maintained by the practice. Obviously, cloud computing carries many potential advantages and disadvantages. Some advantages are the following:

◆ *Reduced cost.* The cost of cloud computing can be significantly lower than the cost involved in maintaining the software, hardware, and related services in the practice. Cloud services often use the latest hardware and software available, which are usually difficult for small and medium-sized practices to afford.

◆ *Increased security.* The physical and cyber security of the practice's IT systems have become an increasing area of concern for most practices. Moving practice IT functions to the cloud reduces the chance of a physical loss of IT assets and may reduce the probability of cyber threats.

◆ *Twenty-four/seven service availability.* Most cloud computing services operate on a round-the-clock basis.

◆ *Backup.* Reputable cloud service companies offer sophisticated backup services to prevent data loss due to catastrophic IT failures.

◆ *Scalability.* Cloud services may be much more scalable than traditional IT systems.

◆ *Expertise.* Most small and medium-sized practices do not have the IT expertise on-site that is available with a cloud computing service.

◆ *Flexibility.* Although most cloud services require a service contract of a specified length, the commitment to any cloud service may be less than the commitment the practice makes when buying the equipment and software and hiring the necessary expertise to operate it.

Disadvantages include the following:

◆ *Variable reliability of the Internet.* Cloud services depend on an Internet connection, and that connection can be a primary point of failure for a medical practice's IT systems. The practice must consider the reliability of its Internet service provider as well as its routers when making the decision to use cloud-based computing services.

◆ *Potential for cloud service provider errors.* Cloud service providers are not perfect. Data may be lost. The company might go out of business or its performance quality might be lower than expected. All these types of issues must be considered, and a thorough understanding of the consequences of SaaS gained, before committing to a cloud-based service.

◆ *Lack of function compatibility.* If the practice does not switch all its IT systems to the cloud-based service, will all the IT functions still be compatible? The practice needs to determine which, if not all, services will be transferred to the cloud, assess the provider's services for compatibility issues, and plan for service gaps before committing to moving to the cloud.

◆ *Negative or skeptical stakeholder temperament toward the cloud.* Some people simply are not comfortable with the idea that their data and important business functions are being handled remotely by a cloud service. **Attitudes** are a rather intangible consideration, but they should be discussed with practice stakeholders to gauge comfort level (Torrieri 2011; Moumtzoglou and Kastania 2014).

Attitude
Mental state indicating level of readiness.

IT GOVERNANCE

Successful adoption of an IT system for a practice requires well-structured IT governance. Forming this structure is the first step in going digital.

IT governance frames the expectations for the practice for how the IT systems being considered will enhance the operations and bring additional value to patients. Like all practice decisions, IT system implementation must be guided by the mission, vision, and values of the practice.

A readiness assessment of the practice should be conducted to analyze how the practice is organized. In this process, each of the following elements should be honestly and realistically assessed (HealthIT.gov 2016):

1. Is adequate support in place for the investment and training in IT systems by the governing board of the practice?

2. What administrative processes are employed by the practice?

3. Are these administrative processes streamlined and documented? (An example is shown in exhibit 3.10.)

4. Are clinical workflows in the practice well understood and documented on flowcharts?

5. Are data collection and reporting processes in the practice well established and documented?

6. What is the level of computer literacy and comfort with IT of practice staff and physicians?

7. Does the practice have access to reliable and adequate IT infrastructure, such as high-speed Internet connectivity?

8. Does the practice have sufficient financial capital to purchase new or additional hardware?

9. Do any clinical priorities need to be considered, such as diabetic care, morbidity from obesity, and other chronic disease? (In specialty practices, a registry is often helpful in following patients with particular diseases or those that have undergone special procedures. A disease registry is a tool and process for tracking the clinical care and outcomes of a specified patient population. Registries are used to support care management of these groups of patients. For example, a disease registry might track all patients with diagnoses of heart disease or diabetes.)

10. Does the practice have specialty-specific requirements?

One of the biggest challenges in introducing medical practices to modern information management systems has been the slow adoption rate. IT adoption in practices has lagged other areas of the healthcare industry for a number of reasons, including the following:

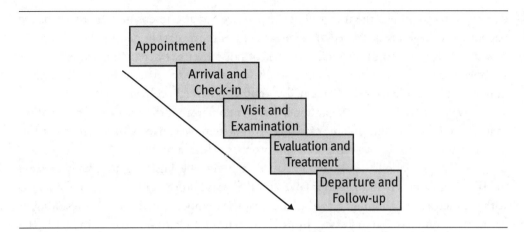

EXHIBIT 3.10
Simple Process
Flowchart for a
Patient Visit

◆ *High cost.* Physicians have long demonstrated efficiency in their ability to use paper records. The cost and inconvenience of conversion have been major impediments to implementing information management systems in the practices.

◆ *Issues surrounding change management.* Although much more efficient than paper records, the adoption curve for an information management system requires changes in process flow and the adoption of new skills. Practitioners are often reluctant to embrace these kinds of changes.

◆ *Lack of interoperability.* Many early medical record systems were proprietary, which often made interconnectivity among systems difficult to achieve, limiting the usefulness of the technology. In addition, the companies that offered these systems were often small and prone to leaving the market, either through merger and acquisition or by going out of business. As a result, practices were left with systems that could not be maintained and therefore had limited usefulness. Although this situation has greatly improved in recent years, the concern lingers and should be considered when evaluating any IT system.

SYSTEM SECURITY AND PRIVACY

The concern for security and privacy in the healthcare environment has never been greater than it is today. According to Gemalto (2015), a cybersecurity analyst firm, 34 percent of cyber breaches taking place in the first half of 2015 occurred in healthcare institutions. Although little information is available about specific breaches related to medical practices, this trend represents an area of great concern. Practices must be vigilant to safeguard their data not only to protect the integrity of the practice but also to ensure the privacy of the patients. The biggest issue related to the breach of healthcare data is identity theft; however, new threats have emerged, including the use of ransomware, whereby malicious software is implanted in the computer system that denies access to the data in the system until a ransom is paid to the hackers. Blackmail is another potential problem.

Whatever the specific threat, most patients do not want their personal information shared with others. In one notable case, Anthem's systems were hacked and as many as 130 million patient records may have been compromised (McCann 2015).

HIPAA violations are also on the rise. As exhibit 3.11 illustrates, the steady increase in HIPAA violations reported and resolved for the years 2003 through 2012 has coincided with the increase in electronic records. Note that the number of investigations resulting in corrective action has also increased, from 17 percent in 2003 to 36 percent in 2012. The most common sources of complaints, according to these data, are impermissible access and disclosure (HHS 2016).

These data are an indicator that, although malicious hacking is a serious source of compromise for healthcare systems, violations of HIPAA and similar data breaches are

Exhibit 3.11

HIPAA Violations

Year	Investigated: No Violation		Resolved After Intake and Review		Investigated: Corrective Action Obtained		Total Resolutions
Partial Year 2003	79	5%	1,177	78%	260	17%	1,516
2004	360	7%	3,406	71%	1,033	22%	4,799
2005	642	11%	3,889	68%	1,162	21%	5,693
2006	897	14%	4,128	62%	1,574	24%	6,599
2007	727	10%	5,017	69%	1,494	21%	7,238
2008	1,180	13%	5,940	63%	2,221	24%	9,341
2009	1,211	15%	4,749	59%	2,146	26%	8,106
2010	1,529	17%	4,951	54%	2,709	29%	9,189
2011	1,302	16%	4,466	53%	2,595	31%	8,363
2012	979	10%	5,067	54%	3,361	36%	9,407

Source: HHS (2016).

more commonly because of careless behavior of individuals in the practice. Some of these behaviors include the following (Zabel 2016):

◆   Lacking or not enforcing Internet use policies.

◆   Not encrypting sensitive information. All information sent through the Internet should be encrypted to prevent malicious use of practice or patient information.

◆   Not training people properly on Internet security. This training should be a standard part of new employee orientation, and refresher training should occur on a regular basis.

◆   Using weak passwords, sharing passwords, or writing passwords in locations where they can be easily found. Another problem related to passwords is that many users fail to change them on a frequent basis.

◆   Clicking on malicious links (known as phishing) and knowingly or unknowingly providing access to cyber criminals.

◆   Not having rule-based access. Everyone working on the practice computer system should be given access based on their need to know specific information and on their roles and responsibilities. Failing the establishment of these measures, if a breach occurs, most access to the system should be limited to some extent.

◆   Having inadequate firewall, malware, and virus protection. A firewall is a network security system designed to prevent unauthorized access to or from a private network. Firewalls and other preventive programs can limit the potential for unauthorized access as well as the introduction of malicious software into the practice's IT systems. They can be software based, hardware based, or a combination of both.

◆   Failing to regularly monitor systems for failure. All IT systems in the practice should be checked regularly for the possibility of breaches, malware, and other malicious activity.

DISCUSSION QUESTIONS

1. What are some of the important purposes of an electronic records system?

2. Discuss some of the reasons that implementing electronic records in a medical practice is so difficult.

3. What is meant by the term *meaningful use*, and what are its components?

4. What are some important considerations for project management in the implementation of an information system?

5. What are some key steps in selecting a medical record system for the practice?

REFERENCES

Agency for Healthcare Research and Quality (AHRQ). 2017. "Health IT Tools and Resources." Accessed May 18. https://healthit.ahrq.gov/health-it-tools-and-resources.

American Medical Association (AMA). 2016. "How to Select a Practice Management System." Accessed June 2. www.ama-assn.org/ama/pub/advocacy/topics/administrative-simplification-initiatives/pms-toolkit.page?.

Centers for Medicare & Medicaid Services (CMS). 2017. "What Are the Value-Based Programs?" Accessed April 23. www.cms.gov/Medicare/Quality-Initiatives-Patient-Assessment-Instruments/Value-Based-Programs/Value-Based-Programs.html.

Cryts, A. 2016. "Ways to Get Physicians to Embrace the EHR." Published July 19. www.physicianspractice.com/ehr/ways-get-physicians-embrace-ehr.

Gemalto. 2015. "Gemalto Releases Findings of First Half 2015 Breach Level Index." Published September 9. www.gemalto.com/press/Pages/Gemalto-Releases-Findings-of-First-Half-2015-Breach-Level-Index.aspx.

Healthcare Information and Management Systems Society (HIMSS). 2016. "What Is Interoperability?" Accessed June 5. www.himss.org/library/interoperability-standards/what-is-interoperability.

HealthIT.gov. 2016. "Frequently Asked Questions: How Do I Conduct a Readiness Assessment?" Accessed March 15. www.healthit.gov/providers-professionals/frequently-asked-questions/394#id64.

———. 2014a. "Health Information Exchange (HIE)." Updated June 5. www.health IT.gov/HIE.

———. 2014b. "What Is HIE?" Updated May 12. www.healthit.gov/providers-professionals/ health-information-exchange/what-hie.

———. 2013. "How to Attain Meaningful Use." Updated January 15. www.healthit.gov/ providers-professionals/how-attain-meaningful-use.

Health Research & Educational Trust (HRET). 2013. "Metrics for the Second Curve of Health Care." Published April. www.hpoe.org/Reports-HPOE/Metrics_Second_Curve_4_13.pdf.

Jones, S., and F. Groom (eds.). 2017. *Information and Communication Technologies in Healthcare*. Boca Raton, FL: CRC Press.

McCann, E. 2015. "Anthem Hack: 'Healthcare Is a Target.'" Published February 6. www. healthcareitnews.com/news/anthem-hack-healthcare-target.

Moumtzoglou, A., and A. N. Kastania. 2014. *Cloud Computing Applications for Quality Healthcare Delivery*. Hershey, PA: IGI Global.

Nelson, R., and N. Staggers. 2018. *Health Informatics: An Interprofessional Approach*. St. Louis, MO: Elsevier.

Torrieri, M. 2011. "Should Your Medical Practice Use Cloud-Based Computing?" Published December 23. www.physicianspractice.com/technology/should-your-medical -practice-use-cloud-based-computing/page/0/5.

US Department of Health & Human Services (HHS). 2016. "Enforcement Results by Year." Accessed June 6. www.hhs.gov/hipaa/for-professionals/compliance-enforcement/data/ enforcement-results-by-year/index.html.

US Government Publishing Office (GPO). 2009. "H. R. 1." Accessed June 3, 2016. www.gpo. gov/fdsys/pkg/BILLS-111hr1enr/pdf/BILLS-111hr1enr.pdf.

Wisconsin Health Information Exchange (WISHIN). 2013. Home page. Accessed June 5, 2016. www.wishin.org.

Zabel, L. 2016. "10 Common HIPAA Violations and Preventative Measures to Keep Your Practice in Compliance." Published June 22. www.beckershospitalreview.com/healthcare -information-technology/10-common-hipaa-violations-and-preventative-measures-to- keep-your-practice-in-compliance.html.

CHAPTER 4

REGULATORY ISSUES, THE LAW, AND PRACTICE MANAGEMENT

Risk comes from not knowing what you're doing.

—Warren Buffett

LEARNING OBJECTIVES

➤ Appreciate the number of regulations affecting the medical practice.

➤ Understand the nature of contracting.

➤ Describe contracting prohibitions for medical practice contracts.

➤ Articulate legal requirements for a valid contract.

➤ Understand the seriousness of Stark law.

INTRODUCTION

Healthcare is one of the most heavily regulated industries in the United States. The need for such extensive regulation is understandable when one considers the impact of healthcare and the medical practice on society (Field 2008). In recent years, calls for additional regulation have increased in the wake of criticism that the US healthcare system and physician practices may place patients at undue risk due to the imbalance of the agency relationship that exists between a physician and his or her patients (Makary 2012).

The medical practice makes decisions and guides patients on matters of great consequence. In addition, providers, unlike almost any other types of professionals, can influence the behaviors and actions of consumers. Most patients have limited knowledge of healthcare, and as a result, they rely on the physician or another provider to serve as their agent in seeking solutions to their healthcare needs (Gafri and Whelan 1998). Some observers argue that the provider–patient relationship constitutes an agency relationship under the law; at the least, the practitioner has an absolute obligation to act in the best interest of the patient (ACP 2016; this resource is a valuable reference that all practice managers and leaders should be familiar with and have available for use in the practice).

This unmatched position of trust also places the healthcare provider in a position to potentially abuse the relationship because he or she has such immense power over the patient.

One issue that emerged as a consequence of the traditional fee-for-service or volume-based care is physician-induced demand (PID). PID is an economic concept whereby the service provider is in a position to create demand for these services for the provider's own benefit. Because medical services have, until recently, been reimbursed entirely on a volume basis such that the more service that is provided, the more the practice is paid, physicians have had an incentive to deliver more services than may be needed (Johnson 2014). Through policy and education, and aided by the growth of reimbursement models based on value rather than volume, practices must defend against self-serving behavior in the practice.

The number of rules and laws regulating healthcare is enormous. The Affordable Care Act (ACA) alone contains more than 11,000 pages of regulations (O'Donnell and Akinnibi 2013). Being aware of, let alone understanding, all the rules and regulations pertaining to healthcare delivery is almost impossible for any practice manager. One way for managers to stay current with new and changing rules and regulations is to regularly check sources such as the following:

◆ The *Federal Register*, at www.federalregister.gov

◆ The US Department of Health & Human Services "Laws & Regulations" web page, www.hhs.gov/regulations

◆ The Centers for Medicare & Medicaid Services (CMS) "Regulations & Guidance" web page, www.cms.gov/regulations-and-guidance/regulations-and -guidance.html

◆ The websites of, briefings by, and seminars offered by professional organizations, such as the American College of Healthcare Executives (www. ache.org), Medical Group Management Association (www.mgma.com), Healthcare Information and Management Systems Society (www.himss. org), Healthcare Financial Management Association (www.hfma.org), and American Group Psychotherapy Association (www.agpa.org)

◆   CMS's Center for Consumer Information & Insurance Oversight website, www.cms.gov/cciio/resources/regulations-and-guidance/

Another recommendation is to have a working relationship with a law firm that specializes in healthcare matters; when in doubt about regulations, seek its opinion. Newsletters published by health law firms can also be helpful in keeping the manager current on new and changing regulations. The American Health Lawyers Association (2017) may be a useful resource in selecting a law firm for the practice.

JURISDICTION

The jurisdiction refers to the governmental unit empowered to make regulations and to enforce those regulations. Medical practices are governed under the laws of local, state, and federal jurisdictions. On occasion, international law may also be relevant.

Legal issues in the practice management realm generally fall into two categories:

◆   General applications of the law, which include most areas of state and federal law that apply to all businesses and all employment situations

◆   Specific applications of the law, which apply to the medical practice and the healthcare environment

LAWS REGULATING THE ORGANIZATION AND GOVERNANCE OF CORPORATIONS

BUSINESS LICENSES

Most cities and municipalities require all businesses, including medical practices, to be licensed. Practice leaders should check with the local city clerk's office for regulations regarding the requirements for business licenses and proceed in accordance with these local requirements.

LICENSING OF MEDICAL PROFESSIONALS AND THE NATIONAL PROVIDER DATA BANK

The licensing of medical professionals is performed at the state level. With that activity falling to the states, national licensing functions are naturally limited. However, a national database, known as the National Provider Data Bank (NPDB), tracks the significant negative occurrences of medical professionals. Prior to the development of the database, practitioners who had serious issues related to their practices could avoid detection by moving to another state. The NPDB, which now contains more than 1.26 million reports, allows any prospective employer or any hospital considering privileging a practitioner to determine if that practitioner has any serious violations in his or her background, regardless of the state of origin.

The database requires that the following events be reported (HHS 2016a):

◆ Adverse actions—negative actions taken against providers related to licensing, privileges, and certifications. Licensing bodies, hospitals, and certification authorities are required by federal law to report these events to the NPDB.

◆ Medical malpractice payments—payments made on behalf of a provider by his or her insurance company for a written claim or judgment against the provider.

◆ Criminal convictions—all criminal convictions handed down by federal or state courts.

Practices must be aware of the NPDB status of its current and prospective providers. These data are available at the NPDB website, www.npdb.hrsa.gov. In addition to making inquiries at the time the practice is vetting new members, practice leaders should query the NPDB annually to check the status of each current provider.

CORPORATE ORGANIZATIONAL DOCUMENTS

Practices can organize in a number of legal forms, as discussed in chapter 1. A provider may choose to practice outside of any legal entity, which is known as a sole proprietorship. Other forms, as shown in exhibit 4.1, require the creation of a legal organization. The exhibit compares the different legal forms of practices on the basis of their prominent features.

Each state has laws in place governing the establishment of corporations and partnerships. In cases other than a simple proprietorship, most states require the medical practice to file organizational documents with the state and to register as a business. These documents include the corporate or partnership name, the business purpose in the case of corporations, the registered agent, and the person responsible for tax and other important notifications regarding the entity. Corporations are also required to indicate the person filing the incorporation documents, including information about the number and type of shares that will be issued. Additionally, many states require the names and addresses of the directors and officers and the legal address of the company.

In most cases, practices wishing to form corporations or partnerships should seek the advice of competent legal counsel and other advisers to be sure that the practice is properly documented and registered.

Exhibit 4.1
Corporate and Partnership Entities and Their Taxation

Issue	C-Corp	S-Corp	Partnership	LLC
Tax treatment	The corporation and the shareholders are taxed on distributions (double taxation)	Expenses and revenues flow through to shareholders	Expenses and revenues flow through to partners	Expenses and revenues flow through to partners
Limit on ownership	No limit on number of shareholders or classes of stock	Limited to no more than 75 shareholders, only one class of stock, and must be a domestic corporation	Can be a partnership of individuals or other entities such as corporations or trusts	Must have at least one owner, but no limitation on the number of owners
Designation of owners	Shareholder	Shareholder	Partner	Manager sometimes referred to as member
Governance	Directors and officers	Directors and officers	Partners	Members or managers
Governing documents	Articles of incorporation, bylaws, and agreements between the shareholders	Articles of incorporation, bylaws, and agreements between the shareholders	Partnership agreements	Articles of organization, operating agreement
Authority to bind entity to contracts	Officers and directors	Officers and directors	Partners	Members or managers
Liability of owners for obligations of the organization	No personal liability, but individuals can be held liable for their own actions	No personal liability, but individuals can be held liable for their own actions	Partners are jointly and severally liable for obligations. This means each partner is liable for all obligations	Members and managers are not liable for obligations of the organization. Individuals can be held liable for their own actions

Finally, following the corporate document requirements regarding meetings, elections of officers, shareholder meetings, voting, and other corporate organizational duties is important. Corporations that fail to do so risk the removal of their corporate status, which results in the loss of all corporate benefits.

SPECIAL ORGANIZATIONAL FORMS FOR PROFESSIONALS

Chapter 2 discusses some of the many ways medical practices are organized and structured. Although the laws vary from state to state, a number of special categories for medical practice corporate forms are common. They are as follows:

◆ Professional corporations (PCs)

◆ Professional associations (PAs)

◆ Professional limited liability corporations (PLLCs)

These organizations have characteristics that differentiate them from other incorporated entities. These characteristics include the following:

◆ The owners must be providers and be licensed by the state.

◆ In many states, the tax year for PCs, PAs, and PLLCs must be based on the calendar year. This requirement helps prevent tax avoidance through shifting income between the owners and the company, as most PCs operate as a vehicle for providing income to the owners.

◆ Taxation is different, as professional corporations are taxed at a flat 35 percent level and distributions are taxed again at the individual level.

◆ Industry-specific rules may apply to the organization regarding its name or how it is otherwise designated. This requirement varies significantly by state; for example, practices that operate in California are prohibited from using a fictitious person's name as part of the organization's name (Medical Board of California 2013).

◆ The owners are required to be the primary producers of the services offered. This regulation is a departure from most corporate structures. The potential hazard in situations whereby the governed are also the governors is that rules and performance standards are less rigorous. The practice manager must continually help the providers understand that the organization provides the structure and framework to fulfill the goals of the physicians.

◆ Special approvals may be required by state medical governing boards of the secretary of state.

Because rules of incorporation for professionals vary by state, practice leaders should familiarize themselves with the laws of the state in which they intend to incorporate.

CONTRACT LAW

Contract law is an important aspect of practice administration and requires special expertise. Depending on the organizational structure of the practice, contracts exist between the physicians and the practice, other providers, outside payers, vendors, and other entities. Examples of entities that contract with medical practices include the following:

◆ Government payers

◆ Commercial payers (insurance companies)

◆ Other healthcare organizations, as when a practice member becomes a hospital's medical director

◆ Medical supply companies

◆ Equipment leasing companies

◆ Real property lessees

◆ Lending institutions, in the form of promissory notes

◆ Staff, in the form of employment agreements

Some aspects of standardized contracts may seem routine, but the practice manager should be cautious about the execution of any contract without expert legal advice.

FEDERAL AND STATE TAXATION

Medical practices are subject to all local, state, and federal rules and regulations on taxation, including property, sales, employment, and income taxes. These taxes vary greatly by state, and special circumstances may apply in any particular jurisdiction, so medical practice managers must understand all the relevant tax issues that pertain to the practice in its location. Complications may arise if the practice operates in more than one jurisdiction, such as practice locations in more than one state, which is increasingly common today.

PCs, PAs, and PLLCs often are taxed differently in many states and are taxed at the highest individual tax rate. This is one reason medical practices often do not retain earnings. In other corporations, **retained earnings** add to owner **equity**, which can ultimately be taxed at a favorable capital gains rate (Harkavy 1953). (In many corporations, retained earnings increase the equity and, therefore, the value of the **stock** of the corporation. When the stock is held for the required period and then sold, that gain can be treated under a favorable capital gain status.) In special corporations such as PCs, these retained earnings may be treated as ordinary income and, again, taxed at the highest individual tax rate.

Practices, especially small ones, often contract with **accountants** and other tax professionals to assist with the many requirements of the tax system and the intricacies of the corporate forms that practices may employ (Anderson 2016).

ANTITRUST LAWS

Recently, antitrust laws have not been as significant an issue for most medical practices as in the past; however, like other businesses, medical practices are subject to antitrust laws. Antitrust laws are intended to prevent the concentration of market power, which could create monopolies that become harmful to individuals and the public at large. Some relevant federal laws governing antitrust are as follows (Legal Information Institute 2016):

◆ The Sherman Act regulates the artificial raising of prices by prohibiting the restriction of supply and other monopolistic practices.

◆ The Clayton Act clarifies and provides additional specifications to the Sherman Act regarding remedies, exceptions, and enforcement strategies.

◆ The Robertson-Patman Act prohibits the establishment of minimum prices as a protection for small business.

◆ The Federal Trade Commission (FTC) Act outlaws unfair trade practices and unfair methods of competition, such as deceptive advertising. The FTC is allowed to investigate and apply financial remedies to violations of the law.

◆ The Hart-Scott-Rodino Act requires large corporations to file a report with the FTC prior to a merger so that the commission can determine if the merger would violate antitrust laws.

In addition, state antitrust statutes may influence the merger and acquisition activity of medical practices.

Although this area of the law has been relatively quiet in recent years for medical practices, the US Department of Justice in 2016 brought an antitrust action against the Carolinas HealthCare System for anticompetitive activities related to its numerous medical practices (DOJ 2016). This recent case demonstrates the importance of practice managers maintaining familiarity with antitrust laws. For in-depth information and full guidance on antitrust issues related to medical practices, see FTC (2017).

Labor Laws

Generally speaking, all labor laws apply to the medical practice, as they do to any employer. Therefore, practice managers must be aware of all of the applicable local, state, and federal laws that apply to employment practices. For example, laws vary in their application on the basis of the number of people employed, highlighting the importance of understanding the nature of each law and how it may apply to the particular organization.

Labor laws deal with fair employment practices, wage and hour rules, and nondiscrimination in hiring and employment. The US Department of Labor (2016b) maintains a helpful website that provides a great deal of information about individual states' employment laws as well as federal regulations.

The Americans with Disabilities Act of 1990 provides definitions and rules regarding the employment of people with disabilities and helps define what constitutes a disability. As with other federal laws regarding employment, this act is enforced by the US Equal Employment Opportunity Commission (EEOC 1990).

The Occupational Safety and Health Administration (OSHA 2016) enforces regulations related to workforce health and safety and investigates potential safety violations and outbreaks of workplace illnesses.

The Family Medical Leave Act and its amendments offer protection for employees requesting a leave of absence to deal with health-related issues. The legislation provides for the following (DOL 2016a):

Twelve workweeks of leave in a 12-month period for:

- the birth of a child and to care for the newborn child within one year of birth;
- the placement with the employee of a child for adoption or foster care and to care for the newly placed child within one year of placement;
- to care for the employee's spouse, child, or parent who has a serious health condition;
- a serious health condition that makes the employee unable to perform the essential functions of his or her job;
- any qualifying exigency arising out of the fact that the employee's spouse, son, daughter, or parent is a covered military member on "covered active duty;" or
- twenty-six workweeks of leave during a single 12-month period to care for a covered service member with a serious injury or illness if the eligible employee is the service member's spouse, son, daughter, parent, or next of kin (military caregiver leave).

These policies are intended to protect workers from being terminated because of an extended leave due to the conditions described above, and they help the organization preserve the employer–employee relationship.

The private inurement doctrine is part of the *Internal Revenue Code* and prohibits private parties from receiving undeserved benefits from a charitable organization as defined under section 501(c)3 of the code. This issue may be relevant for physician practices or for physicians in employment or contractual relationships with not-for-profit organizations, such as hospitals, because it imposes certain compensation restrictions. In general, any compensation received from a charitable organization must be set at market rate. This doctrine often comes into play when practices are acquired by hospital systems or other organizations that are tax-exempt under section 501(c)3 (IRS 2016).

Other laws that have major implications for medical practices include the following:

◆ Health Insurance Portability and Accountability Act (HIPAA), discussed later in the chapter

◆ ACA

◆ Genetic Information Nondiscrimination Act

◆ Health Information Technology for Economic and Clinical Health Act, discussed in chapter 3

FEDERAL LAWS GOVERNING MEDICARE FRAUD AND ABUSE

Fraud and abuse has resulted in billions of wasted dollars each year and is a significant problem for Medicare and Medicaid. Fraudulent billing may amount to 3 percent to 10 percent of the total healthcare spending in the United States, representing $98 billion in 2011 (Goldman 2012). Significant efforts are ongoing to deter fraud and abuse, which in some cases have created difficulties for providers. Many well-intended, law-abiding practitioners have been caught up in the web of regulation due to misinterpretations of these complex rules. Regulations related to fraud and abuse require great attention and focus in the medical practice environment (GAO 2012).

FALSE CLAIMS ACT

The False Claims Act is part of the US Criminal Code. Passed in 1863, the law provides for assignment of liability, including triple damages and penalties, to anyone who knowingly submits or causes the submission of a false claim to the US government. The act was a result of false claims for payment submitted to the government during the Civil War (Showalter 2017).

This law has found new meaning for the medical practice in modern times because it is used to prosecute fraudulent claims for medical services to Medicare and Medicaid. It contains an old legal device known as *qui tam*, a Latin phrase meaning "he who brings a case on behalf of our Lord the king, as well as for himself" (DOJ 2017). The qui tam provision allows whistleblowers to bring cases on behalf of the federal government against providers they believe have engaged in fraudulent billing activities to Medicare or Medicaid. The federal government has encouraged whistleblower activity by providing large bounties in cases where money is recovered from the provider.

ANTI-KICKBACK STATUTE AND PHYSICIAN SELF-REFERRAL LAW

The anti-kickback statute (AKS) and Stark law have similar aims in protecting assets of the Medicare and Medicaid program. Exhibit 4.2 illustrates the comparison between the two sets of laws. Note that the AKS applies to all federal programs and those doing business with the government, whereas the Stark law applies specifically to the Medicare and Medicaid programs.

The Stark law, named for Rep. Fortney Hillman "Pete" Stark Jr., D-CA, who sponsored the initial legislation, is set forth in section 1877 of the Social Security Act. Also known as the physician self-referral law, Stark deserves special consideration by practice leaders because it has an enormous impact on the medical practice. It is intended to prohibit self-referral of designated services (listed in exhibit 4.3) offered by the provider, a family member of the provider, or an entity controlled by the provider or family member. The prohibition stems from PID, as providers create a conflict of interest and the potential for abuse when they refer patients to services in which the providers have an economic interest.

The Stark law is complicated and requires careful attention from practice leaders. It must be taken into consideration in all contracts and dealings with related parties, such as family members or other organizations in which the practitioner has a financial interest (CMS 2015a; StarkLaw.org 2013).

Stark allows for certain exceptions so that the normal activities of the medical practice are not impeded. Those exceptions are noted in exhibit 4.4. Congress provides guidance to CMS in creating these exceptions, which is founded in a quote from Representative Stark (Teplitzky 1999):

What is needed is what lawyers call a bright line rule to give providers and physicians unequivocal guidance as to the types of arrangements that are permissible and the types that are prohibited. If the law is clear and the penalties are severe, we can rely on self-enforcement in the great majority of cases.

EXHIBIT 4.2

Comparison of
the Anti-Kickback
Statute and Stark
Law*

	THE ANTI-KICKBACK STATUTE (42 USC § 1320a-7b(b))	THE STARK LAW (42 USC § 1395nn)
Prohibition	Prohibits offering, paying, soliciting or receiving anything of value to induce or reward referrals or generate Federal health care program business	• Prohibits a physician from referring Medicare patients for designated health services to an entity with which the physician (or immediate family member) has a financial relationship, unless an exception applies • Prohibits the designated health services entity from submitting claims to Medicare for those services resulting from a prohibited referral
Referrals	Referrals from anyone	Referrals from a physician
Items/ Services	Any items or services	Designated health services
Intent	Intent must be proven (knowing and willful)	• No intent standard for overpayment (strict liability) • Intent required for civil monetary penalties for *knowing* violations

Penalties	Criminal:
	  • Fines up to $25,000 per violation
	  • Up to a 5 year prison term per violation
	Civil/Administrative:
	  • False Claims Act liability
	  • Civil monetary penalties and program exclusion
	  • Potential $50,000 CMP per violation
	  • Civil assessment of up to three times amount of kickback
		Civil:
		  • Overpayment/refund obligation
		  • False Claims Act liability
		  • Civil monetary penalties and program exclusion for *knowing* violations
		  • Potential $15,000 CMP for each service
		  • Civil assessment of up to three times the amount claimed

Exceptions	*Voluntary* safe harbors	*Mandatory* exceptions
Federal Health Care Programs	All	Medicare/Medicaid

*This chart is for illustrative purposes only and is not a substitute for consulting the statutes and their regulations.

Source: Reprinted from OIG (2016).

Audit
A careful review of
financial records to
verify their accuracy.

All members of the medical practice who are involved in contracting and developing relationships with third-party providers or considering merger or acquisition activity must be familiar with Stark and the AKS. Also important is that all providers and staff in the practice have a thorough understanding of the provisions of the Stark law that apply to the practice. Policies and procedures need to be in place to safeguard the practice from any violations, and periodic **audits** should be undertaken to ensure that all billing practices and

EXHIBIT 4.3
Designated Health
Services Defined
by the Stark Law

Clinical laboratory services

Physical therapy services

Occupational therapy services

Outpatient speech-language pathology services

Radiology and certain other imaging services

Radiation therapy services and supplies

Durable medical equipment and supplies

Parenteral and enteral nutrients, equipment, and supplies

Prosthetics, orthotics, and prosthetic devices and supplies

Home health services

Outpatient prescription drugs

Inpatient and outpatient hospital services

Source: CMS (2015a).

contractual relationships are in compliance with the Stark law. Even the inadvertent violation of Stark's provisions can result in heavy fines and possibly endanger the practice's existence.

REGULATION OF BILLING IN MEDICAL PRACTICES

The complicated nature of billing and payment processes in the medical practice and the constant addition and revision of billing regulations has made compliance a major issue. Unlike in many industries, erroneous billing of medical services may not only cause unhappy patients but also lead to legal action by state and federal government. The practice manager and leaders must ensure the highest integrity in their billing practices. To meet this expectation, standards for ethical and accurate billing must be established and staff must be well trained not only about the intent of the practice's billing standards but also on the details of the billing process. Innocent mistakes can result in substantial penalties, and willful deceit or careless disregard for proper procedures can lead to criminal enforcement (CMS 2015b).

Medical billing has become a profession unto itself. Wise practice leaders consider employing or contracting with certified professional coders (CPCs) and other billing specialists. CPCs undergo a rigorous training and examination process to reach this professional designation, leading many of them to become among the best qualified individuals to provide coding and billing activities for the practice (AAPC 2017).

Like so many areas, being familiar with the resources that provide guidance and information to organizations on billing, coding, and other management concerns is important

Exhibit 4.4
General Exceptions
to the Stark Law

Physician services (section 411)

In-office ancillary services (section 412)

Prepaid plans (section 413)

Intrafamily rural referrals (section 414)

Academic medical centers (section 415)

Implants furnished by an ASC (section 416.1)

EPO and other dialysis-related drugs furnished or ordered by an ESRD facility (section 416.2)

Preventive screening tests, immunizations, and vaccines (section 416.3)

Eyeglasses and contact lenses following cataract surgery (section 416.4)

Source: LegisWorks (2017).
Note: ASC = ambulatory surgical center; EPO = erythropoietin; ESRD = end-stage renal disease.

because the field changes rapidly and the amount of information available is beyond the scope of any textbook. All practice managers and leaders must continuously seek new knowledge, updates, and information and look for credible websites to follow on a regular basis. Many of these sites offer daily updates that deliver news and information to the practice leadership by e-mail. A few of the many reputable and reliable websites include the following:

◆ www.ache.org (the American College of Healthcare Executives home page)

◆ www.cms.gov (the CMS home page)

◆ www.aafp.org/practice-management.html (the Practice Management page of the American Academy of Family Physicians)

◆ http://medicaleconomics.modernmedicine.com (the Medical Economics website, part of the Modern Medicine Network)

◆ www.medscape.com/resource/medical-practice-management (the Practice Management & Strategy page of the Medscape website)

◆ www.mgma.com (the Medical Group Management Association home page)

◆ www.amga.org (the home page for the organization formerly known as the American Medical Group Association)

In addition to the organization, agency, and reference sites listed, virtually every medical specialty society has practice management information, much of which is specific to the specialty. Choose the sites that serve the particular practice best, as the vast amount of information available can easily be overwhelming, and follow them. Information that is received but unused is of no value; be thoughtful about what you choose to read and digest.

MEDICAL RECORDS REGULATIONS

HEALTH INSURANCE PORTABILITY AND ACCOUNTABILITY ACT

HIPAA was enacted in 1996 by Congress and signed by President Bill Clinton the same year (GPO 1996). The act is among the most important laws affecting the medical practice in the area of patient privacy. HIPAA establishes strict rules and accountability for protecting patient health information (PHI) in any form: written, oral, or electronic (HHS 2016b).

The act allows the sharing of PHI on an as-needed basis in three principal areas (GPO 1996):

1. Treatment: one or more providers may discuss PHI when providing, managing, or coordinating care.
2. Payment: allows the medical practice to disclose PHI in order to receive payment for services rendered.
3. Healthcare operations: this can include a significant number of activities related to the operation of the medical practice including:

   a) quality assessment and improvement activities, including case management and care coordination;
   b) competency assurance activities, including provider or health plan performance evaluation, credentialing, and accreditation;
   c) conducting or arranging for medical reviews, audits, or legal services, including fraud and abuse detection and compliance programs;
   d) specified insurance functions, such as underwriting, risk rating, and reinsuring risk;
   e) business planning, development, management, and administration; and
   f) business management and general administrative activities of the entity, including but not limited to: de-identifying protected health information, creating a limited data set, and certain fundraising for the benefit of the covered entity.

HIPAA PRIVACY BREACH MANAGEMENT

As discussed in chapter 3, HIPAA violations are on the increase, at least in part because of the increased use of electronic records. Criminals no longer have to steal a physical record in order to breach the privacy of a patient; locking the medical records room door is no longer an adequate safeguard of the patient record.

Social media has also provided new ways to breach privacy, often in unintended ways. The innocent posting of a picture, a tweet, or a blog comment can lead to a privacy violation. One of the best ways to prevent privacy breaches is to have in place carefully crafted social media and medical record access policies that are in compliance with HIPAA. Several key privacy principles should be included as part of any such policy (GPO 1996):

◆ Recognition of the professional and ethical responsibility to protect patient privacy

◆ Strict limitation on or prohibition of transmitting patient images

◆ Prohibition of the posting or publishing of any information that could lead to the identification of the patient

◆ Compliance with all practice policies regarding the use of electronic devices

◆ Maintenance of a professional relationship with the patient at all times

RETENTION OF MEDICAL RECORDS

The retention guidelines of a medical record vary by state. The state medical board should be able to provide guidance on this issue. In most cases, the records of children need to be maintained longer than those of adults. New digital technologies make the task of medical record retention easier and less expensive than old paper records. The practice manager should be versed in the medical record retention regulations in the state where the practice is located (AHIMA 2013).

MALPRACTICE

Malpractice can be defined as professional activity that is careless, illegal, or improper. In medicine, malpractice is a special type of personal liability related to professional practice and the physician–patient relationship, which is considered an implied contractual relationship. Although in the eyes of the law the physician–patient relationship is contractual, it is different from those in many other aspects of our lives (e.g., the purchase of a car or home). It is essentially an agreement between the physician and the patient that the physician will provide the patient with treatment.

Furthermore, the law has very specific definitions of treatment. Malpractice law varies by state, so, as with each area of law considered in this chapter, the practice leader must be knowledgeable about the laws of the state where the practice is located.

These state laws, as well as additional federal legislation, regulate the operations of the medical practice and, importantly, the relationship of the medical practice with its physicians and with third parties. Examples of the third parties affected by malpractice laws and regulations include the following:

◆ Federal contracts, such as those with Medicare and Medicaid and other government payers

◆ Commercial insurance contracts

◆ Provider agreements with hospitals and other healthcare organizations

The most common contract in the medical practice is the provider agreement between the physicians of the practice and the organization.

THE MEDICAL PRACTICES ACT

The federal Medical Practices Act requires that all physicians who practice in the United States be licensed. It sets out general definitions of professional and unprofessional conduct and creates licensing bodies to regulate medical practice. The act prohibits the splitting of bills for services between providers and generally regulates such aspects of medical practices as marketing management relationships; fee sharing; and related arrangements between physicians, their practice, and other parties.

ADDITIONAL MEDICAL PRACTICE LEGISLATION: MORE ON THE HEALTH INSURANCE PORTABILITY AND ACCOUNTABILITY ACT

Although the HIPAA patient privacy provisions tend to receive the most attention, the law was passed with this main purpose (GPO 1996):

[T]o amend the Internal Revenue Code of 1986 to improve portability and continuity of health insurance coverage in the group and individual markets, to combat waste, fraud, and abuse in health insurance and healthcare delivery, to promote the use of medical savings accounts, to improve access to long-term care services and coverage, to simplify the administration of health insurance, and for other purposes.

Medical practices must be sure to maintain policies and procedures that protect the privacy of their patients. These should include having private spaces available to discuss personal issues related to their financial obligations, treatment plans, and scheduling of procedures to ensure that others cannot see or hear the reason for other patients' visits.

Information visible on computer screens and tablets and documents used at the appointment desk or nurses' station must also be protected if it contains personal health information.

CERTIFICATE-OF-NEED LAWS

Some states require a **certificate of need** be granted for hospital or health system building projects that expand the capacity of the practice. Certificate-of-need (CON) laws are intended to encourage effective allocation of healthcare resources. In most states that require a CON for expansion of services, the state's health plan indicates the level of need for certain services on the basis of specific community and population characteristics. Some states have repealed their CON laws, so the practice must understand CON as it relates to its jurisdiction and maintain awareness of political shifts that may influence CON decisions.

RISK ASSESSMENT

Assessing risk is an important aspect of practice management. Risk occurs in a number of domains, and all should be considered when creating a risk mitigation program:

- ◆ Malpractice risk
- ◆ Risk due to the physical environment
- ◆ Employee safety and security
- ◆ Financial risk
- ◆ Compliance risk

Additional areas of risk, including emergency management and cybersecurity, are discussed in detail in chapter 11.

INSURING AGAINST RISK

Although they may expend great effort to act prudently in all respects of their operations, many practices purchase insurance against many of the risks that may arise. Types of insurance include the following:

- ◆ General business liability insurance, which protects against a variety of risks that can occur at the medical practice. Examples are a visitor falling in the waiting room or an accident occurring in the parking lot.

◆ Business property insurance, which protects against the loss of equipment or damage to the practice building.

◆ Business income protection, which provides coverage for a loss of income to the practice for reasons such as the building being damaged by fire.

◆ Data breach protection insurance, a new line of insurance that provides assistance and economic protection from the consequences of a data breach.

◆ Officers and directors insurance, which provides protection against actions by the officers and directors of the practice that may result in lawsuits such as employment discrimination or wrongful dismissal.

Medical practice leaders must have a firm grasp of the terms of all insurance policy coverage and ensure that the practice is adequately protected from the hazard intended to be covered. Specifically, most policies contain exclusions and limitations of coverage that need to be understood before purchasing the policies. Also important is to deal with reputable agents and insurance companies; in the end, the protection will only be as good as the company behind the policy.

MEDICAL MALPRACTICE INSURANCE

Malpractice is a special category of insurance of particular interest to medical practices. Malpractice insurance is offered in three primary forms:

◆ *Claims made coverage.* This type of coverage pays for claims and the defense of claims taking place during the time that the policy is in force. For example, for a policy issued on January 1, 2016, and expiring on December 31, 2016, only those claims made in 2016, and only for actions occurring during that time leading to the claims made, would be covered. The advantage of this type of policy is that the premiums are relatively inexpensive; however, the practice needs to make sure its coverage does not lapse without an extended policy endorsement.

◆ *Occurrence coverage.* This type of coverage pays for any claim that occurred during the policy. For example, if a policy was issued on January 1, 2016, and expired on December 31, 2016, any alleged malpractice that occurred during that time would be covered regardless of when the claim of that malpractice was made.

◆ *Extended reporting endorsement.* These policies are offered to providers and medical practices to extend the coverage of claims made policies. They essentially convert a claims made policy into an occurrence policy so that any alleged act of malpractice that occurred during the policy is covered. This type of coverage can be helpful when considering changes in employment, practice arrangements, retirement, or other situations that may cause a claims made policy to expire. Whether to purchase an extended reporting endorsement for a provider can be a significant point of discussion during contract negotiations because of the expense of these policies.

The practice must carefully consider the type of malpractice coverage it purchases for the protection of its providers, including the potential consequences triggered by providers joining and leaving the organization.

COVERAGE LIMITS FOR MALPRACTICE INSURANCE

When contemplating coverage limits for malpractice insurance, the risk of claims and the historical amount of claim settlements should be considered. Historically, obstetrics and gynecology, neurosurgery, and orthopedic surgery are the higher-risk specialties. Claims tend to be more frequent for these specialties, and settlements tend to be more substantial, than for other types of practice. Because of this history, practices specializing in these areas often purchase higher limits of coverage than practices specializing in areas that are considered less of an insurance risk, such as pediatrics and family medicine.

Premiums can vary dramatically from state to state on the basis of the tort laws that govern malpractice claims and adjudication. In states where damages are limited, malpractice costs tend to be lower than in states that do not place a cap on damages. Each practice needs to consider malpractice coverage options in the context of its state's laws.

Medical malpractice coverage should be obtained for both the practice and the individual practitioners. Medical practice liability cannot be shielded by any corporate form from malpractice liability; this point differentiates malpractice from other types of liability. Finally, the majority of medical malpractice claims are brought against a relatively small number of providers, and this number is closely correlated with the number of patient complaints received by those providers (Hickson et al. 2002).

RISK MITIGATION PROGRAMS

As the old saying goes, "An ounce of prevention is worth a pound of cure." That maxim holds true in medical malpractice. In this arena, prevention is typically carried out through risk mitigation programs. Risk mitigation requires (1) active and continuous monitoring by the practice manager of the behavior of all members of the practice and (2) intervention when violation of expected behavior occurs. Hickson and his colleagues at Vanderbilt

University School of Medicine have undertaken substantial work on the factors that influence malpractice claims and how they can be prevented (Vanderbilt Center for Patient and Professional Advocacy 2017). Disruptive behavior and the lack of professionalism have been found to be two causes at the root of malpractice cases (Reiter, Pichert, and Hickson 2011; Catron et al. 2015; Pichert et al. 2013).

An effective risk management program for reducing malpractice claims and improving the patient experience is founded on the following principles (Hickson, Moore, and Pichert 2012):

◆   Professionals are willing to engage in all aspects of the job—tedious or otherwise—to the best of their ability.

◆   Professionals commit to

— technical and cognitive competence,

— clear and effective communication,

— being available,

— modeling respect, and

— self-awareness.

◆   Professionalism demands self- and group regulation.

Another important benefit of a risk management program is improved employee satisfaction. Medical practices are stressful enough without having additional tensions imposed by the detrimental behaviors of practice members. Additional information about managing staff issues is found in chapter 8.

DISCUSSION QUESTIONS

1. Discuss some of the major regulations and laws that govern contracting for medical practices.

2. What are designated health services, and what is their significance to the medical practice?

3. What are some exceptions to the Stark law?

4. What components of a contract are required for it to be legally binding?

5. Why are "claims made" malpractice insurance policies so popular?

REFERENCES

AAPC. 2017. "Certified Professional Coder (CPC®)." Accessed April 30. www.aapc.com/certification/cpc.

American College of Physicians (ACP). 2016. *ACP Ethics Manual*, 6th ed. Accessed July 22. www.acponline.org/clinical-information/ethics-and-professionalism/acp-ethics-manual-sixth-edition-a-comprehensive-medical-ethics-resource/acp-ethics-manual-sixth-edition.

American Health Information Management Association (AHIMA). 2013. "Retention and Destruction of Health Information (2013 Update)." Published October. http://library.ahima.org/doc?oid=107114#.V5EcN7grIuU.

American Health Lawyers Association. 2017. Home page. Accessed April 29. www.healthlawyers.org/Pages/home.aspx.

Anderson, K. 2016. *Prentice-Hall's Federal Taxation 2016: Corporations, Partnerships, Estates and Trusts*, 16th ed. New York: Prentice-Hall.

Catron, T. F., O. D. Guillamondegui, J. Karrass, W. O. Cooper, B. J. Martin, R. R. Dmochowski, J. W. Pichert, and G. B. Hickson. 2015. "Patient Complaints and Adverse Surgical Outcomes." *American Journal of Medical Quality* 31 (5): 415–22.

Centers for Medicare & Medicaid Services (CMS). 2015a. "Physician Self Referral." Modified January 5. www.cms.gov/medicare/fraud-and-abuse/physicianselfreferral/index.html.

———. 2015b. "Protecting Yourself & Medicare from Fraud." Revised August. www.cms.gov/Outreach-and-Education/Outreach/Partnerships/Downloads/ProtectYourselfFromFraudAug2015.pdf.

Federal Trade Commission (FTC). 2017. "Competition in the Health Care Marketplace." Accessed April 29. www.ftc.gov/tips-advice/competition-guidance/industry-guidance/health-care.

Field, R. 2008. "Why Is Health Care Regulation So Complex?" *Pharmacy and Therapeutics* 33 (10): 607–8.

Gafri, A., and C. Whelan. 1998. "The Physician-Patient Encounter: The Physician as a Perfect Agent for the Patient Versus the Informed Treatment Decision-Making Model." *Social Science & Medicine* 47 (3): 347–54.

Goldman, T. R. 2012. "Eliminating Fraud and Abuse." Published July 31. www.healthaffairs.org/healthpolicybriefs/brief.php?brief_id=72.

Harkavy, O. 1953. "The Relationship Between Retained Earnings and Common Stock Prices for Large Listed Corporations." *Journal of Finance* 8 (3): 283–97.

Hickson, G., C. Federspiel, J. Pichert, C. Miller, J. Gauld-Jaeger, and P. Bost. 2002. "Patient Complaints and Malpractice Risk." *Journal of the American Medical Association* 287 (22): 2951–57.

Hickson, G. B., I. Moore, and J. W. Pichert. 2012. "Balancing Systems and Individual Accountability in a Safety Culture." In *From Front Office to Front Line*, 2nd ed., edited by S. Berman. Oakbrook Terrace, IL: Joint Commission Resources.

Internal Revenue Service (IRS). 2016. "1990 EO CPE Text: C. Overview of Inurement/Private Benefit Issues in IRC 501(c)3." Accessed June 8. www.irs.gov/pub/irs-tege/eotopicc90.pdf.

Johnson, E. M. 2014. "Physician-Induced Demand." In *Encyclopedia of Health Economics*, vol. 3, 77–82. Cambridge, MA: Elsevier.

Legal Information Institute. 2016. "Antitrust: An Overview." Updated June. www.law.cornell.edu/wex/antitrust.

LegisWorks. 2017. "Public Law 89-97–July 30, 1965." Accessed June 20. www.legisworks.org/GPO/STATUTE-79-Pg286.pdf.

Makary, M. 2012. *Unaccountable: What Hospitals Won't Tell You and How Transparency Can Revolutionize Health Care*. New York: Bloomsbury.

Medical Board of California. 2013. *Guide to the Laws Governing the Practice of Medicine by Physicians and Surgeons*, 7th ed. Sacramento, CA: Medical Board of California.

Occupational Safety and Health Administration (OSHA). 2016. "OSHA Law & Regulations." Accessed June 8. www.osha.gov/law-regs.html.

O'Donnell, J., and F. Akinnibi. 2013. "How Many Pages of Regulations Are in the Afford- able Care Act?" Published October 23. www.usatoday.com/story/opinion/2013/10/23/ affordable-care-act-pages-long/3174499.

Office of Inspector General (OIG). 2016. "Comparison of the Anti-Kickback Statute and Stark Law." Accessed June 9. http://oig.hhs.gov/compliance/provider-compliance-training/ files/StarkandAKSChartHandout508.pdf.

Pichert, J. W., I. N. Moore, J. Karrass, J. S. Jay, M. W. Westlake, T. F. Catron, and G. B. Hick- son. 2013. "An Interventional Model That Promotes Accountability: Peer Messengers and Patient/Family Complaints." *Joint Commission Journal on Quality and Patient Safety* 39 (10): 435–46.

Reiter, C. E., J. W. Pichert, and G. B. Hickson. 2011. "Addressing Behavior and Performance Issues That Threaten Quality and Patient Safety: What Your Attorneys Want You to Know." *Progress in Pediatric Cardiology* 33 (1): 37–45.

Showalter, J. S. 2017. *The Law of Healthcare Administration*, 8th ed. Chicago: Health Admin- istration Press.

StarkLaw.org. 2013. "Stark Law—Information on Penalties, Legal Practices, Latest News and Advice." Accessed June 9. http://starklaw.org.

Teplitzky, S. V. 1999. Testimony Before the Subcommittee on Health of the House Commit- tee on Ways and Means: Hearing on Medicare "Self-Referral" Law. Published May 13. https://waysandmeans.house.gov/Legacy/health/106cong/5-13-99/5-13tepl.htm.

US Department of Health & Human Services (HHS). 2016a. "National Practitioner Data Bank." Accessed July 22. www.npdb.hrsa.gov.

———. 2016b. "Summary of the HIPAA Privacy Rule." Accessed June 9. www.hhs.gov/ hipaa/for-professionals/privacy/laws-regulations.

US Department of Justice (DOJ). 2017. "False Claims Act Cases: Government Intervention in Qui Tam (Whistleblower) Suits." Accessed April 23. www.justice.gov/sites/default/files/ usao-edpa/legacy/2011/04/18/fcaprocess2_0.pdf.

———. 2016. "Justice Department and North Carolina Sue Carolinas Healthcare System to Eliminate Unlawful Steering Restrictions." Published June 9. www.justice.gov/opa/

pr/justice-department-and-north-carolina-sue-carolinas-healthcare-system-eliminate-unlawful.

US Department of Labor (DOL). 2016a. "Wage and Hour Division (WHD): Family and Medical Leave Act." Accessed June 8. www.dol.gov/whd/fmla.

———. 2016b. "Wage and Hour Division (WHD): State Labor Laws." Accessed June 8. www.dol.gov/whd/state/state.htm.

US Equal Employment Opportunity Commission (EEOC). 1990. "Titles I and V of the Americans with Disabilities Act of 1990 (ADA)." Published July 26. www.eeoc.gov/laws/statutes/ada.cfm.

US Government Accountability Office (GAO). 2012. "Medicare Program Integrity: CMS Continues Efforts to Strengthen the Screening of Providers and Suppliers." Published April. www.gao.gov/assets/600/590006.pdf.

US Government Publishing Office (GPO). 1996. "Health Insurance Portability and Accountability Act of 1996." Washington, DC: GPO.

Vanderbilt Center for Patient and Professional Advocacy. 2017. Home page. Accessed May 1. ww2.mc.vanderbilt.edu/cppa/45374.

CHAPTER 5

STRATEGIC PLANNING, PROJECT MANAGEMENT, AND MARKETING IN PRACTICE MANAGEMENT

Strategy without tactics is the slowest route to victory, tactics without strategy is the noise before defeat.

—Sun Tsu

LEARNING OBJECTIVES

➤ Understand why medical practices market their services.

➤ Discuss the reasons practices add ancillary services.

➤ Appreciate and describe the nature and aspects of strategic planning in the medical practice.

➤ Appreciate and describe the nature of project management in the medical practice.

INTRODUCTION

Strategic planning, project management, and marketing are all essential elements for modern-day practice management. As illustrated in exhibit 5.1, the cycle of practice development starts by considering the overall mission of the practice. The next step is engaging in a strategic planning process and then deciding whether to offer new services

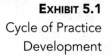

Exhibit 5.1
Cycle of Practice
Development

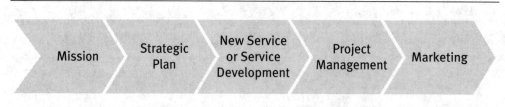

or improve existing services. Finally, a project management approach is used to develop the tactics for implementing the strategic plan decisions and to market the new or improved services in an appropriate way. This chapter examines the elements involved in this process.

Strategic Planning

Strategy is a set of actions and policies that provide the blueprint for achieving an overall aim. Strategic planning is defined as the process by which an organization develops and makes decisions about its strategy, or direction, which often involves the allocation of resources and a commitment to implement those decisions (Ginter 2013).

Once the mission of the organization has been examined as a starting point, the strategic product planning process can begin. Exhibit 5.2 shows one approach to the strategic planning process for the medical practice. A number of important steps need to be acted on. First, the practice leaders must obtain input from all stakeholders. This input may be gathered by administering surveys, examining market data, and collecting competitor information, such as where their patients come from, the hospitals they use, the services they offer, and the payment methods accepted. At this point, the practice leaders should also consider any regulatory issues to be addressed, such as certificate of need (discussed in chapter 4).

The next step is to conduct a self-examination of the practice. This process, which is discussed in detail in a later section, should include an internal and external assessment of the practice.

In exhibit 5.2, notice how the importance of communication to the strategic planning process is emphasized. Input from a broad base of stakeholders is essential, as is clarifying and reviewing that input and making sure all stakeholders understand the decisions that are made and why. A good communication strategy helps ensure acceptance of the decisions and engagement in the tactics for implementation. This communication strategy is an essential part of overcoming resistance to change and provides an opportunity for feedback that can improve the planning process and the success of implementation. People do not support what they do not believe, and lack of agreement leads to half-hearted efforts by members of the practice.

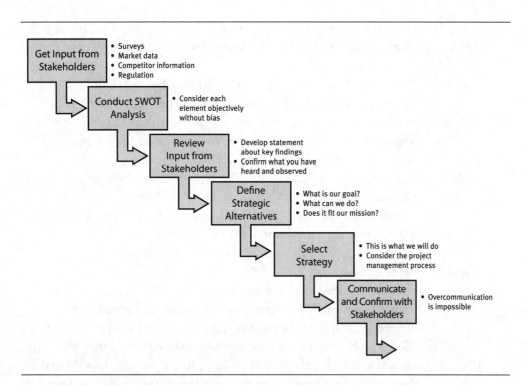

EXHIBIT 5.2
Strategic Planning
Process

DEVELOPING A COMMUNICATION PLAN

As indicated in the previous section, the success of any project or implementation of new strategy depends in large part on the effectiveness of the communications related to the effort. Therefore, each project or implementation strategy must include a communication plan. Several important steps are involved in developing an effective plan:

Step 1: Title your communication plan in a way that specifies the project or strategy being discussed.

Step 2: State the overall objectives of the communication plan. This step may sound simple, but it is necessary to prevent confusion about the nature of the communication.

Step 3: Determine the audience. Identifying the individuals who receive the communications influences the level of detail, language, and format of the communication.

Step 4: Establish the specific issues that must be addressed. In other words, what is the message? How much should be communicated at any given opportunity? Although overcommunication is probably not a concern, people can be overloaded with information at any one time. Consider how much and what level of detail should be given on a topic.

Large, important projects may require a series of communications to effectively convey all the information that needs to be understood by the audience.

Step 5:   Determine the channel of communication to be used. Many possibilities are available, including a paper memo, an e-mail, face-to-face meetings in large or small groups, individual meetings, a press release, or a newsletter or blog. The effectiveness of the message may depend on how it is delivered. High-impact messages, on the one hand, may require face-to-face delivery in a venue where people can ask questions to deal with their concerns. On the other hand, an announcement of moderate or low impact, such as regarding a shift in routine, may only require an e-mail or a paper memo. General news can be effectively distributed by a newsletter or a blog.

Step 6:   As the old saying goes, "Old news is no news." Information must be communicated in a timely fashion to afford little opportunity for misinterpretation or for rumors and distortions to circulate among members and staff of the practice. Often, practice managers and leaders take an undue amount of time to communicate because they are focused on crafting the perfect message. In the process, they fail to get the communication out immediately, creating unnecessary anxiety or allowing a distorted sense of reality to develop through the rumor mill, which then requires tremendous effort to correct.

This may be an opportune time to address a pervasive presence in every office setting, including the medical practice: the rumor mill or grapevine. The rumor mill is an informal channel of communication in which information courses quickly through the organization, but it is information that is often inaccurate, incomplete, or intended to distort the truth. Effective practice managers are conscious of the rumor mill or grapevine and provide accurate, timely communication to prevent people from using the rumor mill as their primary source of information.

Having a communication plan helps ensure that people are informed, feel included, and are able to deflect rumors with facts.

SWOT
A strategic planning technique that systematically looks at a company's strengths, weaknesses, opportunities, and threats.

STRENGTHS, WEAKNESSES, OPPORTUNITIES, AND THREATS ANALYSIS

Among the most useful tools in strategic planning is the **SWOT**, which stands for strengths, weaknesses, opportunities, and threats. A SWOT analysis is a self-examination of these attributes from an internal and external stakeholder perspective. This process can be difficult to perform effectively because it is often hard to critically examine oneself without introducing bias, such as overestimating one's strengths, underestimating weaknesses, exaggerating opportunities, and minimizing threats. Therefore, the SWOT facilitator is a valuable participant who establishes proper ground rules for conducting the exercise in a way that provides the most useful information. Simply trying to confirm the excellence of the practice is not useful in moving forward. Recognizing and capitalizing on strengths is important, but equally important is to be realistic about all the SWOT elements.

The SWOT analysis is often conducted as a face-to-face activity. SWOT sessions are designed to be versatile and thus can be appropriate for the overall performance of the practice or can address a specific area of concern. The steps of an effective face-to-face SWOT analysis are as follows:

1. If desired, the group selects an outside facilitator versed in organizational development techniques.

2. Select a tool such as nominal group technique or affinity charting to be sure all input is received and captured.

   a. Nominal group technique is a method for group brainstorming that encourages contributions from every participant (CDC 2006).

   b. The affinity chart organizes many ideas into their relationships. It encourages teams to be creative and use their intuition. It was developed in the 1960s by Japanese anthropologist Jiro Kawakita (ASQ 2017).

3. Decide which individuals should attend the session, and be as inclusive as practical so that a number and variety of stakeholder views can be included.

4. Schedule this SWOT session for a time that enables maximum participation.

5. Plan the meeting such that it follows good meeting protocol, as discussed in chapter 9. For example, distributing some or all of the information listed in step 6 to participants prior to the exercise may be helpful.

6. Prepare for the SWOT analysis. This activity may include collecting key data from

   a. surveys;

   b. practice metrics;

   c. market data;

   d. demographic data;

   e. competitor information;

f.   changes to the practice environment, such as new regulations; and

g.   results of interviews, minutes, discussions, or other sources of potentially important information.

7.   On the day of the exercise, establish ground rules for the activity. Any meeting should feature a safe environment so that people can speak freely without fear of repercussions and the respectful participation and careful attention of all attendees. Additional ground rules may be established using the following tactics:

a.   Ask all participants to be engaged and be present for the full duration of the exercise. Fulfilling this request requires that clinical staff have adequate coverage and that pagers, cell phones, and other devices be turned off.

b.   Ask all participants to state their expectations for the exercise. The facilitator, the practice manager, or another practice leader should record these expectations and review them at the end of the exercise to determine whether they were met.

c.   Let the participants know that issues not specifically related to the SWOT analysis that may emerge will be added to a designated "parking lot" (a meeting technique that allows the facilitator to record important information to be addressed later).

d.   Discuss plans for follow-up, such as how information will be distributed and an expected time frame for resolving issues or completing other follow-up activity.

e.   Always ask the participants if they have any conditions to add to the list of ground rules and then seek agreement.

8.   Conduct the SWOT analysis. The SWOT exercise involves the following steps:

a.   Ask participants to consider questions about the strengths, weaknesses, opportunities, and threats facing the practice.

b.   Record each participant's input on a flip chart or another recording medium that is visible to all participants. This activity is typically performed by the facilitator, who should take care to solicit input from all participants. Certain participants may be more dominant than others, and the facilitator should be adept at ensuring each participant has an opportunity to provide input. (Even if the practice contracts with an outside firm for facilitation, the skills required to facilitate such events are worth acquiring by the practice leaders, as they are essential for effective practice management in general. Leaders should consider taking a class or workshop in organization development and practicing the learned skills by conducting a session themselves.)

c.   Complete a SWOT analysis matrix such as that shown in exhibit 5.3. Once each segment of the matrix is filled in, the facilitator should summarize the key points and solicit additional input. If the list of items seems too large to discuss in a manageable way, the facilitator may engage the participants in prioritizing the list.

d.   Reinforce a realistic mind-set about solutions. The practice should recognize which resolutions are in its control and which are not when addressing the issues that arise from the analysis. For example, an increase in the number of patients with high-deductible health plans may be seen as a practice threat, but the practice may have few or no options to change that trend. A better focus for the practice in this case may be on helping patients manage the cost of their plan by enhancing the financial counseling it provides.

FORCE FIELD ANALYSIS

Much of what takes place in today's practice management environment is in response to the changing external healthcare environment. Change management is discussed in detail

EXHIBIT 5.3
SWOT Analysis

Strengths	**Weaknesses**
• Resources • Providers • Staff • Location • Services	• Lack of capacity • Old equipment • Waiting times • Community awareness
Opportunities	**Threats**
• New services • Increase market share • Better management • Affiliations • Mergers or acquisitions	• Affordable Care Act/ regulations • Nontraditional competitors • Aging workforce • Financial constraints

in chapter 8; here, we introduce one tool that is of particular importance in the context of the strategic planning process: force field analysis (Berg 2004).

Force field analysis, created by Kurt Lewin as a tool to take the SWOT process a step further, helps medical practices understand the barriers to implementing ideas or changes identified in the SWOT analysis. Exhibit 5.4 illustrates the force field analysis process.

When the forces seeking to push a change forward are equal to the forces that push against the change, the situation will not change. To overcome that deadlock, the forces that seek change must be greater than the forces that oppose it. Force field analysis provides a useful visual tool to examine the forces that encourage and oppose change.

Participants in the force field analysis discussion can use a template such as the one in exhibit 5.4 as a framework to discuss the barriers creating resistance to change and to design interventions that help to overcome that resistance. One example is the resistance to adopting electronic health records. Barriers reinforcing the resistance might be lack of training on the use of the new system. An obvious solution is to increase the amount of training that users receive to improve their confidence in their ability to operate the system correctly. Another example is the difficulty in recruiting providers. One barrier might be lack of assistance for paying student loans. The solution may be for the practice to enhance its salary and benefit package by providing this additional benefit.

EXHIBIT 5.4

The Future State of the Practice

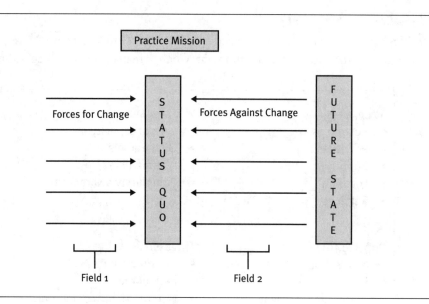

A force field analysis is an effective way for stakeholders to collectively examine a barrier and devise plausible solutions to overcome it.

ECONOMIC ANALYSIS OF NEW OR IMPROVED SERVICE

Often a strategic analysis indicates the need for the practice to offer a new service. The decision to add a service typically involves answering several questions such as those that follow:

◆   Does the service add to the business of the practice?

◆   Does the service fill a strategic need for the practice, such as a service identified by a community needs assessment?

◆   Does the service offer a competitive advantage?

◆   Will the new service bring a new group of patients to the practice that it has not seen before?

◆   Will the revenue from the new service justify the investment?

◆   Is a certificate of need required?

◆   Does the practice have the existing capability to perform the new service in a high-quality way, or will it involve acquiring new talent?

Some additional considerations related to offering a new service include the following:

◆   Cost of new space or of adapting existing space

◆   Personnel costs or professional fees

◆   Equipment cost or capital cost

◆   Financing cost

◆   Incremental costs, for example, regularly needed supplies

◆   Expected incremental revenue

When contemplating a new service, practice leaders must be realistic in the estimation of revenue and be clear about the basis for their financial projections. Some approaches to determining the expected volume of service include the following:

◆ Conduct a market assessment, which includes

— performing a focused SWOT analysis related to the specific service under consideration by comparing the practice to competitors, for example, in terms of whether nontraditional competitors are entering the market;

— examining referrals and other data elements captured by the practice management system over the past two to three years by source of the referral: physician, physician assistant or nurse practitioner, or group;

— reviewing the payer mix, which is the percentage of payment received from each payer, over the past two or three years, and noting any changes in employers or insurance carriers in the market; and

— collecting and compiling the data, and sharing it with key stakeholders.

◆ Base decisions on data while being aware of bias and oversimplifications of the results, as new services represent significant investments of time, talent, and other resources.

◆ Ask providers to account for the number of services ordered in a given time frame by recording the number of services ordered.

◆ Examine payer information such as Medicare data (see, e.g., Engelberg Center 2014), and determine the frequency of services.

◆ Consult specialty societies for information about a particular service.

◆ Employ a consultant to evaluate the business case for the new service.

Present value
A concept that compares the value of money available in the future with the value of money in hand today. Used to analyze investment opportunities that have a future payoff. For example, $78.35 invested today in a 5 percent savings account will grow to $100 in five years. Thus, the present value of $100 received in five years is $78.35.

ANALYSIS OF A CAPITAL INVESTMENT

Many computer programs that perform capital investment analysis are available and inexpensive, including Microsoft Excel (Veney, Kros, and Rosenthal 2009; Marcinko and Hetico 2012). Exhibit 5.5 shows four primary methods for determining the financial viability of a capital investment:

1. Breakeven analysis

2. Payback analysis

3. Net **present value** (NPV) analysis

4. Internal rate of return (IRR) analysis

Exhibit 5.5
Capital Investment Analysis Methods

Method	Advantages	Disadvantages
Breakeven analysis	• Very easy to calculate • Easy to interpret • Easy to communicate	• No time frame for breakeven • Depends on knowing volume of service expected
Time to payback	• Very easy to calculate • Easy to interpret • Easy to communicate	• Answers not financial in terms • Future cash flows after payback not included in analysis • Does not consider the TVM or profitability
Net present value	• Results in dollars • Accounts for all cash expenses for the life of the project • Includes the time value of money (TVM)	• The selection of the discount rate is very speculative • Rate conditions likely to change over the life of the project
Internal rate of return (IRR)	• Accounts for all cash expenses for the life of the project • Includes the TVM • Commonly used method, so most stakeholders recognize it	• Assumes reinvestment at the IRR • Can get more than one answer

Fixed cost
A cost that does not change as sales volume changes (in the short run). Normally includes such items as rent, depreciation, interest, and any salaries unaffected by increases or decreases in sales.

Variable cost
A cost that changes as sales or production changes. If a business is producing nothing and selling nothing, the variable cost should be zero.

Breakeven point
The amount of revenue from sales that equals the amount of expense. Often expressed as the number of units that must be sold to produce revenues equal to expenses. Sales above the breakeven point produce a profit; sales below produce a loss.

Breakeven Analysis

A breakeven analysis allows the practice manager or the financial manager of the practice to determine the number of services needed to break even, considering **fixed costs** and **variable costs**. This exercise can be especially useful when the expected service volume is known. A breakeven analysis uses the following formula (SBA 2016):

$$\text{Breakeven point} = \frac{\text{Fixed costs}}{\text{Unit selling price} - \text{Variable costs}}$$

Exhibit 5.6 shows the results of a breakeven analysis graphically. Note that assuming constant fixed cost, the **breakeven point** is where total revenue equals total cost.

EXHIBIT 5.6
Breakeven Analysis

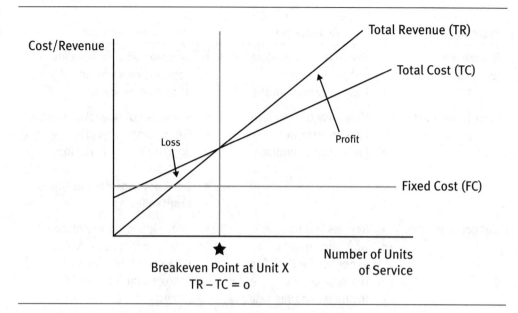

PAYBACK ANALYSIS

Payback analysis has some similarities to breakeven analysis in that both are easy to calculate and interpret. However, unlike a breakeven analysis, a payback analysis gives an answer in terms of time rather than monetary units. The formula for payback analysis is

$$\text{Payback period in years} = \text{Intitial investment} \div \text{Annual cash flow} =$$
$$\text{Years to pay back intital investment.}$$

For example, the payback period of an initial investment of $500,000 given annual **cash flow** of $50,000 per year is

$$\text{Payback} = \frac{\$500,000}{\$50,000} = 10 \text{ years.}$$

This analysis requires careful consideration of cash flow, which is operating revenue minus operating cost. It does not take profitability into account.

Cash flow
The amount of cash generated by business operations, which usually differs from profits. Calculated as operating revenue minus operating cost.

NET PRESENT VALUE

NPV provides information about viability in financial terms. The formula for calculating the NPV of an investment is as follows:

$$\text{NPV} = R \times \frac{1 - (1 + i)^{-n}}{1} - \text{Initial investment},$$

where

R is the net cash inflow expected for each period, with net cash flow equal to total revenue minus total expenses;

i is the required rate of return per period, which may be established by the practice as a reasonable **return on investment** or may be the **interest** rate the practice must pay to borrow money for the capital investment; and

n is the number of periods during which the project is expected to operate and generate cash inflows.

One consideration related to required rate of return is the best use of funds. For example, is investing in the practice preferred to using the money for other purposes, such as distribution as income? These issues can be determined by comparing alternative rates of return on the investment and deciding what is an adequate rate.

An example of a work sheet for an NPV calculation is shown in exhibit 5.7.

In this example, the practice is purchasing an electrocardiograph machine for $5,000 to perform electrocardiograms (EKGs). The practice leader expects the machine to be

Return on investment
A measure of the effectiveness and efficiency with which managers use the resources available to them, expressed as a percentage.

Interest
A charge assessed for the use of money.

EXHIBIT 5.7
Calculation of the Net Present Value of Electrograph

Years	0	1	2	3	4	5
Initial investment	($5,000)					
Projected net cash flow		$1,000	$1,000	$1,000	$1,000	$1,000
Discount rate		8.0%	8.0%	8.0%	8.0%	8.0%
Present value factor		.9259	.8573	.7938	.7350	.6806
Annual present value of cash flow		$926	$857	$794	$735	$681
Total present value of cash flow	$3,993					
Net present value of project	($1,007)					

useful for five years and the practice to receive a net cash flow of $1,000 in each year. The practice's desired rate of return is 8 percent. To determine the NPV of the practice's cash flow, the practice leader or financial manager must find the appropriate NPV factor (PVF). The PVF can be found in NPV tables published in many sources, including financial textbooks. Exhibit 5.8 illustrates the section of the NPV table of interest in this example. It shows corresponding PVFs for 8 percent, 9 percent, and 10 percent rates of return for periods 1, 2, 3, 4, and 5.

The total NPV of cash flows from the project are calculated to be $3,993. After subtracting the initial investment of $5,000, the resulting NPV of the project is a loss of $1,007. If the project is being contemplated strictly on a financial basis, it would not be considered viable.

Adjustments can be made to improve the financial status of the project, such as increasing the annual cash flow by increasing the use of the machine or purchasing a less expensive piece of equipment. Perhaps the machine lasts longer than anticipated and produces cash flows for a longer period. One weakness of NPV analysis is that it does not take into account cash flows after the initial period of the investment.

The practice manager needs to be cautious in calculating the NPV of a project because it is easy to overestimate cash flow, underestimate cost, and use unrealistic return rates. The project, and the assumptions being made in the calculations, should be discussed with all appropriate stakeholders in the practice. In particular, the providers who will be ordering the studies (EKGs in the previous example) and the technical staff who will perform them using the equipment should be consulted to understand what the likely volume and capacity of the equipment will be.

In the case of very new technology, practice leaders are encouraged to review the literature on the application of these technologies and understand how likely they are to change from their current state. This review will help the practice decide the rate of return needed to make the project practical. If the technology is likely to change quickly, a higher rate of return is required.

EXHIBIT 5.8
Present Value
Factors

Periods	8%	9%	10%
1	.9259	.9174	.9091
2	.8573	.8417	.8264
3	.7938	.7722	.7513
4	.7350	.7084	.6830
5	.6806	.6499	.6209

In cases where the equipment is essential to the proper care and standard convenience of patients, the NPV of the project is less important. The NPV may also be less important in cases where the equipment is needed for the convenience of the practitioners or for marketing reasons. For example, a practice that does not have certain equipment is likely sending patients to other locations to obtain those services, potentially delaying treatment or putting the patients off from getting the service; patients may even change practices because of the inconvenience of having to go to multiple locations.

All these considerations need to be taken into account when discussing the possibility of offering a new service or purchasing new equipment for the practice. Leaders must be sure that all stakeholders have a clear understanding of the expectations and possible consequences from the decisions made.

INTERNAL RATE OF RETURN

IRR is another often-used method of evaluating a capital investment, albeit a significantly more complicated approach than the other methods discussed in this chapter.

The formula for calculating IRR is

$$0 = P_0 + \frac{P_1}{(1 + IRR)} + \frac{P_2}{(1 + IRR)_2} + \frac{P_3}{(1 + IRR)_3} + \ldots + \frac{P_n}{(1 + IRR)_n},$$

where P_0, P_1, ... P_n equals the cash flows in periods 1, 2, ... n, respectively, and *IRR* equals the project's internal rate of return.

The problem with this formula is that one must use trial and error to determine the IRR because the equation cannot be solved without knowing the IRR. Of course, computer resources are now available that allow for easy and specific calculations. Nowicki (2018) is a valuable resource for practice managers performing capital investment analysis.

PROJECT MANAGEMENT

Regardless of the decision the practice makes regarding a given plan or project, the success of the endeavor greatly depends on how well it is managed. Project management skills are essential for the effective practice manager. The necessary skills for high-quality project management have been defined in a number of ways by different authors; however, a few have been acknowledged as important by most authors:

◆ *Communication.* Virtually every aspect of the management of a medical practice requires excellent communication skills, and this notion holds true of project management. The nature of the project, why the project is important, why it is being undertaken, expectations and timelines for the project, and the roles and responsibilities of the project team all must be communicated clearly.

◆   *Scope.* Scope is an important constraint of a project. It refers to the parameters of the project, and the practice manager must clearly define those boundaries to prevent "scope creep," the tendency of a project scope to increase in size as it is being implemented.

◆   *Initiation.* Getting a project started is an obvious necessity; and getting it off to a good start is important as well to ensure a smooth overall process. Confusion about roles and scope early on often lead to miscommunication and lack of understanding about what needs to be accomplished.

◆   *Quality management.* Careful monitoring throughout the project is required to ensure that the project is progressing as planned. When contracting with external vendors to complete projects, the practice leader must oversee the project to make sure it is implemented according to the contract's terms, according to the stated specifications, and at the requested level of performance.

◆   *Organization management.* Often, projects are disruptive to the organization undertaking them, so the practice manager must anticipate disruptions and involve those who will be affected in the process of mitigating those disruptions.

◆   *Time management.* Projects are notorious for getting off schedule, sometimes for reasons that are unforeseen. Often, however, they veer off schedule because the time frames were unrealistic or the project was poorly managed. Plan the timeline of projects carefully. Consider what might cause delays. The more complicated the project, the more people are involved and the more likely delays occur.

◆   *Project integration management.* This strategy is helpful when multiple projects occur simultaneously or when a new project will be integrated into established procedures or activities of the practice. Examples include integration of a new laboratory system into the electronic health record, management of projects that involve changes in the physical structure of the practice, or addition of equipment, procedures, or service lines.

◆   *Cost management.* Cost overruns can be a serious problem in project management. They can be avoided by ensuring that the original project is properly specified, either in the contract of outside vendors or by the practice as it anticipates the implementation of the project. Careful planning and specification of any project is a fundamental aspect of success.

♦ *Risk and issue management.* No matter how carefully one plans, any project will encounter unanticipated events that need to be managed to achieve the optimum outcome. Carefully determined timelines, budgets, and other project specifications help offset risk from the beginning, and comparing the plans to actual outcomes frequently helps ensure that the project is running as anticipated. The more specific the timelines and budgets are, the more carefully they can be managed and issues anticipated.

Projects that involve physical construction or disruptions to service may not only pose special risk to the financial health of the practice but also create hazards that must be avoided. Considerations need to be made regarding patient flow, workplace safety, and any effects on the practice during project implementation, as practices rarely cease operations to implement changes.

The project management process is illustrated in exhibit 5.9, emphasizing some important aspects. For example, all major projects should emanate from the strategic planning process so that the practice remains true to its mission, vision, and values. Planning and design, project execution, and project management form a triangle of recursive interactions. For the project to function in an optimal way, the plan and design may need to be refined or adjusted while the project is being executed and managed.

The final step is closeout and reflection. Each time a practice implements a new project, its leaders should take time at the end to reflect on what went well and what could be improved. Projects represent an opportunity not only to develop a new aspect of the

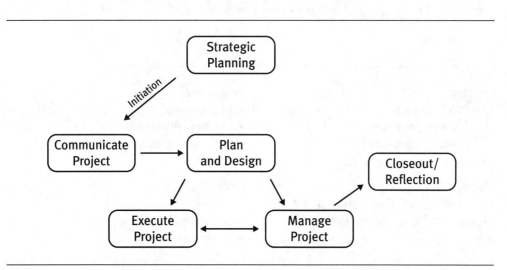

EXHIBIT 5.9
Project
Management
Process

practice but also to learn how to execute projects more effectively. Each project is a unique learning experience—a viewpoint that the practice manager should encourage among staff and members (Schwalbe and Furlong 2013).

WHAT IS MARKETING?

Marketing is often defined in the context of the so-called four Ps, as depicted in exhibit 5.10. They include the following categories:

◆ *Product*—Identifying, selecting, and developing the service.

◆ *Price*—Determining the price of the service or, in the case of many payers, determining the usual and customary payment for the service.

◆ *Place*—Determining the distribution channel for the service. Making this determination is no longer a simple exercise because it often involves more than considering simply where the office will be located. In today's world, place may even be virtual, so practices must consider how patients wish to receive the practice's services and how those services can be provided in a safe and effective manner.

◆ *Promotion*—Determining what strategies will be used to promote the services of the practice.

Preparing a marketing plan can involve a SWOT analysis or a situational 2 × 2 matrix. An example of a matrix is shown in exhibit 5.11, which considers the macroenvironment, consumers, the market, and internal practice factors.

EXHIBIT 5.10
The Four Ps of
Marketing

Product
- SWOT analysis
- Survey information
- Strategic plan(ning)
- Differentiation of service

Place (Distribution)
- Services available at the practice
- Location(s) of the practice

Promotion
- Advertising
- Community events
- Informative events

Price (Positioning)
- Noneconomic factors
- Accepted insurance plans
- Case mix

Macroenvironment	**Market Analysis**
What does your practice do well?	*Where are the opportunities for practice?*
• Excellent leadership	• Untapped market for new procedure
• Excellent physicians	• Hiring new physicians
• Good reputation	• Need for geriatric care in community
• Capacity to serve	• Underserved areas of community
• Great staff	
Consumer Analysis	**Internal Practice Analysis**
What part of your practice needs improvement?	*What is happening in your area that could threaten your practice?*
• High nurse turnover	• New regulation (e.g., Affordable Care Act)
• Locations of practices	• Growing elderly population
• Reduced capacity due to physician retirement	• Complexity of business services
• Provision of geriatric care	

EXHIBIT 5.11
Marketing Plan
Situational Analysis
Two-by-Two Matrix

Often, people think of marketing as equivalent to advertising. Although advertising is an important component of the marketing effort, no amount of advertising can ensure a successful practice without the proper product offered at a reasonable price in a reasonable location that is accessible to patients.

Marketing in healthcare has changed dramatically in recent years. Not long ago, healthcare marketing was considered unprofessional and unethical. Now, we see many health-related goods and services aggressively marketed to the public and other purchasers of healthcare services.

Physician practices are no exception. Many practices engage in marketing as a fundamental part of their business operation. Of course, marketing can serve not only the practice but also the public. It allows the practice to potentially expand services, and it provides the public with needed information about the availability of healthcare services.

The following story, written by an unknown author and retold in Oetjen and Oetjen (2006), offers a simple and humorous way to think of medical practice marketing:

If the circus is coming to town and you paint a sign saying, "Circus is coming to Fairgrounds Sunday," that's advertising. If you put that sign on the back of an elephant and walk it through town, that's promotion. If the elephant walks through the mayor's flower bed, that's publicity. If you can get the mayor to laugh about it, that's public relations. And, if you plan the whole thing, that's marketing.

MARKETING THE MEDICAL PRACTICE

Rising consumerism has caused a significant shift in the expectations of patients and presents new challenges to the medical practice. They are the direct result of an increase in managed care imposing restrictions on patients' access to care, the growing cost of care, and the lack of involvement of patients and families in their care, all leading to the rise of the patient-centered medical care practice. Patients also have access to more information than ever before and feel more comfortable discussing their care in detail (Petri, Walter, and Wright 2015; Laidman 2012).

Generational issues play an important role in how practices should be marketed. Understanding them also helps determine which services are important to the different generational groups as well as how those services are delivered. Generational segmentation may be a very important aspect of medical practice marketing, but the extent to which it applies depends on the nature of the practice. For example, although pediatric practices serve the healthcare needs of children, they must market to appeal to parents and grandparents. Practices need to take generational characteristics into consideration and think about who they are actually marketing to when deciding on strategies.

Some insights into generational differences include the following (Fry 2016; MGMA 2009; Taylor and Pew Research 2016):

- ◆ The traditionalists, ages 70 to 87, also known as the silent generation, rely heavily on primary care practices for their medical care and consume traditional media, such as television and newspapers. They often have great respect for authority and tend to defer to physicians readily regarding medical decision making, thereby making direct contact between the patient and a trusted provider an effective tool for marketing.

- ◆ The baby boomers, ages 51 to 69, are self-directed. They like to research and verify recommendations given to them by their providers. Relevant media, such as web-based information about disease and treatment options, can be effective with boomers.

- ◆ Members of generation X, ages 35 to 50, tend to take an active role in determining their care. They see healthcare providers more as educational resources to leverage their own healthcare decisions than as care providers, they are influenced by branding, and they switch providers without hesitation. Successful marketing strategies include those that suggest a high level of provider engagement while still allowing the patient to take an active role in his or her care. Patient-centered care has special appeal to generation X.

- ◆ Members of the millennial generation, ages 18 to 34, often enter the healthcare system through urgent care or the emergency department.

Millennials have an affinity for communication technology, such as social media and smartphone or tablet apps; however, they do not necessarily appreciate medical technology.

Not all attributes apply to every member of his or her respective generation, but practice leaders should consider generational differences when creating strategies to appeal to the practice's patient base or the patients it wishes to attract.

The first step in marketing a medical practice is to create a marketing plan. A marketing plan includes the following components:

1. Analysis of the relevant market and the practice's objectives

2. Key strategic issues

3. Milestones to the primary objectives

4. Budget and media decisions

5. Timeline

These components are described in exhibit 5.12.

Exhibit 5.13 illustrates the tactical and strategic nature of marketing as it relates to time and effort for each step of the strategic marketing process. The steps include the following:

1. *Mission.* The practice managers and leaders should consider the mission of the practice and be sure that marketing efforts support that mission.

EXHIBIT 5.12
Marketing Plan: Executive Summary

The executive summary of the practice's marketing plan should address the following key elements:

1. What are the dominant issues discovered in the practice's SWOT analysis?
2. What are the key objectives the practice seeks to achieve? Be specific and concise.
3. What, in one or two sentences, is the practice's marketing strategy to achieve those objectives?
4. What other issues unique to the practice should be addressed?

Answers to these questions comprise the body of the marketing plan; therefore, the executive summary cannot be written until the plan has been completed. It is a snapshot of what the practice aims to accomplish with regard to strategy and marketing.

EXHIBIT 5.13
Tactical and
Strategic Nature of
Marketing in Terms
of Time and Effort
for Each Step of
the Process

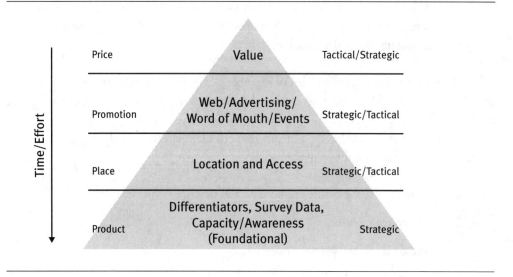

2. *Situation analysis.* An analysis such as SWOT should be conducted to determine the status of the practice in relation to its competitors and the market it serves.

3. *Establishment of objectives.* What are the desired outcomes the marketing plan should achieve? An example is to increase the practice's financial stability.

4. *Strategies and tactics.* The approaches and tools to achieve objectives are determined, such as growing the practice (strategy) by adding providers and services (tactics).

5. *Evaluation.* Good management involves the evaluation of the process to determine if the objectives have been met. The evaluation should be performed against criteria established when the process was implemented. Too often, practices lack discipline in evaluating their actions and define success differently once they have implemented the plan. Evaluations should be used to adjust the tactics or even change the strategy.

The foundation of good marketing is a meaningful examination of the services offered by the practice and the practice features that differentiate the practice from others. These foundations emanate from the strategic plan and are a key to practice success. Regardless of how well promoted, conveniently located, or reasonably priced a practice is, it will not be successful unless those services offer the patients value and are in keeping with their expectations.

In general, services can be described in terms of high-involvement consumption or low-involvement consumption. Healthcare services involve high-involvement consumption, which entails complex services and products that require a substantial investment of money and time to process information or that may be risky in nature. Medical services are an example of high-involvement consumption. Low-involvement consumption involves services and products that are more routine and of less importance to the consumer; therefore, they require less information processing and are likely to be less expensive and less risky. Buying a newspaper is an example of low-involvement consumption. Medical practices must focus on high-involvement marketing to capture the nature of this complex service and engage patients in understanding the benefits of the practice.

MEDIA SELECTION AND PROMOTION

Practices can promote their services using many types of media. As with services, media are often described in terms of how much effort, or involvement, is required by the consumer to engage in the medium.

High-involvement media require a substantial amount of attention and information processing on the part of the consumer. Examples include the following:

- Direct mail

- E-mail direct ads

- Phone calls

- Newspaper ads

- Community events

- Internet ads, banners, and paid postings

Low-involvement media require little effort on the part of the consumer. They are often graphic or pictorial in nature and designed for a passive audience. Examples are as follows:

- Television ads

- Radio ads

- Billboards

- Internet

Notice that the Internet appears in both types of media. The nature of the Internet allows for both passive and active involvement by the consumer.

We live in a time such that many factors affect the marketing of the medical practice, and the Internet is one of the most influential of these factors. According to a 2012 Pew Research Center study on the Internet and healthcare, 59 percent of adults surveyed had looked for health information on the Internet in the previous year. In addition, 35 percent had attempted to determine their condition using information on the Internet, the so-called "Internet diagnoses," and 53 percent of those individuals discussed their findings with their clinician. In 41 percent of those cases, the Internet diagnosis was confirmed by the clinician (Pew Research Center 2012).

The informed patient is more assertive and willing to make more demands on the clinician than the passive consumer of old. The new consumer-patient wants to be seen as an integral contributor to the care team and seeks convenience and improved access to care, including access at work, at home, and via the Internet.

Another important aspect of practice promotion involves event marketing. Practices can engage in local or regional events that support a cause and provide exposure for the practice in the process. Exhibit 5.14 lists key considerations when engaging in event marketing.

The medical practice often does not take full advantage of its marketing opportunities or does not carefully weigh the costs or benefits of opportunities. This short-sighted approach results in an ineffective marketing strategy. The practice manager and leaders should thoughtfully craft its marketing plan to produce the most effective outcome. Practices may consider engaging an outside firm to provide marketing expertise (Berkowitz 2011).

EXHIBIT 5.14
Marketing Event
Considerations

Exposure
Duration—one-time event vs. multiple vs. ongoing

Audience
Size and composition—who are we trying to reach?

Messaging
What are we saying, how are we saying it, and what promises are we making?

Alignment
Are we promoting the practice as a whole or a specific service?

DISCUSSION QUESTIONS

1. Describe and discuss the development cycle for the medical practice.

2. What is a SWOT analysis and how is it used in strategic planning?

3. What are the four Ps of marketing?

4. Describe and discuss the various methods of determining return on investment.

5. Describe and discuss force field analysis and how it is used in strategic planning.

REFERENCES

American Society for Quality (ASQ). 2017. "Affinity Diagram." Accessed May 2. http://asq. org/learn-about-quality/idea-creation-tools/overview/affinity.html.

Berg, B. 2004. *Quantitative Methods for Social Sciences*, 5th ed. New York: Pearson.

Berkowitz, E. 2011. *Essentials of Healthcare Marketing*, 3rd ed. Sudbury, MA: Jones & Bartlett Learning.

Centers for Disease Control and Prevention (CDC). 2006. "Gaining Consensus Among Stakeholders Through the Nominal Group Technique." Published November. www.cdc.gov/ healthyyouth/evaluation/pdf/brief7.pdf.

Engelberg Center for Health Care Reform at Brookings. 2014. "Online Health Care Data Sources." Published December 1. www.brookings.edu/wp-content/uploads/2014/11/ Online-Health-Care-Data-Resources.pdf.

Fry, R. 2016. "Millennials Overtake Baby Boomers as America's Largest Generation." Published April 25. www.pewresearch.org/fact-tank/2016/04/25/ millennials-overtake-baby-boomers.

Ginter, P. 2013. *The Strategic Management of Health Care Organizations*, 7th ed. San Francisco: Jossey-Bass.

Laidman, J. 2012. "Patient Dissatisfaction Increases with Delays, Short Visits." Published February 13. www.medscape.com/viewarticle/758566.

Marcinko, D. E., and H. R. Hetico. 2012. *Hospitals & Healthcare Organizations: Management Strategies, Operational Techniques, Tools, Templates and Case Studies*. New York: Productivity Press.

Medical Group Management Association (MGMA). 2009. "Conquering Generational Issues in Healthcare Organizations." Published July 16. www.mgma.com/blog/conquering-generational-issues-in-health-care-organizations.

Nowicki, M. 2018. *Introduction to the Financial Management of Healthcare Organizations*, 7th ed. Chicago: Health Administration Press.

Oetjen, R., and D. Oetjen. 2006. *Medical Practice Management Body of Knowledge Review: Planning and Marketing*. Englewood, CO: Medical Group Management Association.

Petri, R. P., Jr., J. A. G. Walter, and J. Wright. 2015. "Integrative Health and Healing Practices Specifically for Service Members: Self-Care Techniques." *Medical Acupuncture* 27 (5): 335–43.

Pew Research Center. 2012. "Internet and Health." Published February 12. www.pewinternet.org/2013/02/12/the-internet-and-health.

Schwalbe, K., and D. Furlong. 2013. *Healthcare Project Management*. Minneapolis, MN: Schwalbe Publishing.

Taylor, P., and Pew Research Center. 2016. *The Next America: Boomers, Millennials, and the Looming Generational Showdown*. New York: PublicAffairs.

US Small Business Administration (SBA). 2016. "Breakeven Analysis." Accessed April 3. www.sba.gov/content/breakeven-analysis.

Veney, J. E., J. F. Kros, and D. A. Rosenthal. 2009. *Statistics for Health Care Professionals: Working with Excel*, 2nd ed. San Francisco: Jossey-Bass.

CHAPTER 6

THIRD-PARTY PAYERS, THE REVENUE CYCLE, AND THE MEDICAL PRACTICE

Even small healthcare institutions are complex, barely manageable places . . . large healthcare institutions may be the most complex organizations in human history.

—Peter Drucker

LEARNING OBJECTIVES

➤ Articulate the function of medical financing.

➤ Appreciate the complexity of medical billing.

➤ Understand the medical billing process.

➤ Recognize the complexities of the medical reimbursement system.

➤ Appreciate the effects of the Affordable Care Act on medical financing.

INTRODUCTION

If you were to ask virtually anyone in practice management about the most difficult aspects of their work, they would likely mention dealing with third-party payers and the revenue cycle. Many aspects of billing and receiving payment for medical services are complicated and often confusing. Medicare, Medicaid, and other government payers as well as the various commercial payers—collectively known as third-party payers—all have different rules and requirements for billing medical services. New plan structures also have added levels of complexity, including bundled payments, pay-for-performance strategies, and compensation changes for providers (Barr 2016; Lagarde and Blaauw 2017).

Approximately 35 large health insurance carriers operate in the United States, though it may seem like many more because each company has many brands, subsidiaries, and plans. Some of the major companies are listed below (Insurance Providers 2016):

◆ AARP, a product of UnitedHealthcare

◆ Aetna

◆ American National Insurance Company

◆ Assurant

◆ Blue Cross Blue Shield Association

◆ Cigna

◆ Health Net

◆ Highmark

◆ Humana

◆ Kaiser Permanente

◆ Medical Mutual of Ohio

◆ Molina Healthcare

◆ UnitedHealth Group

ROLE AND SCOPE OF FINANCING HEALTHCARE

Private health insurance carriers are the primary mechanism through which individuals obtain healthcare coverage. For many years, the private payer system has held a great deal of influence over the way healthcare is delivered and the types of services provided. In fact, financing often determines who has access to healthcare, as people are often reluctant to purchase services they cannot afford. Without health insurance, out-of-pocket costs are prohibitively high, not only because the individual pays the entire fee but also because individuals do not enjoy the discounts afforded to health insurers. As a result, uninsured people seek less care or avoid care altogether. The converse situation can also be true: A classic RAND study established that the demand for healthcare is often higher with comprehensive health insurance (Manning et al. 1988).

This latter phenomenon is an example of what economists call moral hazard. If the cost is relatively low to obtain medical services, individuals seek more care than perhaps they need. Important to note is that, with the advent of high-deductible health plans (HDHPs), patients have more cost shifted to them, with the likelihood that they will use more discretion when consuming services. Traditionally, patients who had health insurance were unconcerned about the cost because the third-party payer paid most or all of the bill. A problem with the traditional payer system is that it has contributed to the rising cost of health insurance premiums (Nyman 2004).

One way to understand the nature of this consequence is by applying the notion of supply and demand. Financing influences supply. Practices create supply if patients are willing to purchase and receive services. Not surprisingly, new services proliferate when they are covered by insurance, leading to additional healthcare costs.

The special nature of provider services, however, invites more regulation of supply in healthcare than in other industries. Much of healthcare is publicly financed, and its utilization has a direct impact on state and federal budgets, so many constituencies have an interest in trying to control cost. Regulation of healthcare supply has also been implemented because patients are poorly equipped to determine their exact medical needs, making provider-induced demand (PID) a concern for policymakers. PID exists when the physician (or another provider) unduly influences a patient's demand for care, even when this demand goes against that physician's interpretation of the patient's best interests (McGuire 2000).

Finally, healthcare cost as related to demand also influences the diffusion of technology. If a new technology comes to the medical practice and no third parties are willing to pay for it, that technology is unlikely to be adopted because patients are typically unwilling or unable to pay for the new service ushered in by the technology. A finding by Cain and Mittman published in 2002 holds true today: Practices tend not to adopt technologies that are not covered by third-party payers.

MANAGEMENT DECISIONS

By necessity, then, management decisions are influenced by payment sources. For example, if a treatment or procedure is not reimbursed as an inpatient service but is paid for as an outpatient service, that treatment is most often delivered on an outpatient basis. This financial engineering means services are more lucrative for the practice when offered on an outpatient basis than are the identical services provided on an inpatient basis. It also creates competition among providers for the revenue from services that are offered in different venues. For example, an echocardiogram can be provided in either the hospital's outpatient department or the medical practice. The vagaries and peculiarities of the reimbursement system, including the variations of payment for the same service depending on location of delivery, have significantly affected the distribution of services because these services tend to move to the location where they are reimbursed at the highest rate.

The source of funding affects the supply of healthcare professionals as well. Providers tend to practice where they can make a living. Physicians and other healthcare professionals are more concentrated in urban areas than in rural areas. This pattern is one reason rural and other underserved areas experience shortages of healthcare professionals. Lower-economic-status patients tend to live in these areas and generate a lower wage for the practitioner than in urban or other adequately served areas. In addition, some providers are unable to use their training and skill base in rural areas, making practice in those locations infeasible. Take, for example, a pediatric neurologist. The incidence of conditions treated by this specialist is small, so a rural community would not have enough cases to justify acquiring the equipment or bringing the specialist on staff in that location.

Finally, the cost of malpractice coverage has been shown to be an important factor in the supply and location of healthcare professionals, with areas having lower malpractice cost attracting physicians more easily than those with high malpractice costs (Chou and Sasso 2009).

INSURANCE CONCEPTS

Insurance offers a basic protection against risk. The fundamental issue is knowing whether or how much insurance to purchase for a particular aspect of living in the world.

The general rule is that people should be insured against risks they cannot adequately assume by themselves. Would you insure your coffee cup? Not likely, because coffee cups are typically so inexpensive that you would not need to cover its replacement by buying insurance should the cup become unusable, and the process of buying and selling insurance on a coffee cup would cost more than the value the insurance provides.

But what amount of risk can the patient afford to take? If an individual breaks her coffee cup, she can go out and buy a new one without undue hardship. But most patients facing a $50,000 heart surgery would experience significant financial hardship without insurance to cover the procedure. Insurance is a means to protect against a risk that one cannot afford to accept for oneself.

What, then, is risk? It is the possibility of a substantial financial loss from some event. The fact that this possibility is small is an important concept; the low probabilities of substantial financial loss allow for insurance companies to pool that risk and spread it over its many subscribers, as not everyone who buys insurance will access the insurance pool.

The following definitions are helpful to know when embarking on a discussion about insurance:

◆ *Insured*—the individual protected by the insurance.

◆ *Insurer*—the agency or carrier that assumes the risk.

◆ *Underwriting*—the process of evaluating the risk through actuarial procedures, which are highly mathematical and model driven. Underwriting has become less important with the passage of the ACA, as insurance applicants can no longer be rejected because of preexisting conditions; in the past, this was a primary function of underwriting and allowed the insurance carrier to reject patients who would undoubtedly use their insurance and incur significant costs. Today, the primary method of underwriting is a community-based rating system that takes into account the probable utilization of the entire population of a specified area or community.

◆ *Indemnity plan*—a now virtually extinct type of insurance policy that indemnifies, or compensates, the insured against the cost of medical care up to the policy limits.

◆ *Discounted fee-for-service*—an arrangement by which payments are made to providers on the basis of a negotiated discount off the physician's usual and customary fee schedule.

◆ *Prospective fee schedule*—an arrangement by which payments are made to providers on the basis of a negotiated price set in advance that does not necessarily correspond to the physician's stated fees or fee schedule.

◆ *Retrospective payment*—a now rarely used arrangement by which payments are set after the services have been provided, such as a cost-plus arrangement whereby the physicians are paid their cost to provide the care plus a margin for profit.

◆ *Physician capitation*—an arrangement, known as per member per month, by which payments are made to providers on a per capita basis, meaning a payment is set for each patient at a negotiated price. The **capitation** rate typically is expressed in terms of a specific group or class of services, such as primary care, and may even be expressed in the provider–payer contract as specific Common Procedural Terminology codes.

◆ *Pay for performance*—an arrangement by which at least a portion of the payment made to the physician is based on the outcome of the service or on meeting specific, predetermined performance goals. Pay for performance is often provided as part of a payment arrangement in which the entire payment is not at risk for underperformance.

Capitation
Payment to the provider as a fixed amount for each patient he or she agrees to treat, regardless of whether or not those patients seek care. Payment is typically based on a set number of dollars per member per month.

◆ *Shared savings plan*—an arrangement by which the physician is given an opportunity to share in the cost savings to the health plan, calculated using a predetermined cost-savings formula and achieved by fulfilling specified conditions, including clinical performance.

◆ *Bundled payment*—an arrangement by which the payer provides to the physician a single payment for all activities related to delivering a specific clinical service. These clinical services are often surgical in nature, such as heart transplantation or cardiac bypass surgery. Two difficulties for practices in contracting for bundled payment are

1. convincing all the physicians and other providers to agree on the fees they will receive and

2. managing the distribution of payments to the multiple providers involved.

◆ *Coinsurance*—the portion of the medical claim that the patient is required to pay, usually expressed as a percentage. For example, a policy that calls for 20 percent coinsurance requires the patient to pay $20 of a $100 fee.

◆ *Deductible*—total amount of payment required by the patient for all services before the insurance plan begins to pay for any services. For example, if the patient's plan has a $1,000 deductible, the patient must pay the first $1,000 of services before any payment is made by the plan. Once the $1,000 deductible has been met, the patient still pays any coinsurance and copayment (see below) specified by the plan (as the deductible feature operates independently of copayments and coinsurance), and the plan pays the balance of the fee.

◆ *Copayment*—a fixed portion of the bill that the patient is required to pay for a service. For example, the policy may require the patient to pay a $20 copayment for each office visit. This amount is payable in addition to the coinsurance and deductible as specified by the policy.

◆ *In network*—a term referring to a physician who has negotiated fees with the health plan and has by contract agreed to accept this fee as full payment.

◆ *Out of network*—a term referring to physicians who have no prior agreement with the health plan and therefore are not required to accept the plan's reimbursement as full payment for their services. Some plans do not reimburse out-of-network providers at all.

TYPES OF HEALTH COVERAGE

PRIVATE COMMERCIAL INSURANCE

The majority of Americans obtain their healthcare coverage through their employer, and at one time most policies provided coverage for virtually 100 percent of medical costs. This type of insurance is known as first-dollar coverage and arose from post–World War II competition for employees due to wage and price controls. Employers were allowed to provide benefits to employees in lieu of increasing salaries. This approach to attracting and compensating employees was further popularized by a court decision making health insurance premiums tax deductible (Scofea 1994).

Some observers argue that the concept of first-dollar coverage is flawed because most people can absorb some amount of healthcare costs on their own. First-dollar plans also proved unsustainable, as patients' demand for healthcare services outmatched insurers' ability to cover all health-related expenses over the long term (Shortridge et al. 2011). Gradually, deductibles and coinsurance were added as a demand-side regulator in an attempt to reduce rapidly increasing healthcare costs (Hoffman 2006).

HIGH-DEDUCTIBLE HEALTH PLANS

HDHPs have been offered by insurers for many years; however, they have only become popular in recent years as the cost of insurance has continued to escalate and as employers and patients alike have sought ways to reduce their insurance costs. In general, as the name implies, these plans provide insurance protection to the insured but carry a significant deductible that must be funded by the patient or responsible party. These deductibles are currently subject to limits imposed by the Affordable Care Act (ACA).

HEALTH SAVINGS ACCOUNTS

Health savings accounts (HSAs) are vehicles by which patients may set aside tax-free funds for future medical expenses. The patient establishes and owns the account; therefore, it is portable and is never taxed as long as the funds are used for specified medical and health services (although the services and products for which the money is used may be taxed). Employer contributions are optional.

HEALTH REIMBURSEMENT ACCOUNTS

Similar to HSAs, health reimbursement accounts are pretax fund accounts that can be used to pay for future medical expenses. In contrast to HSAs, health reimbursement accounts are owned by the employer that establishes them; therefore, they are not portable for the employee.

THE ACA AND COMMERCIAL INSURANCE

The ACA is discussed in other sections of the text; here, the discussion highlights some features that the ACA has brought to the commercial insurance environment. For the most part, the ACA does not affect Medicare, Medicaid, or other government payers (aside from its attempt to expand Medicaid coverage for the working poor who are unable to obtain coverage under the commercial provisions of the act, which was struck down by a Supreme Court ruling in 2012 [Rosenbaum and Westmoreland 2012]).

The act does request that states develop insurance exchanges, which allow for commercial carriers to provide a competitive marketplace for individuals and families to purchase health insurance that is not available to them in their workplace or by other means. The ACA also provides subsidies to improve the affordability of health insurance on a sliding income scale.

Commercial insurance carriers play a major role in carrying out the terms of the ACA through their participation in the healthcare exchanges. These companies offer qualified plans to individual purchasers, who can shop and compare the plans to determine which best fits their needs.

Many states did not establish healthcare exchanges of their own. In those situations, the federal exchange, HealthCare.gov (2016), provides the exchange to those seeking to purchase coverage. States chose not to establish exchanges for a number reasons, mostly political (Desilver 2013).

Four levels of plans are typically available on the exchange: platinum, gold, silver, and bronze. They cover a specified percentage of the insured patient's costs as shown in the following:

- ◆ Bronze = 60 percent coverage and a 40 percent coinsurance up to the out-of-pocket maximum

- ◆ Silver = 70 percent coverage and a 30 percent coinsurance up to the out-of-pocket maximum

- ◆ Gold = 80 percent coverage and a 20 percent coinsurance up to the out-of-pocket maximum

- ◆ Platinum = 90 percent coverage and a 10 percent coinsurance up to the out-of-pocket maximum

The out-of-pocket maximums are defined under the ACA. In 2015, coinsurance for ACA health insurance exchange plans could not exceed $13,200 for a family plan and $6,600 for an individual plan.

The ACA has also defined specific services that must be covered in these packages. This provision is designed to make sure everyone participating in the exchange has access to sufficient coverage. Individual and small-group plans must include items and services in the following 10 categories (Small Business Majority 2016; HealthCare.gov 2016):

◆ Ambulatory patient services

◆ Emergency services

◆ Hospitalization

◆ Maternity and newborn care

◆ Mental health and substance use disorder services and behavioral health treatment

◆ Prescription drugs

◆ Rehabilitative and habilitative services and devices

◆ Laboratory services

◆ Preventive and wellness services and chronic disease management

◆ Pediatric services, including oral and vision care

Exhibit 6.1 shows the average medical deductible for the four plan categories available on the exchanges. For those individuals who purchase bronze and silver plans, deductibles are significantly higher than they have typically been in the past when offered through the employer. As a result, practices may experience a significant increase in bad debt, as the average patient encounter effectively has no coverage under the bronze and silver plans.

Exhibits 6.2, 6.3, and 6.4 show the average coinsurance rates for primary care physician visits, specialty physician visits, and inpatient services by physicians, respectively. Again, the differences in coverage among the bronze, silver, gold, and platinum plans is dramatic. Most people selecting insurance plans on the exchange choose the bronze and silver plans because of their lower-cost premiums.

According to the 2015 Gallup Healthways Well-Being Index survey, the ACA has had a significant impact on the number of uninsured in the United States, producing significant increases in lives covered by Medicaid as well as the number of individuals purchasing plans for themselves and their family members (Gallup 2015).

These data are summarized in exhibit 6.5.

EXHIBIT 6.1
Average Medical
Deductible,
in Plans with
Combined Medical
and Prescription
Drug Deductibles

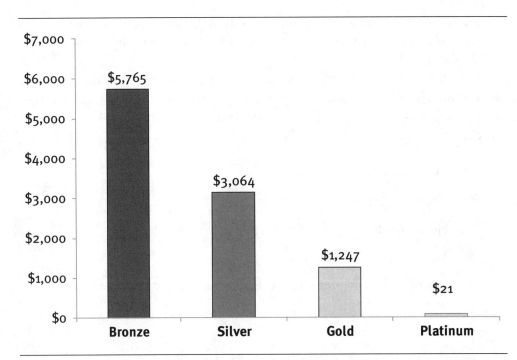

Source: Kaiser Family Foundation analysis of marketplace plans in the 38 states with federally facilitated or partnership exchanges in 2016 (including Hawaii, New Mexico, Oregon, and Nevada). Data are from HealthCare. gov health plan information for individuals and families available at www.healthcare.gov/health-plan-information/.

EXHIBIT 6.2
Average
Copayments for
Primary Care
Physician Visits
(includes plans
with copayment or
both copayment
and coinsurance)

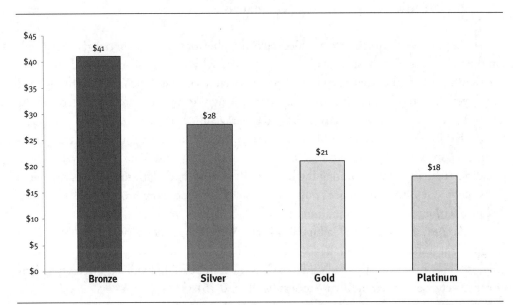

Source: Kaiser Family Foundation analysis of marketplace plans in the 38 states with federally facilitated or partnership exchanges in 2016 (including Hawaii, New Mexico, Oregon, and Nevada). Data are from HealthCare. gov health plan information for individuals and families available at www.healthcare.gov/health-plan-information/.

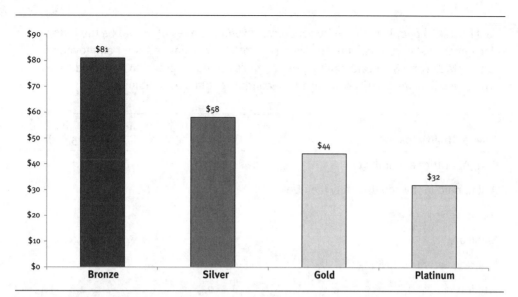

EXHIBIT 6.3
Average Copayments for Specialist Physician Visits (includes plans with copayment or both copayment and coinsurance)

Source: Kaiser Family Foundation analysis of marketplace plans in the 38 states with federally facilitated or partnership exchanges in 2016 (including Hawaii, New Mexico, Oregon, and Nevada). Data are from HealthCare.gov health plan information for individuals and families available at www.healthcare.gov/health-plan-information/.

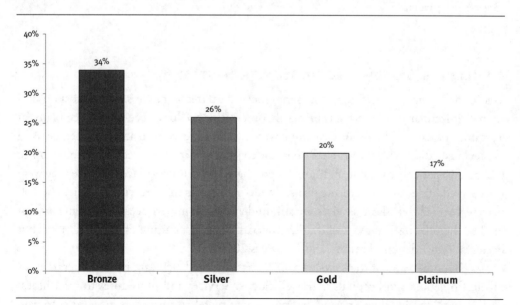

EXHIBIT 6.4
Average Coinsurance Rates for Inpatient Physician Services (includes plans with coinsurance or both copayment and coinsurance)

Source: Kaiser Family Foundation analysis of marketplace plans in the 38 states with federally facilitated or partnership exchanges in 2016 (including Hawaii, New Mexico, Oregon, and Nevada). Data are from HealthCare.gov health plan information for individuals and families available at www.healthcare.gov/health-plan-information/.

Exhibit 6.5
Results of Survey
on Type of
Insurance Held by
US Residents

Gallup asked people in the United States between the ages of 18 and 64 the following question: "Is your insurance coverage through a current or former employer, a union, Medicare, Medicaid, military or veteran's coverage, or a plan fully paid for by you or a family member? (Primary and secondary insurance combined)"

Type of Health Insurance	Q4 2013 (%)	Q1 2015 (%)
Current or former employer	44.2	43.3
A plan paid for by self or family member	17.6	21.1
Medicaid	6.9	9.0
Medicare	6.1	7.3
Military/veteran's coverage	4.6	4.7
A union	2.5	2.6
Something else	3.5	4.2
No insurance	20.8	14.5

Source: Gallup (2015).

AN ILLNESS SYSTEM, NOT A HEALTH SYSTEM

Traditionally, the US healthcare system has focused on treating illness. Now, most observers recognize that it should focus primarily on creating wellness. Fee-for-service plans, at least until passage of the ACA, have not covered wellness services to any great degree. And as previously discussed, if insurance does not cover a service, most people are reluctant to purchase it; patients have not traditionally purchased preventive services because they were not covered under their healthcare plans. The ACA requires that preventive services be 100 percent covered, but those services are still underutilized, in part because patients are not used to them being covered and, frankly, in part because a culture of prevention has not been realized (Adepoju, Preston, and Gonzales 2015).

The other side of the services coin is that so-called sick care is more lucrative for medical practices and hospitals than well care is. Services and procedures to treat illness cost more to provide than preventive services cost; therefore, providers have more to gain financially from delivering sick care. This point is not made to suggest that physicians and hospitals are acting with nefarious intentions. Rather, the policies and payment systems of the US healthcare system have valued and encouraged sick care over prevention. This unintentional bias toward sick care is one reason current reforms focus on keeping people well and creating incentives and payment structures that help keep people healthy by encouraging well care. Accountable care organizations (ACOs) and value-based purchasing, discussed later in the chapter, are two examples of new delivery and reimbursement structures designed to encourage well care.

FLAWS IN FEE-FOR-SERVICE

The fee-for-service system has no controls over utilization, which creates a moral hazard on both the provider side and the patient side. This is a very important concept in medical economics: Because insured patients do not pay the cost of care directly, they tend to use more services than they need. Consumer-directed health plans reduce moral hazard because much of the cost is out-of-pocket for those consuming the services.

Think about the concept this way: If I offer to buy you a car and say that I will pay the cost regardless of which car you choose, would you buy the cheapest car available? The answer is most likely "no." You might not buy the most expensive car, but you would buy the car you either like the most or perceive to be the best. In this same way, overutilization of specialty care is prevalent in the fee-for-service world.

PID is another important economic concept. As noted earlier, the provider's pen is the most expensive instrument in the healthcare system because the provider orders or provides most of the services patients receive. This is how the system operates, but it is not the ideal operational scenario because it encourages providers to order and deliver services to benefit their own interest and not the interest of the patients. Although the vast majority of providers are honest and do not intentionally promote the overutilization of services or make other decisions simply for their own financial gain, the absence of impediments to over-ordering—or of any incentives not to do so—supports supplier-induced demand. The fear of litigation has also contributed to overutilization, as providers worry they could miss an underlying health issue and be sued, even though the probability of a positive result on a test might be small. Compounding these physician-oriented factors, patients often want more, not less, service, and they equate level of service with degree of quality or healthfulness (Segal 2012).

Inefficiencies that plague the US healthcare system can be absorbed by insurance companies raising premiums. Insurers often determine their costs using actuarial methods and then pass those costs along to the patients. But simply passing along a higher premium only covers up the most severe problems with fee-for-service. In fact, this approach to insuring patients is more of a cost management system than a managed care system. The price of overutilization is hidden in the raising of patients' insurance premiums. In this way, the cost of operational inefficiencies that otherwise should be addressed is passed along to the consumer with the excuse of rising healthcare costs. While healthcare costs are, in fact, increasing more rapidly than inflation, this increase is not so much due to growth in the true cost of care itself as to providers' inability to manage the healthcare system effectively and efficiently. Medical practices should engage in education and dialogue around PID, and provide necessary peer review to help ensure that it is not an issue for the practice.

Managed Care

Managed care has fundamentally transformed the delivery of healthcare, and other countries have adopted some of its features because they determined that fee-for-service does not serve their populations well.

In the United States, early attempts at changing payment mechanisms to control cost have not been well received because they effectively restricted access to care, and, as we know, Americans do not like to have restrictions placed on their decision making. In the course of using evolving versions of managed care, the ability to control costs has not achieved the outcomes it was originally expected to.

Some core features of managed care are as follows:

◆   Information technology is a primary means by which to integrate the functions of billing, collection, and account management.

◆   An insurance mechanism is used to provide payment coverage and benefit design.

◆   A main goal is to streamline delivery of and payment for care.

◆   It formally controls patient utilization.

◆   It offers behavioral incentives to providers and patients to change behaviors that will decrease cost and improve health, such as placing more emphasis on wellness and prevention.

Types of Managed Care Plans

The most prominent types of managed care plans are health maintenance organizations (HMOs), **preferred provider organizations (PPOs)**, and **point-of-service (POS) plans**.

HMOs are organizations that provide care to a specific group of patients for a contracted rate of payment. Two types of HMOs predominate in the market:

◆   *Open panel*—Under this arrangement, a physician and other providers may maintain an independent practice contract with the HMO (in-network providers) to see HMO patients as well as non-HMO patients. Patients are

---

Preferred provider organization (PPO)
A health insurance plan with an established provider network ("preferred providers") that covers maximum benefits when members visit a preferred provider.

Point-of-service (POS) plan
A health insurance plan in which members do not have to choose how to receive services until they need them. The most common use of the term applies to a plan that enrolls each member in both an HMO (or HMO-like) system and an indemnity plan. These plans provide different benefits depending on whether the member chooses to use plan providers or go outside the plan for services.

usually required to select a primary care physician among those contracted by the HMO and may seek care with that HMO's other physicians and providers as well. In some cases, an open-panel HMO allows the member to receive care from an out-of-network provider, but benefits from the plan are usually paid at a lower rate.

◆ *Closed panel*—Under this arrangement, the physicians and other providers typically are employees of the HMO or under exclusive contract to see only HMO patients. The patient is required to seek all care in-network with the HMO and, except for special circumstances, such as an out-of-area emergency, may receive no plan benefits if they go out-of-network for care.

The exact structures of organization and benefit packages vary widely and may differ from these general definitions.

PPOs are networks, or groups of providers, who contract with an insurance company or other third-party payer to provide services at an agreed-on, usually discounted, price, which may be paid on a fee-for-service or capitated basis. A PPO is usually not exclusive to any health plan and, in fact, may contract with several different payers or patients as well. In many ways, PPOs resemble open-panel HMOs.

POS plans are health plans that are a hybrid of HMOs and PPOs. They allow a wide range of options to the patient in seeking care, but they pay for these benefits at different levels, depending on whether or not the service was delivered by an in-network provider.

EVOLUTION OF MANAGED CARE

How did managed care come about? Although much history and many noteworthy events have occurred in the development of managed care, one of the first applications of managed care began in 1929 at Baylor University. Baylor may have been the first organization to pay for the healthcare of teaching staff using what we would now call a prepayment model. The university created a capitated contract with local providers stating that patients were to pay a certain sum (a capitation) at the beginning of each month in return for receiving medical care (Momanyi 2010). Some people have asserted that this contract was the precursor to the Blue Cross Blue Shield program.

Sometime after Baylor's adoption of this model, other employers became active purchasers of health insurance using managed care mechanisms and the managed care companies operating at the time. As a result, employers began to wield enormous buying power. In response, different types of organizations emerged to balance the supply and demand of care, leading to organizational integration of payment with delivery.

The supply-and-demand economics of managed care works like this: Supply-side regulators can both have availability and restrict availability of services. The certificate-of-need rules, for example, are a supply-side regulator. Demand-side regulation, such as actions to increase the cost of a service or to make a service less available, thereby decreasing patient demand, is a function of managed care through the implementation of copayments and deductibles.

Managed care began to grow because of the flaws in the fee-for-service system. The cost appeal of managed care in the early days was significant. Costs were lower because most of the contracts that were in place provided deep discounts to billed charges and imposed some restrictions on access. Most managed care organizations (MCOs) use a large provider panel, which may include practically every provider in the community. Subtle differences may be seen among MCO contracts, but the terms are similar.

The fact that most provider contracts are managed care contracts in some sense weakens the economic position of the provider because the ability to access a large pool of patients—say, the members of a Blue Cross Blue Shield plan—requires financial compromise. A practice that does not have access to Blue Cross Blue Shield patients will likely have few patients. The desire on the part of the practice to include these patients gives the MCO an advantage in negotiations.

The only large, open-access insurance plan operating today is Medicare. Traditional Medicare beneficiaries can visit any provider they choose as long as that provider accepts Medicare, which most do. Medicare pays any enrolled provider the allowable fee-for-service. Under Medicare Part C, private insurance replaces traditional Medicare with a commercial plan that provides managed care benefits to the Medicare recipient. The advantage for the recipient is often a reduced-cost plan that may have expanded benefits, but the recipient is also required to follow the restrictions of the plan, which may include a restriction on which providers the recipient may see.

Managed care plans, including Medicare Part C, often develop a PPO. These physician networks agree to care for the insurer's patients at a set price and under certain terms and conditions. Medicare and other government insurance programs are discussed in more detail later in the chapter.

PREPAID PLANS AND THE HMO ACT

A significant piece of legislation that further enabled the development of managed care was the Health Maintenance Organization Act of 1973, which provided federal funds to start new HMOs. This law was akin to the ACA of the time, as the industry was attempting to figure out ways to control costs and provide better care (Mueller 1974). The law introduced a new way of thinking about care delivery and prompted providers to think about prevention as a model.

INTEGRATION OF THE QUAD FUNCTIONS

A true managed care environment involves an integration of the quad functions of health-care (Shu and Singh 2015):

◆ Delivery of healthcare service

◆ Financing

◆ Insurance

◆ Payment

In a managed care environment, financing is negotiated between employers and the MCOs, whereby the quad functions are wrapped into one mechanism. This system is a continuum in that the functions and structures overlap. Different degrees of overlap are evident in the US healthcare delivery system.

For example, for the insurance function, the MCO assumes the risk, as an insurance company does. Thus, in theory, the need for insurance companies has been eliminated by the MCO system. However, traditional insurance companies such as Blue Cross Blue Shield, UnitedHealth Group, and Aetna have shifted their focus to sell mostly managed care products. In this way, the MCO and the insurance company are becoming indistinguishable, so the practice manager likely does not need to spend too much time determining their differences.

Another managed care feature is shared risk, such that often the financial risk is shared between the MCO and the provider. Risk sharing has been used in earlier financing models, via capitation, and many capitation or similar prepayment arrangements will be seen in the future as payment mechanisms evolve and new systems emerge.

ACOs, which were defined in the ACA, set a foundation for MCOs that assume more financial risk for patient care. They are now responsible for more of the cost of patient care and are also required to place more focus on quality and outcomes than in the past to be reimbursed.

On the delivery side, a comprehensive array of services is needed for an organization to function as an MCO. Most MCOs contract with their own providers, although some large medical practices have been able to create a viable MCO through organic growth and acquisitions, developing the extensive menu of medical services needed to support the MCO structure. Kaiser Permanente and Geisinger Health are two examples of large medical practices that are also MCOs. In these organizations, the physician practices serve as both the insurers and the provider of services. They collect premiums from companies and individuals, and, in return, they deliver the care. The insurance functions of their business in the MCO perform the actuarial work and other administrative functions.

COST CONTROL METHODS

A number of mechanisms have been devised to decrease costs in the managed care system. Chief among these are restrictions on the choices beneficiaries have, particularly in the area of which providers patients are allowed to see.

Limiting provider choice has been seen as a controversial approach. Some physicians may be more economically efficient than others. By visiting the less economically efficient physician, patients may be causing additional resources to be used. Notably, these more expensive physicians are not necessarily the higher-quality physicians.

Gatekeeping

The gatekeeper concept is one mechanism used in managed care to discourage patients from visiting any specialist they choose, also known as self-referral, potentially to so-called nonpreferred specialty providers. The gatekeeper in this model is the primary care physician (PCP). The approach was villainized because the patient was required to visit the PCP before going to a specialist.

In many ways, the gatekeeper system makes sense from a care perspective, as many patients do not fully understand their medical needs. Why not see the PCP first to discuss the possibility of additional care? The reason for the intense dissatisfaction among patients with the gatekeeper system is rooted in the way it was carried out. Many patients felt disrespected by this restriction, as if they had no idea what they needed for their own health.

Interestingly, the patient-centered medical home (PCMH), a highly respectable concept that is deemed to be attuned to patients' rights and autonomy, also employs the gatekeeper concept. The patient begins addressing the medical episode with the medical home and then moves along to an appropriate specialist chosen on the basis of the medical home's determination. The difference between the PCMH and the MCO is that the medical home concept is founded on a patient-first notion and is not simply instituted as a mechanism to reduce referrals. Patients get to know the providers, and the providers get to know the patients, making the PCMH the preferred place for medical care. The patient comes to see the medical home as the most appropriate place to go for any medical need, knowing that his or her best interest will be served in the long term.

Case Management

Case management is another managed care concept that, if properly executed, can be a great benefit to a patient undergoing a complex series of medical treatments. Case managers facilitate recovery by ensuring patients are in a safe and appropriate environment. For example, In the case of a hip replacement, the patient's case manager may evaluate the patient's home to makes sure it is a safe and proper environment in which to receive postsurgical care. The case manager removes any loose rugs on the floor to prevent falls, verifies that someone is in the home to help the patient, makes sure a path is clear to the bathroom, and takes other precautions. Those patients whose home is not safe for the patient's recovery, as is often the case with elderly people, may need to be admitted to a nursing home for a supportive environment. In the wake of continued cost escalation, new efforts to develop additional home-based services and innovative technologies to monitor patients in the home are becoming commonplace.

Chronic Disease Management

Disease management is an important process for patients with chronic disease that has been used intermittently over the past few decades by providers and practices. For example, the long-term treatment and care of an individual with diabetes, a high-incident disease in US society, requires a provider who can monitor and help the patient manage the disease over a long period so that it does not spiral out of control. Disease management is becoming common and proving useful in healthcare environments to both improve care and manage the rising cost of chronic disease.

Utilization Review and Tiered Benefits

Utilization review is typically a retrospective look at what care has been provided and whether it has made appropriate use of services on the basis of trends, benchmarks, customary practices, and other metrics considered in determining the quality of healthcare.

Practices are often profiled by MCOs through utilization review. Some physicians simply "cost more" than others because of the way they practice without necessarily demonstrating a higher quality of care. Because of this differentiation, MCOs have introduced payment tiers. Tiers are created by ranking physicians according to their costs and quality. The payer may provide reimbursement commensurate with the practitioner's rank. For example, physicians in tier 1, the highest tier, may be paid 100 percent of the allowable reimbursement for the services they provide. A tier 2 physician who ranks higher in costs and lower in quality may only be paid 80 percent of the allowable reimbursement; a tier 3 physician may be paid at an even lower rate. Some plans allow for no payment to be provided if certain benchmarks are not met.

This tier structure gives the patients an incentive to choose physicians who have demonstrated, according to their profile, that they provide higher quality at lower cost. This approach is controversial because the validity of the structure depends on an accurate profiling system, which some observers believe is not always in place.

> **Utilization review**
> An organized procedure carried out through committees to review admissions, duration of stay, and professional services furnished and to evaluate the medical necessity of those services and promote their most efficient use.

EFFICIENCIES, AND QUALIFICATIONS, OF MANAGED CARE

Much of the discussion on managed care thus far has been provided to help the reader understand its intended enhancements to the healthcare system. Now, we move on to consider how managed care has performed. Fundamentally speaking, the managed care model has not worked as smoothly or as well as expected. Instead, managed care quickly became managed cost.

To say that managed care is efficient offers an idealized view of the model. It has not realized all the envisioned benefits or kept all the promises that some observers claimed it would. That said, efficiencies have occurred under managed care. It eliminated insurance and payer intermediaries and brought them together under one organization, the MCO. It also implemented risk sharing with providers, which helped to reduce PID. For example, a physician practice that receives only a set sum of money each month to care for a patient tends to think twice about ordering a test unless it is necessary.

Of course, in addition to the inefficiencies ushered in by managed care, discussed in the next subsection, the potential consequence of capitation is that it creates incentives to not provide a service that is needed. Providers are human, and we all respond to incentives and are susceptible to issues that may influence us to make a decision that, in an ideal world, we would not make (Johnson 2014). Prudent delivery of healthcare—thinking about what is best for the patient—is the goal. MCOs produced the first real effort to collect data and manage the care of patients on the basis of that evidence. However, the amount and type of data, and the systems to support their analysis, are inadequate via the MCO, and the decision making required for good patient-based judgments may suffer.

INEFFICIENCIES IN MANAGED CARE

One major inefficiency of the current managed care financing system is the level of complexity for providers who contract with multiple plans. In addition, the MCO's medical policies are often at odds with what the provider perceives to be in the best interest of the patient, leading to denial of payment. Furthermore, appeals of payment denials can be lengthy. New organizational structures and payment mechanisms may help to align services and payment systems in a way that reduces the complexity and increases the efficiency of the system.

GOVERNMENT HEALTH INSURANCE PROGRAMS

Medicare and Medicaid were created by an amendment to the Social Security Act in 1965 as titles XVIII and XIX, respectively. These programs were part of the Great Society initiative of the Johnson administration.

Prior to 1965, the only health insurance coverage available was through private insurers, with the exception of a few targeted government programs that provided coverage for the poor and elderly. Medicare and Medicaid represented a major step forward in the "Great Society," the vision of the Johnson administration. Its importance in providing medical services for the poor and elderly is hard to overestimate. Following the implementation of Medicare and Medicaid, these underserved groups had access to healthcare services as never before, and the availability of services was no longer left to the charitable inclinations of the providers. Because more people were demanding services from the delivery system, Medicare and Medicaid spurred more rapid development of medical services.

In general, Medicare covers those who are aged 65 or older or who have permanent disabilities; Medicaid is a means-tested program intended to cover the poor (Cohen and Ball 1965). The table that follows lists some important features of the Medicare and Medicaid programs.

Features	Medicare	Medicaid
Eligibility	Those over age 65 and the permanently disabled; no means testing.	Means tested, which varies by state.
Funding	Payroll taxes and premiums.	State and federal funding.
Benefits	Standardized throughout the country.	Vary by state, with minimum federal standards. States may apply for waivers to create innovative programs.

MEDICARE

Medicare has four distinct components. Part A provides coverage for inpatient care and some skilled nursing and rehabilitation facility charges but typically does not pay for medical practice services. Any US resident who has worked for at least 40 quarters and paid payroll taxes into the Health Insurance Trust automatically receives Medicare after reaching age 65. Part A is subject to an annual deductible.

Part B provides coverage for outpatient services, which include medical practice services. It is a voluntary program funded through Part B premiums, which are adjusted on the basis of household income. Part B typically pays 80 percent of charges, leaving 20 percent to be paid by the patient.

Part C, also known as **Medicare Advantage**, came into effect with the 1997 Balanced Budget Act. Part C does not add new benefits to Medicare Parts A and B but packages them in a managed care plan, which is offered by a number of insurance companies. Part

Medicare Advantage
Program established by the Balanced Budget Act of 1997 whereby an eligible individual may elect to receive Medicare benefits through a managed care organization. Formerly called Medicare+Choice and still informally known as Medicare Part C.

C often combines Parts A, B, and D and Medigap coverage (see next subsection) under one umbrella policy.

Part D provides coverage for prescription drugs and requires payment of the monthly premium to Medicare in addition to Part B premiums. This coverage is offered through stand-alone plans and through the Medicare Advantage program.

MEDIGAP COVERAGE

Medigap
A supplemental health insurance policy sold by private insurance companies that is designed to pay for healthcare costs and services not paid for by Medicare or any private health insurance benefits.

Even when all four Medicare programs are used together, they do not cover 100 percent of healthcare costs for beneficiaries. Many Medicare recipients choose to purchase additional coverage, known as **Medigap** coverage, which pays the Part A deductible and the 20 percent that is not paid by Part B. This coverage is typically purchased from a commercial insurance carrier or managed care company.

MEDICAID

Medicaid, also referred to as Title 18 of the Social Security Act, is primarily intended to provide coverage for services to low-income US residents. It is a means-tested program that is operated jointly by the state and federal governments. Because of this joint-funding arrangement, benefits vary widely from state to state but are subject to a minimum threshold established by the federal government.

DUAL ELIGIBILITY

Low-income individuals who qualify for Medicare may also qualify for Medicaid. If they receive both Medicare and Medicaid benefits, they are considered dual eligible. Typically, Medicare is the primary payer for their medical services, and Medicaid pays the deductibles, coinsurance, and other medical expenses, much as a Medigap policy does.

OTHER FEDERAL HEALTH INSURANCE PROGRAMS

Additional federal health insurance programs offer insurance coverage for specific population groups. Two of these, the Indian Health Service (IHS) and TRICARE, are discussed here.

Indian Health Service

The IHS is the principal federal healthcare provider of a comprehensive delivery system for American Indians and Alaska Natives. Its mission grew out of the special government-to-government relationship between the federal government and federally recognized Indian tribes (IHS 2016).

TRICARE

TRICARE is a program sponsored by the federal government that provides a wide range of health services to active and retired members of the military and their families. Because private practitioners are often involved in the care of military personnel and their families, many practices need to bill and receive reimbursement from TRICARE for services provided (Defense Health Agency 2017). A solid understanding of the TRICARE system is helpful for managers of these practices. Please visit www.tricare.mil for more details and resources.

THE REVENUE CYCLE

The revenue cycle for a medical practice is illustrated in exhibit 6.6. Whether for a small proprietary practice or a large multispecialty practice in or outside of a large healthcare organization, most of these activities are performed by all practices because the processes represented in the revenue cycle do not change according to the size of the organization. The technology and procedures may differ, but the steps in the process do not.

The revenue cycle is focused on two fundamental aspects of practice management. In managing the revenue cycle, the practice aims to (1) increase collections and the collectability of patient revenue sources and (2) improve its cash position. To achieve these goals, the practice must focus on timeliness in performing all activities, as well as the following:

1. Pricing, which likely relates to how well the practice has negotiated its managed care insurance contracts

2. Coding the medical services

3. Capturing charges correctly

4. Managing the denial of payment by insurance carriers and MCOs

5. Managing any underpayment of billed services

6. Having a properly integrated fee schedule system that is maintained on a regular basis

7. Managing **accounts receivable**

Accounts receivable
Amounts owed to the practice by its customers.

Much of this work depends on having properly trained staff and a modern practice management system that can handle many of these processes electronically. Some practices outsource receivables management to a firm or an individual who specializes in that activity. This decision often depends on the size of the practice and its ability to attract qualified accounts receivable staff.

EXHIBIT 6.6
The Revenue Cycle

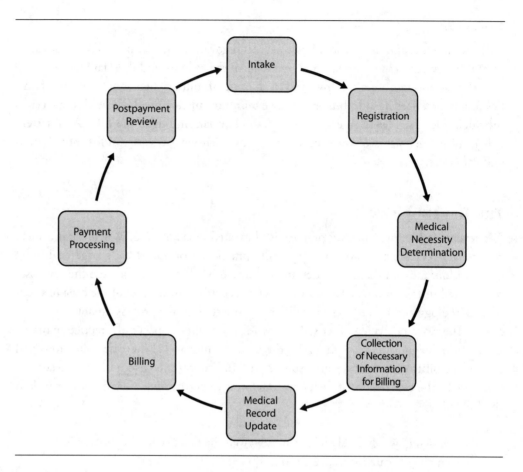

SCHEDULING AND INITIAL PATIENT CONTACT

In most cases, the patient makes the first contact with the physician practice. In some instances, the patient is referred from another practice and that organization may initiate the appointment process.

Patient contact occurs in three stages: registration, check-in, and provision of services.

Patient Registration

The registration process is as follows:

1. Patient intake, or preregistration, is performed prior to the patient's visit to collect all necessary medical and insurance or other payment information. Some insurance plans require preauthorization for services, which must be received before the services are provided. The preregistration process helps ensure a smooth visit.

2. Registration takes place at the time of the patient visit. Relevant patient information is gathered, including demographics, such as age; address and other contact information; emergency contact information; and payment information, such as insurance and other potential forms of payment.

    Often the registration process also includes collecting a patient history and other relevant background information about the medical condition.
    During this registration process, the practice should assess the financial status of the patient and help the patient access assistance if needed. Some activities that may occur in assisting patients in this way may include the following:

    ◆ Helping the patient recognize the expectation for payment and understand the potential liability if he or she fails to pay for services. As we have discussed, healthcare is often very expensive, and those new to accessing the healthcare system may be unaware of the extent of their liability. The need for this type of patient education is increasing, even for those with health insurance, because the number of HDHPs has grown.

    ◆ Determining if the patient is eligible for any charity or discount programs.

    The practice may also offer a plan that allows patients to make periodic payments for the services.

Patient Check-In

Check-in is a straightforward function whereby the patient is received by the practice. Information is verified, including the patient's identity, and any updates to patient information are made.

Provision of Patient Services

In most practices, for this stage the patient is escorted by one of the clinical personnel to the appropriate service or to the examination room. One critical step in the revenue cycle depends on the proper capture of charges for services provided. Charge capture is usually performed either by completing a form called a super bill or by using an electronic system to capture the charges into the medical record.
    We dedicate the next section to discussion of coding as part of charge capture.

CODING AND CLAIMS

The proper coding of the services provided by a medical practice is crucial not only to maximize legitimate revenue but also to avoid compliance issues and concerns. Medical coding specialists are valuable members of the practice and provide expertise in managing the preparation of insurance claims. Any practice is well served by ensuring that the medical coders who prepare claims for the practice, whether internal or external, are certified by the American Association of Professional Coders and hold the designation of CPC, indicating that they have successfully completed the training and certification process required of a professional coder (AAPC 2017).

Also of note, every practice should have systems in place to audit and verify that all charges have been captured and that they have been captured correctly.

International Classification of Diseases

The International Classification of Diseases (ICD), now in its tenth revision, is a system used by US healthcare providers to record and code all symptoms discussed, diagnoses made, and procedures performed during patient visits. ICD-10 replaced ICD-9-CM (for Clinical Modification) in 2015 and consists of 68,000 codes that are three to seven characters in length. Exhibit 6.7 lists some differences between ICD-9-CM and ICD-10.

Current Procedural Terminology

Current Procedural Terminology (CPT), currently in its fourth version, is a coding product that is maintained and sold by the American Medical Association (AMA 2017a). It is used to indicate in the patient's medical record any procedures provided by the medical practice.

As with ICD-10 codes for diagnoses, a proper CPT-4 code is required for filing claims for reimbursement of the procedures provided by the practice.

Submission and Processing of Claims to Payers

Today, virtually all claims for reimbursement are submitted electronically to payers using the billing functions of the practice management system. Smaller practices may use billing services, to which the practice submits its claims online, with the billing service then processing and submitting the claim on the practice's behalf.

Review and Management of Claim Denials

As previously noted, medical billing is complicated, and the opportunity for errors and incorrect processing is significant. Therefore, practices must review all reimbursed claims to ensure that they have been paid in accordance with the contract in place with the third-party payer. In addition, they need to review and manage any claims denied. In the digital age, most of this process can be performed electronically. Programs are available to compare

	ICD-9-CM	**ICD-10 Code Sets**
Procedure	3,824 codes	71,924 codes
Diagnosis	14,025 codes	69,823 codes

ICD-10 Code Structure Changes (selected details)

	Old	**New**
Diagnosis Structure	ICD-9-CM • 3–5 characters • First character is numeric or alpha • Characters 2–5 are numeric	ICD-10-CM • 3–7 characters • Character 1 is alpha • Character 2 is numeric • Characters 3–7 can be alpha or numeric
Procedure Structure	ICD-9-CM • 3–4 characters • All characters are numeric • All codes have at least 3 characters	ICD-10-PCS • ICD-10-PCS has 7 characters • Each can be either alpha or numeric • Numbers 0–9; letters A–H, J–N, P–Z

EXHIBIT 6.7
Differences
Between
ICD-9-CM and
ICD-10 Code Sets

Source: Medicare Learning Network (2016).

the practice's fee schedule for a particular payer against the payments received and generate an exception report indicating those payments that appear to be inaccurate.

Finally, practices must reconcile accounts by **posting** payments against charges and applying applicable discounts and adjustments.

Post
To enter a business transaction into a journal, a ledger, or another financial record.

BAD DEBT AND CHARITY CARE

An important aspect of revenue management is the consideration of bad debt and charity care. The practice should develop policies on how it manages bad debt and its position on providing charity care. Bad debts are uncollectible fees that the practice had expected to be paid. Charity care is care provided without the expectation of payment.

If bad debt and charity care are not managed correctly by writing those services off as uncollectible and removing them from accounts receivable, the accounts receivable balance of the practice provides an unrealistic view of its potential collectible revenue. Failure to account for bad debt and charity care also skews performance metrics by making the practice's accounts receivable appear more valuable than they are.

REVENUE CYCLE FAILURES

Revenue cycle management is a critical aspect of physician practice management, but it is fraught with difficulties and often represents a primary failure point for practices. Each step of the revenue cycle process can be vulnerable to errors, such as those that follow (Trew 2010):

1. Lack of proper insurance information or failure to verify the information

2. Incomplete or erroneous registration data

3. Failure to capture charges

4. Failure to post charges correctly

5. Application of improper diagnostic codes

6. Significant delays in posting charges (most insurance companies have time limits on when claims can be made)

7. Ineffective denial management

8. Failure to manage underpayments on a timely basis

MEASURES OF REVENUE CYCLE PERFORMANCE

Resource-based relative value scale (RBRVS)
Means by which to determine the rate at which Medicare reimburses physicians on a fee-for-service basis. Calculated using the costs of physician labor, practice overhead, materials, and liability insurance, with the resulting amounts adjusted for geographical differences.

Measuring and monitoring the performance of a practice's revenue cycle performance is essential to ensure that the process is proceeding as anticipated and to provide benchmarks for improving performance in the future. Exhibit 6.8 illustrates some important metrics that should be measured to monitor revenue cycle performance. The practice manager must focus on the metrics that do not meet the standard set by the practice and consider steps to improve performance.

RESOURCE-BASED RELATIVE VALUE SCALE

The **resource-based relative value scale (RBRVS)** is a fundamental aspect of healthcare funding. It was originally developed by the federal government for the Medicare and Medicaid programs but has been widely adopted by virtually all payers. RBRVS seeks to provide a consistent methodology for valuing medical services on a relative basis, taking into account the amount of work involved as well as the resources used.

Measure	Metric
Preregistration count	98%
Upfront collection rate	5%
Denial rate due to registration errors	2%
Coding failures	1%
Charge entry delays	48 hours
Percentage of claims filed electronically	100%
Accounts receivable greater than 90 days	less than 5%
Unposted receipts	5 days
Payment-to-billing ratio	30%

EXHIBIT 6.8
Revenue Cycle
Performance
Measures

The formula used to calculate RBRVS is shown in exhibit 6.9.

Three separate relative value units (RVUs) are associated with calculating a payment under the Medicare Physicians Fee Schedule (PFS).

◆ The Work RVU reflects the relative time and intensity associated with providing a Medicare PFS service.

◆ The Practice Expense RVU reflects the costs of maintaining a practice (e.g., office space, supplies and equipment, staff).

◆ The Malpractice RVU reflects the costs of malpractice insurance.

Geographic Practice Cost Indices (GPCIs) are used for each of the three RVUs to account for geographic variations in the costs of practicing medicine in different areas of the country. Each RVU component has a corresponding GPCI adjustment.

$$Payment = CF \times [(RVU_w \times GPCI_w) + (RVU_p \times GPCI_p) + (RVU_m \times GPCI_m)]$$

CF = conversion factor

RVU = relative value unit, w = work, p = practice cost, m = malpractice

GPCI = Geographic Practice Cost Index

EXHIBIT 6.9
Resource-Based
Relative Value
Scale Payment
Formula

Finally, the Conversion Factor (CF) is applied to determine the payment for a service, which is then added to the GPCI-adjusted RVUs multiplied by the CF in dollars. This formula converts the work and other identified factors involved in providing medical services to monetary terms. The calculations seek to determine a fair price for each service (AMA 2017b; CMS 2017; McCormack and Burge 1994).

MEDICARE ACCESS AND CHIP REAUTHORIZATION ACT

The Medicare Access and CHIP Reauthorization Act (MACRA) is a significant piece of legislation for medical practices. Enacted in 2015, MACRA created a new provider incentive structure and affected other aspects of financing.

First, it repealed the sustainable growth rate (SGR) methodology, which was previously used for updating the Medicare PFS and created an unpopular process for physician payments adjustments. Many in the industry saw it as a flawed approach, and political pressure built up over the years to repeal it. The SGR adjusted payments on the basis of the overall volume of services provided as a way to control cost. It was thought that by controlling unnecessary services (see the discussion on PID earlier) in this manner, providers would alter their behavior. Unfortunately, medical care is too complicated to be effectively managed by such mechanisms, and the SGR was repealed in 2015 (US Congress 2015).

MACRA also established annual positive or flat-fee adjustments to the Medicare PFS through 2025 and instituted new fee updates beginning in 2019. Importantly, it also established new merit-based incentives that consolidated all of the existing Medicare quality programs into the Merit-Based Incentive Payment System (MIPS). Pathways for physicians not already in another Medicare alternative payment structure, such as an ACO, were instituted by MACRA to participate in MIPS as Alternative Payment Models (APMs). The APMs are designed to reward practitioners who outperform others in delivering high-quality, coordinated, and efficient care, whereas the MIPS process focuses more on performance reporting than on actual outcomes; however, the goals of improving quality and reducing cost are the same.

MIPS Timeline

2016 through 2019: Each year, a 0.5 percent update will be made to the Medicare PFS.

January 2019: Physicians may choose the APM track or the MIPS track, depending on their eligibility and qualifications.

2020 through 2025: Fee schedules for Medicare physicians stay at 2019 levels (no updates).

MIPS payment for practices and physicians participating in MACRA will be based on a composite score created from the following quality-based programs: Physician Quality Reporting System, Value-Based Payment Modifier, and Meaningful Use (AAFP 2016).

One of the big differences between MIPS and APM is that APM requires practices to take on more financial and technological risk than MIPS, and it goes further toward the goals of high quailty and efficient care by examining actual outcomes.

Practitioners must be one of the following to participate in MIPS:

◆ Physician

◆ Physician assistant

◆ Nurse practitioner

◆ Clinical nurse specialist

◆ Certified registered nurse anesthetist

The final rule for MACRA exempts practices that report $30,000 or less in Medicare Part B charges or have 100 or fewer Medicare patients from reporting requirements in 2017. In addition, it exempts practitioners in their first year of Medicare participation.

Although MACRA only applies to Medicare, many commercial payers follow Medicare's lead in terms of reimbursement, so understanding how MACRA will affect a practice or group is important. As demonstrated by the discussion that follows, the law is complicated. The American College of Physicians has prepared a number of informational documents on MACRA that provide details and a crosswalk between SGR and MACRA (ACP 2015).

MACRA Requirements

The new law is complex and includes many new requirements. The five criteria for participation starting in calendar year 2018 are the following:

◆ Protection of patient health information and documentation that a security risk analysis has been performed.

◆ Electronic prescribing.

◆ Coordination of care through patient engagement. The patient should be able to view, download, transmit, correspond via secure messaging, and have access to patient-generated health data and communicate with the physician electronically through a secure messaging application.

◆ Health information exchange and patient care record exchange, with the ability to request and accept patient care records and to perform clinical information reconciliation.

◆ Public health and clinical data registry reporting, including to immunization registries.

These criteria essentially revolve around

◆ quality;

◆ resource use;

◆ technology, specifically electronic health records (EHRs); and

◆ clinical practice improvement activities.

Consider this example of a measure of patient engagement. In the case of secure messaging, at least one unique patient seen by the MIPS-eligible practitioner during the performance period receives a secure message using the electronic messaging function of a certified EHR. This message could also be sent to the patient-authorized representative, or it could be sent in response to a secure message sent by the patient or representative.

The practice (the physicians or other MIPS-eligible practitioners) must perform the following while continuing to practice medicine:

1. For the period January 1, 2017, to December 31, 2017, use a 2014 or 2015 edition certified EHR.

2. Report on either eight stage 2 or six stage 3 advancing care information objectives and measures.

   a. Attest to their cooperation in good faith with the surveillance of the Office of the National Coordinator for Health Information Technology (ONC).

   b. Undergo ONC direct review of the EHR, including the attestation to their support for health information exchange and the prevention of information blocking.

APMs require participants to bear a certain amount of financial risk in the form of reduced rates, withheld payments, or penalties assessed by CMS when actual expenditures exceed expected expenditures. Payments are based on evidence-based, reliable, and valid quality measures rather than MIPS quality performance categories.

In addition, participants are required to use certified EHR technology. As proposed, 50 percent of practitioners must use certified EHR technology to document and communicate patient care information.

Medical practices must make a number of decisions about MACRA, especially for years beyond 2017. Avoiding penalties in 2017 is expected to be fairly easy, but practices must consider the direction they will take for years 2018 and beyond. Deciding to go in the direction of MIPS or APMs is an important question to be considered on a practice-by-practice basis. Each practice needs to weigh its options and consider the risks and potential rewards, its technological sophistication, and its level of commitment to further technological development. Some practices may consider becoming a certified PCMH, as PCMHs will "automatically" receive full credit for improvement activities, which accounts for 15 percent of the score.

Other practices may band together to achieve economies of scale in administration, contracting, billing, reporting, and technology. The trend toward consolidation will certainly be supported by MACRA. For example, they may join an ACO or a clinically integrated network (CIN). A CIN is a group of physicians, hospitals, and other providers coming together with the goal of improving patient care and reducing overall cost of care.

The rules in the healthcare arena are rarely static. Practice managers and leaders need to follow the developments related to MACRA carefully so that the best decision for the individual practice can be made. Monitoring the CMS website (www.cms.gov) is one important activity, and checking for updates from organizations such as the Medical Group Management Association and the American College of Healthcare Executives can be helpful as well.

DISCUSSION QUESTIONS

1. Illustrate and discuss the steps in the revenue cycle.

2. What has been the impact of high-deductible health plans on the revenue of medical practices?

3. What are the four parts of Medicare? Discuss each of their functions.

4. What are ICD codes? How has ICD-10 changed from ICD-9?

5. What choices do practice managers have in selecting performance metrics for the revenue cycle?

6. Define the term *relative value unit* and describe the components of the resource-based relative value scale.

REFERENCES

AAPC. 2017. "Medical Billing and Coding Certification." Accessed April 23. www.aapc.com/certification.

Adepoju, O. E., M. A. Preston, and G. Gonzales. 2015. "Health Care Disparities in the Post–Affordable Care Act Era." *American Journal of Public Health* 105 (Suppl. 5): S665–S667.

American Academy of Family Physicians (AAFP). 2016. "Frequently Asked Questions: Medicare Access and CHIP Reauthorization Act of 2015 (MACRA)." Updated December. www.aafp.org/practice-management/payment/medicare-payment/faq.html#alternative.

American College of Physicians (ACP). 2015. "Medicare Access and CHIP Reauthorization Act (MACRA), H.R. 2: The End of the SGR—What Do Internists Need to Know?" Published April. www.acponline.org/system/files/documents/advocacy/where_we_stand/assets/macra_handout_hr2_2015.pdf.

American Medical Association (AMA). 2017a. "CPT®: Learn About Current Procedural Terminology (CPT®), the Code Set Used to Bill Outpatient and Office Procedures." Accessed April 23. www.ama-assn.org/practice-management/cpt.

———. 2017b. "RBRVS Overview." Accessed April 23. www.ama-assn.org/rbrvs-overview.

Barr, D. 2016. *Introduction to U.S. Health Policy: The Organization, Financing and Delivery of Health Care in America.* Baltimore, MD: Johns Hopkins University Press.

Cain, M., and R. Mittman. 2002. "Diffusion of Innovation in Health Care." Published May. Oakland, CA: California Health Care Foundation.

Centers for Medicare & Medicaid Services (CMS). 2017. "Physician Fee Schedule." Updated January 11. www.cms.gov/Medicare/Medicare-Fee-For-Service-Payment/PhysicianFeeSched/Index.html.

Chou, C.-F., and A. Sasso. 2009. "Practice Location Choice by New Physicians: The Importance of Malpractice Premiums, Damage Caps, and Health Professional Shortage Area Designation." *Health Services Research* 44 (4): 1271–89.

Cohen, W. J., and R. M. Ball. 1965. "Social Security Amendments of 1965: Summary and Legislative History." Published September. www.ssa.gov/policy/docs/ssb/v28n9/v28n9p3.pdf.

Defense Health Agency. 2017. TRICARE home page. Accessed April 23. www.tricare.mil.

Desilver, D. 2013. "Most Uninsured Americans Live in States That Won't Run Their Own Obamacare Exchanges." Published September 19. www.pewresearch.org/fact-tank/2013/09/19/most-uninsured-americans-live-in-states-that-wont-run-their-own-obamacare-exchanges.

Gallup. 2015. "Well-Being Index." Accessed December 1. www.gallup.com/topic/well_being_index.aspx.

HealthCare.gov. 2016. "Need Health Insurance?" Accessed January 5. www.healthcare.gov.

Hoffman, B. R. 2006. "Restraining the Health Care Consumer: The History of Deductibles and Co-payments in U.S. Health Insurance." *Social Science History* 30 (4): 501–28.

Indian Health Service (IHS). 2016. "Agency Overview." Accessed January 10. www.ihs.gov/aboutihs/overview.

Insurance Providers. 2016. "How Many Health Insurance Companies Are There in the United States?" Accessed June 14. www.insuranceproviders.com/how-many-health-insurance-companies-are-there-in-the-united-states.

Johnson, E. M. 2014. "Physician-Induced Demand." In *Encyclopedia of Health Economics*, vol. 3, 77–82. Cambridge, MA: Elsevier.

Lagarde, M., and D. Blaauw. 2017. "Physicians' Response to Financial and Social Incentives: A Medically Framed Real Effort Experiment." *Social Science & Medicine* 179: 147–59.

Manning, W., J. Newhouse, N. Duan, E. Keeler, B. Benjamin, A. Leibowitz, S. Marquis, and J. Zwanziger. 1988. *Health Insurance Demand for Medical Care: Evidence from a Randomized Experiment.* Santa Monica, CA: RAND.

McCormack, L., and R. Burge. 1994. "Diffusion of Medicare's RBRVS and Related Physician Policies." *Health Care Financing Review* 16 (2): 159–73.

McGuire, T. 2000. "Physician Agency." In *The Handbook of Health Economics*, vol. 1, 462–535, edited by A. Culyer and J. Newhouse. Cambridge, MA: Elsevier.

Medicare Learning Network. 2016. "ICD-9-CM, ICD-10-CM, ICD-10-PCS, CPT, and HCPCS Code Sets." Accessed June 14. www.cms.gov/Outreach-and-Education/Medicare-Learning-Network-MLN/MLNProducts/Downloads/ICD9-10CM-ICD10PCS-CPT-HCPCS-Code-Sets-Educational-Tool-ICN900943.pdf.

Momanyi, B. N. 2010. "Blue Cross and Blue Shield of Texas." Published June 12. www .tshaonline.org/handbook/online/articles/djbcz.

Mueller, M. S. 1974. "Health Maintenance Organization Act." Published March. www.ssa. gov/policy/docs/ssb/v37n3/v37n3p35.pdf.

Nyman, J. A. 2004. "Is Moral Hazard Inefficient? The Policy Implications of a New Theory." *Health Affairs* 23 (5): 194–99.

Rosenbaum, S., and T. M. Westmoreland. 2012. "The Supreme Court's Surprising Decision on the Medicaid Expansion: How Will the Federal Government and States Proceed?" *Health Affairs* 31 (8): 1663–72.

Scofea, L. A. 1994. "The Development and Growth of Employer-Provided Health Insurance." *Monthly Labor Review* (March): 3–10.

Segal, J. 2012. "How Defensive Medicine Has Caused Healthcare Costs to Rise." Published May 25. http://medicaleconomics.modernmedicine.com/medical -economics/news/modernmedicine/modern-medicine-now/how-defensive-medicine -has-caused-healthca.

Shortridge, E. F., J. R. Moore, H. Whitmore, M. J. O'Grady, and A. K. Shen. 2011. "Policy Impli- cations of First-Dollar Coverage: A Qualitative Examination from the Payer Perspective." *Public Health Reports* 126 (3): 394–99.

Shu, L., and D. Singh. 2015. *Delivering Healthcare in America: A Systems Approach*, 6th ed. Burlington, MA: Jones and Bartlett Learning.

Small Business Majority. 2016. "Plan Characteristics and Types." Accessed June 14. http://healthcoverageguide.org/reference-guide/coverage-types/plan-characteristics -and-types.

Trew, F. 2010. "10 Ways to Improve Your Bottom Line by Analyzing the Data from Your Practice Management System." Published August 15. http://managemypractice.com/ ten-ways-to-improve-your-bottom-line-by-analyzing-the-data-from-your-practice -management-system.

US Congress. 2015. "H.R.1470—SGR Repeal and Medicare Provider Payment Modern- ization Act of 2015." Introduced March 19. www.congress.gov/bill/114th-congress/ house-bill/1470.

CHAPTER 7

FINANCIAL MANAGEMENT AND MANAGERIAL ACCOUNTING IN THE PHYSICIAN PRACTICE

It's not only how much money you make. It's what you do with it that determines your financial condition.

—Sandra S. Simmons

LEARNING OBJECTIVES

➤ Appreciate the nature of cost behavior in the medical practice and why understanding it is important.

➤ Understand the importance of financial management in the medical practice.

➤ Describe the nature and purpose of budgeting.

➤ Articulate the use of variance analysis and metrics in the review of financial statements.

➤ Understand the complexities of physician compensation.

INTRODUCTION

Financial management and accounting involve financial planning, collection of financial data, and reporting of financial information about the practice for internal and external stakeholders. This process allows the practice to determine its financial position and make decisions accordingly.

Financial and management accounting are important disciplines unto themselves; however, the modern practice manager needs a basic knowledge of managing the financial aspects of the practice and to become a good consumer of financial information. Today, the collection and production of the various financial documents are often accomplished by using accounting packages that are commonly available in practice management systems or other accounting software. Depending on the practice size, accounting functions may be handled by contracting with outside accounting firms or financial management organizations to assist in the preparation of the documents described in this chapter. In addition to saving the medical practice the labor-intensive task of completing financial management functions, this approach provides a degree of oversight and guidance that can be reassuring. Regardless of the exact approach the practice takes in managing its financial activities, they must be carried out on a consistent and disciplined basis to prevent erroneous over- or understatements of the fiscal well-being of the practice, which can lead to significant regulatory and fiscal issues.

Cost Behavior

A fundamental aspect of managing a medical practice's finances is understanding cost behavior. As shown in exhibit 7.1, different costs behave differently over time. Understanding cost behavior is essential to properly manage and predict costs in relation to practice operations. Without this understanding, errors in planning will occur and projecting these costs will be flawed; this could mean the difference between a successful project or service and a failed one. Careful understanding is also important to assist others in the practice who may be less familiar with finance concepts and therefore may make incorrect assumptions about what supplies, services, and other outlays cost.

Three general terms are used to describe how costs behave:

◆ *Variable costs* vary on the basis of the volume of services and include items such as medical supplies (e.g., examination table paper, tongue depressors).

◆ *Fixed costs* vary only within a given range on the basis of volume of services (e.g., the cost for building rent or the mortgage payment would not change just because the practice saw a few additional patients, but it would change if the practice needed to acquire new space).

◆ *Step-variable costs* are fixed over a specific range of services, but increase when the variable cost range for a service exceeds its limit (e.g., a receptionist who effectively manages 30 patient check-ins per hour cannot keep pace when the

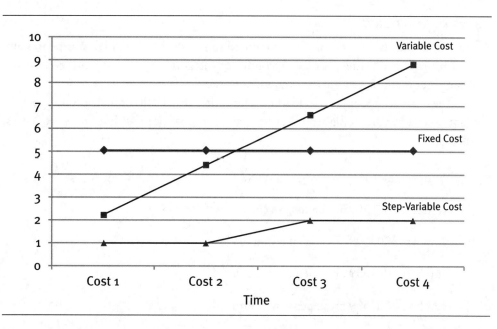

EXHIBIT 7.1
Cost Behavior

practice begins seeing 45 patients per hour, so an additional receptionist is needed).

TYPES OF COSTS

Costs can also be described by two types:

◆ *Direct costs* are directly related to the production of services (e.g., supplies, direct labor, medications).

◆ *Indirect costs* are not specifically attributed to a service but necessary for the operation of the practice in the production of services (e.g., practice manager's salary).

Costs such as rent and utilities charges can be accounted for in a variety of ways, such as allocating them by square foot to a service area and thereby treating them as a direct cost or simply attributing them as an indirect cost of the practice. The way these costs are handled often depends on the level of allocation the practice wishes to employ: The more specific the level of allocation, the more time and effort the practice must invest to provide an accurate accounting. Many practices find that allocating costs to a portion of the practice as direct costs is not worth the expense and effort to do so.

CHART OF ACCOUNTS

A **chart of accounts** is an accounting tool used to list all the categories of expenses and revenue sources used by the practice. Accounts are categories of expenses and revenue that help the accountant determine how transactions should be recorded.

The chart of accounts includes the account title and details of that account, and the accounts are customarily assigned by a systematic coding process with number sequences, as follows:

Numbers 001–199 are asset accounts

Numbers 200–299 are liability accounts

Numbers 300–399 are capital accounts

Numbers 400–499 are revenue accounts

Numbers 500–599 are expense accounts

The Medical Group Management Association (MGMA) has developed a standard chart of accounts that is used by some medical practices that have not established their own. It provides a specific set of accounts for the practice and is available for a nominal cost from MGMA (Gans, Andes, and Gold 2014). Using a standard chart of accounts helps the practice manager make meaningful comparisons against operating benchmarks without the need for significant adjustments to make the data comparable.

ACCOUNTING METHODS

One decision a medical practice needs to make is which accounting method to use for reporting income, for reporting expenses, and for tax purposes. Two commonly used methods of accounting that are recognized under generally accepted accounting principles are the cash-basis accounting system and the accrual accounting system.

CASH-BASIS ACCOUNTING

Many small medical practices use the **cash accounting system**, which resembles the accounting process most of us use in our personal lives.

The cash-basis accounting system recognizes income when it is received and expenses when they are paid. So, as the term *cash basis* implies, a recordable transaction occurs when cash is received or spent. Under this system, accounts receivable are not recorded as income.

ACCRUAL ACCOUNTING

The **accrual accounting system** recognizes income when it is earned (but not necessarily received) and expenses when they are incurred (but not necessarily paid). Under this system, accounts receivable are recorded as income, with an offsetting adjustment that recognizes the probability that all receivables will not be collected.

COMPARING THE ACCOUNTING METHODS

Each method has its advantages and disadvantages. In some respects, the cash-basis system is simpler and more readily understood, whereas the accrual system may recognize the reality of practice operations more accurately. For example, in a cash-basis system, receiving a large check at the end of the month for services rendered in the past inflates the income for that **accounting period**, providing an inaccurate picture of the activity that occurred in the operations. Similarly, paying a large expense during any given period may overinflate expenses. Another concern with the cash-basis system is that it can be manipulated by moving expenses and income from one period to another, especially near the end of accounting periods, again resulting in an unrealistic or inaccurate financial picture.

The accrual system may provide less variation from month to month but requires additional bookkeeping activities to record financial scenarios such as estimating bad debt. Matching expenses and income realistically may provide a better understanding of practice operations.

Regardless of the accounting system chosen by the practice, the practice manager is expected to help all stakeholders (including providers and other staff) understand how the system used by the practice works and provide the most realistic view into practice operations possible.

BUDGETING

One of the most important aspects of managing the medical practice is an effective budgeting process. The budget is a financial blueprint for the practice, and it is set by the strategic plan for the organization. The strategic plan elements needed for the budget include goals for the year, metrics to evaluate progress, formulation of the budget itself, means by which to implement the plan, and the process for measuring and monitoring the budget.

The budget is an operational as well as a governing document, and it serves many purposes, including the following:

◆   It is a way to quantify the goals of the organization in dollars.

◆   It is a communication document that allows all members of the practice to understand the financial objectives of the organization.

Accrual accounting system
An accounting system that records revenues and expenses at the time the transaction occurs, not at the time cash changes hands.

Accounting period
The period of time over which profits are calculated. Normal accounting periods are months, quarters, and years (fiscal or calendar).

◆   It is a way for the practice to express its mission in terms of dollars and units of service.

◆   It is a way to monitor and report results so that corrections may be made throughout the budget cycle. The budget period is typically one year, and, in the case of medical practices that are privately owned, by law the practice year is the calendar year.

In cases where the practice has not developed a strategic plan, the budget is based on events and activities the practice expects to occur during the next budget period. Examples include adding a service, bringing a new provider on board, or anticipating an increase in patients due to a change in insurance plans accepted by the practice.

THE BUDGET CYCLE

Exhibit 7.2 illustrates the budget cycle for the typical medical practice. All key stakeholders must participate in budgeting to help ensure that the budget is accurate, accepted, and seen as credible. Budgeting revenue-to-income ratios is among the most difficult aspects of medical practice budgeting. Although the topic is beyond the scope of this text, special attention should be paid to estimating this part of the budget.

METHODS OF BUDGETING

The three commonly used methods of budgeting are the following:

◆   *Zero-based budgeting* starts each new budget cycle by examining each expense and requiring justification for the expense in the coming year. The advantage of the zero-based budget is that it allows scrutiny on all aspects of the budgeting process, some of which may be overlooked in other circumstances. A major disadvantage is that it is time-consuming, and the level of detail may not always be warranted.

◆   *Incremental budgeting* begins with the previous budget from which to make adjustments on the basis of anticipated changes to expenses and income. One major advantage of the incremental budgeting process is that it takes less time to complete than zero-based budgeting. When major changes in the practice are not anticipated, incremental budgeting may be the more reasonable approach. The incremental budget is static and does not adjust to changes that occur during the budget period.

◆   *Flexible budgeting* is a sophisticated form of budget that adjusts as the volume of services varies. One key advantage of this budgeting form is that, as the

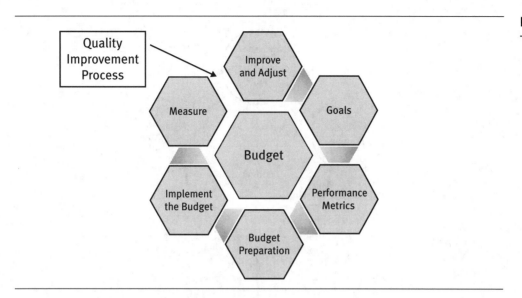

EXHIBIT 7.2
The Budget Cycle

term *flexible* implies, it is adaptable to changes in the circumstances of the practice, such as adding a provider. Flexible budgeting requires disciplined monitoring so that adjustments are not made simply to correct for inaccurate budget preparation.

As suggested by the last bullet point above, precision is an important consideration in budgeting. The practice must decide the level of detail to apply in preparing its budget. Accuracy and detail are always a trade-off in determining the exactness of the final budget. Carefully prepared budgets can take a good deal of time and effort to complete; some small practices do not make a budget at all. Instead, they use the "sum sufficient" approach: simply making purchasing decisions as necessary and maintaining the practice operations at the optimum level of productivity, given factors such as vacations and other scheduling restrictions. This method may be desirable because it does not produce pressure to spend a set budgeted amount and it is a common, sensible, and understandable way to think about spending. However, it may not anticipate the practice's needs as well as a budget can.

COMPONENTS OF THE BUDGETING PROCESS

Exhibit 7.3 shows the multiple components involved in creating an effective operating budget.

The overall budgeting process requires the creation of several individual budgeting categories, or separate "budgets," which include the following:

EXHIBIT 7.3
Budget
Components

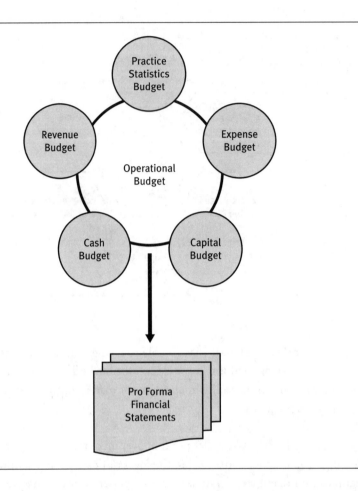

- *Statistical budget*—Sometimes located in a data warehouse (Inmon 2005), the statistical budget contains all the relevant data needed to complete the budget process. These data include the estimated number of procedures, resource-based relative value units, number of employees, salary information, benefit information, expected capital **expenditures**, supply costs, plant and equipment costs, and other expenses and sources of revenue.

- *Revenue budget*—The revenue budget contains an estimate of the services the practice will provide and the expected revenue from those services. In many ways, developing a revenue budget may be the most difficult aspect of budgeting because so many variables must be taken into consideration. For example, estimating the number of services to be provided is challenging because it can vary greatly from year to year depending on several factors, such as the number of provider days worked, fluctuations in demand for services as changes in the community occur, severity of illnesses that are

Expenditure
Occurs when an item
is acquired for a busi-
ness, an asset is pur-
chased, salaries are
paid, and so on.

presented, shifts in competitive position, and changes resulting from new or declining services.

◆ In addition, revenue projection is difficult for professional services such as medical care because appointment slots are ephemeral and gone forever if not used when available—appointments cannot be stored for future use. Thus, demand for services can be highly variable. Historical records of high-volume and low-volume periods may be useful in this part of the budgeting process. One example of an extreme-volume period is flu season, when primary care practices see an unusually high number of patients and may need to accommodate additional patients. When possible, these types of trends should be recognized in the budget for both expenses and income.

◆ *Expense budget*—The expense budget is straightforward in that it can be predictable because it is based on the number of employees and other expenses of the practice. If the medical practice has a good understanding of its expenses and the relationship between its expenses and the volume of services provided, this aspect of budgeting may be the most accurate and easiest to perform.

◆ *Cash budget*—The cash budget is a prediction of the cash flow that will be received by the practice and is an analysis of services provided and the expected income from those services. Some of the variables that go into considering cash budgets are as follows:

— The payers, which are major revenue sources for the practice, and the history of their payment practices

— Expected payment for each service from the payers

— The relative volume of services to be billed to each payer

The practice may develop an average reimbursement per service on the basis of historical payment patterns. This average is determined by dividing the total revenue from a service by the total number of individual units of that service provided.

Total revenue by service ÷ Total number of services =
Average revenue per service

This calculation can be performed by modern practice management systems. The amount may need to be adjusted in consideration of volume and payment changes from payers during the budget process.

Depreciation
An expense that is intended to reflect the loss in value of a fixed asset.

◆ *Capital budget*—The capital budget reflects the **depreciation** costs from existing equipment as well as the expected purchase and depreciation of new equipment. These costs are based on the depreciation methods adopted.

◆ *Operating budget*—The operating budget is the combination of the previously described budgets. It provides the financial operating plan for the practice and can be used to predict the practice's financial performance in the form of the pro forma financial statements. A pro forma is the predicted result from the elements considered in the budgeting process.

FINANCIAL STATEMENTS

Effective financial management of the practice requires the production of a number of important financial documents used to determine the financial position of the practice and to manage the practice in accordance with its mission, vision, values, and goals. Exhibit 7.4 shows some of the principal financial statements needed by the practice and major components that comprise each statement. Note that all financial documents are created for a given time frame, such as monthly, quarterly, or annually. Except for pro forma statements, which are forward looking, all represent financial transactions and events that occurred in the past.

Profit
The amount left over when expenses are subtracted from revenues. Also referred to as *income, net income,* or *earnings*.

PROFIT-AND-LOSS STATEMENT

The profit-and-loss (P&L) statement, also called the income statement, provides an accounting of the revenue, expenses, and resulting **profits** or losses from the activities of the practice.

EXHIBIT 7.4
Financial
Statements

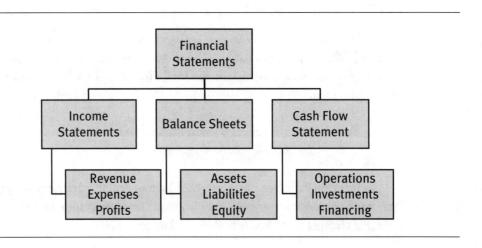

Exhibit 7.5 illustrates a simple income statement for Happy Practice XYZ for the period ending March 31, 2016. Notice the important components:

- Patient revenue

- Major categories of expenses

- Total operating expenses

- Income

Physician or provider compensation is often considered separately as a line item on the income statement, as are physician or provider expenses. The practice often serves as an income vehicle for the practice owners, and that function should be captured in a way that separates actual operating cost for the practice from those expenses that represent owner income.

March 31, 2016			
Revenues			
Patient Revenue			$165,000
Operating Expenses			
Advertising	$5,310		
Wages	$ 30,500		
Utilities	$ 1,080		
Depreciation	$ 800		
Repairs	$ 4,260		
Insurance	$ 600		
Interest	$ 100		
Supplies	$ 3,900		
Total Operating Expenses		$46,500	
Physician Compensation			$118,450
Physician Expenses	$115,000		
Net Practice Income			$ 3,450

EXHIBIT 7.5
Happy Practice XYZ Income Statement

In addition, note the net income line, which is the profit or loss that the practice produced after all expenses and compensation have been paid. Practice income can be used for bonus distribution or for reinvestment in the practice. It can also be retained by the practice, creating additional equity in the practice for the owners.

Exhibit 7.6 illustrates a simple month-by-month practice financial report in the form of a spreadsheet, which shows the elements of the income statement. Tracking income monthly allows the practice manager to monitor the practice's financial performance over time.

STATEMENT OF CASH FLOWS

The statement of cash flows provides useful documentation and a process for analyzing the sources and outlays of the cash coming into the practice. Exhibit 7.7 illustrates a simple cash flow statement for Happy Practice XYZ. Following are some important features to note:

◆ The amount of cash brought into the practice through operations, often known as cash flow, can be positive or negative depending on how much is spent in relationship to cash received.

◆ Other sources of cash can be proceeds from a bank loan or the sale of stock investments.

◆ A major use of cash is for the purchase of equipment.

◆ Payments on loans represent a reduction in cash.

Cash flow results in an increase or decrease in the practice's cash. An important practice management function is ensuring that cash flow is reflected accurately on the statement of cash flows. In addition, practice leaders should help the practice evaluate its use and sources of cash for future operational considerations to avoid being unprepared for cash needs.

BALANCE SHEET

The **balance sheet** is a statement of assets, **liabilities**, and capital at a point in time and reflects all the financial transactions that have occurred in that time frame. Exhibit 7.8 illustrates a simple balance sheet for Happy Practice XYZ. Note the following in particular:

◆ **Current assets** are cash and items that can quickly be turned into cash, such as marketable securities and **inventory**.

Balance sheet
A statement of the financial position of a practice at a specific time, often at the close of business on the last day of the month, quarter, or year.

Liability
An amount owed by a practice to an individual or entity.

Current asset
An asset that is expected to be turned into cash within a year, including cash, marketable securities, accounts receivable, and inventory.

Inventory
The supply or stock of goods and products that a practice has for sale.

EXHIBIT 7.6

Practice Financial Report

Statistic	Jan	Feb	Mar	Apr	May	Jun	Jul	Aug	Sep	Oct	Nov	Dec	Yr to Date
1 Total Charges	$1,000	$1,000	$1,000	$1,000	$1,000	$1,000	$1,000	$1,000	$1,000	$1,000	$1,000	$1,000	$12,000
Avg Daily Charges	$ 32	$ 36	$ 32	$ 33	$ 32	$ 33	$ 32	$ 32	$ 33	$ 32	$ 33	$ 32	$ 33
Total Charges Physician #1	$ 500	$ 500	$ 500	$ 500	$ 500	$ 500	$ 500	$ 500	$ 500	$ 500	$ 500	$ 500	$ 5,500
Total Charges Physician #2	$ 200	$ 200	$ 200	$ 200	$ 200	$ 200	$ 200	$ 200	$ 200	$ 200	$ 200	$ 200	$ 2,400
Total Charges Physician #3	$ 180	$ 180	$ 180	$ 180	$ 180	$ 180	$ 180	$ 180	$ 180	$ 180	$ 180	$ 180	$ 2,160
Total Charges Other	$ 20	$ 20	$ 20	$ 20	$ 20	$ 20	$ 20	$ 20	$ 20	$ 20	$ 20	$ 20	$ 240
2 Total Payments (or Receipts)	$1,000	$1,000	$1,000	$1,000	$1,000	$1,000	$1,000	$1,000	$1,000	$1,000	$1,000	$1,000	$12,000
3 Total Refunds	$ 10	$ 10	$ 10	$ 10	$ 10	$ 10	$ 10	$ 10	$ 10	$ 10	$ 10	$ 10	$ 120
4 % Copayments Collected	50.00%	50.00%	50.00%	50.00%	50.00%	50.00%	50.00%	50.00%	50.00%	50.00%	50.00%	50.00%	600.00%
5 Total Accounts Receivable (A/R)	$ 900	$ 900	$ 900	$ 900	$ 900	$ 900	$ 900	$ 900	$ 900	$ 900	$ 900	$ 900	$10,800
Total over 90 days	$ 10	$ 10	$ 10	$ 10	$ 10	$ 10	$ 10	$ 10	$ 10	$ 10	$ 10	$ 10	$ 120
% over 90	1.11%	1.11%	1.11%	1.11%	1.11%	1.11%	1.11%	1.11%	1.11%	1.11%	1.11%	1.11%	1.11%
6 Gross collection ratio	98.00%	98.00%	98.00%	98.00%	98.00%	98.00%	98.00%	98.00%	98.00%	98.00%	98.00%	98.00%	100.00%
7 Net Receipts—Budget	$1,100	$1,100	$1,100	$1,100	$1,100	$1,100	$1,100	$1,100	$1,100	$1,100	$1,100	$1,100	$13,200
Net Receipts—Actual	$1,000	$1,000	$1,000	$1,000	$1,000	$1,000	$1,000	$1,000	$1,000	$1,000	$1,000	$1,000	$12,000
8 Operating Expenses—Budget	$ 500	$ 500	$ 500	$ 500	$ 500	$ 500	$ 500	$ 500	$ 500	$ 500	$ 500	$ 500	$ 6,000
Operating Expenses—Actual	$ 490	$ 490	$ 490	$ 490	$ 490	$ 490	$ 490	$ 490	$ 490	$ 490	$ 490	$ 490	$ 5,880
9 Net Income	$ 610	$ 610	$ 610	$ 610	$ 610	$ 610	$ 610	$ 610	$ 610	$ 610	$ 610	$ 610	$ 7,320
10 Total encounters	600	600	600	600	600	600	600	600	600	600	600	600	7,200
11 Total new patient visits	30	30	30	30	30	30	30	30	30	30	30	30	360
% new patient visits	5.00%	5.00%	5.00%	5.00%	5.00%	5.00%	5.00%	5.00%	5.00%	5.00%	5.00%	5.00%	5.00%
Full-time equivalent staff	4.00	4.00	4.00	4.00	4.00	4.00	4.00	4.00	4.00	4.00	5.00	6.00	4.25

Exhibit 7.7

Practice Cash Flow
Statement

Cash Flow Statement for Happy Practice XYZ
For the period ending May 31, 2016

Cash from Operations

+ Cash from collections	$5,000
− Cash to suppliers and employees	(4,000)
Net cash from operations	$ 1,000

Cash from Investments

− Equipment purchase	(1,000)
Net cash from investment	−1,000

Cash from Financing

+ Loan from bank	+2,000
− Payment on loan	−500
Net cash from financing	+1,500

Net Increase or Decrease in Cash for the Period	**$ 1,500**

Exhibit 7.8

Balance Sheet,
Happy Practice
XYZ, PC,
December 31,
2015

Assets			Claims on Assets		
Current Assets			Current Liabilities		
Cash	$123,000		Accounts Payable	$100,000	
Marketable Securities	$200,000		Notes Payable	$150,000	
Accounts Receivable	$345,000		Total Current Liabilities	$250,000	
Inventories	$100,000		Long-Term Note	$300,000	
Total Current Assets		$ 768,000	Total Liabilities		$ 550,000
Long-Term Assets			Owners' Equity		$ 843,000
Building (Gross)	$350,000		Total Claims		**$1,393,000**
− Accumulated Depreciation	$−50,000				
Net Building	$300,000				
Land	$325,000				
Total Long-Term Assets		$ 625,000			
Total Assets		**$1,393,000**			

◆ Happy Practice XYZ uses an accrual method of accounting; this is evident because accounts receivable are reflected as a current asset. On a cash-basis system, this item would not appear in the balance sheet.

◆ Long-term assets, including the building minus its accumulated depreciation and the value of the land, are reflected.

◆ Total assets equal current assets plus long-term assets.

◆ Claims against assets are the liabilities of the practice.

◆ Current liabilities include **accounts payable**, which typically include items that have been purchased on **credit** liabilities for which payment is due upon receipt of the invoice or in a short time hence.

◆ Long-term liabilities are reflected as long-term notes, which are obligations to pay (in this case $300,000) at some future date; these are not considered current obligations.

◆ Total liabilities are calculated, and the difference between total assets and total liabilities is the equity in the practice. Equity can be reflected by a simple formula:

Equity = Total assets – Total liabilities.

Accounts payable
Amounts owed by the practice for the goods or services it has purchased from outside suppliers.

Credit
An accounting entry on the right or bottom of a balance sheet usually reflecting an increase in liabilities or capital or a reduction in assets.

The balance sheet can be important for establishing the net value of the practice and may be used by financial institutions in determining creditworthiness. In for-profit practices, income retained in the practice is taxed as business income and again as personal income when it is distributed to the owners. This process is known as double taxation. To avoid double taxation, practice owners often elect to distribute all income as bonuses, which leads to little, if any, retained earnings.

MONITORING FINANCIAL PERFORMANCE

All the financial statements, and the effort expended to prepare them, are of little value unless they are monitored carefully. Monitoring involves careful variance analysis and review of metrics and ratios that reflect the goals of the practice. These measures vary from practice to practice and may be based on the specific concerns of the practice, such as poor cash flow or high expenses.

VARIANCE ANALYSIS

The financial statements must be accompanied by application of variance analysis to effectively monitor the financial progress of the practice. This process allows the practice manager to determine why a variation has occurred between the budgeted amount and the actual results. Variances may be reviewed in terms of metrics and ratios or in absolute terms, and the practice may wish to establish a performance band, or range, of acceptable performance. For example, if, on the one hand, the practice budgeted to collect $1,000 per month and the actual performance was $999, because the variance is small, no analysis is likely necessary. Now let's say that, on the other hand, utility expenses were budgeted to be $500 per month and the actual cost was $1,000, this variance—100 percent of the expected result—warrants investigation. Several possible reasons could explain the outcome, such as the following:

◆   The variance may have occurred in a summer month when the weather was particularly hot, requiring additional utility services.

◆   The budget may contain an average utility cost per month that varies dramatically from month to month; therefore, the practice might see much lower bills at other times of the year. In this case, the practice manager should note the variance and document the likely reasonable explanation.

◆   If no reasonable explanation can be found, a budgeting error may be the cause, meaning the expenses were not estimated correctly. This finding should be noted so that special attention can be paid to this item when preparing the following year's budget to improve its accuracy.

◆   Further investigation may indicate errors of meter readings on the part of the utility company or changes in the practice's operation, such as extended hours causing an increase in volume and therefore utility cost.

Establishing criteria for the review of variances and quickly investigating those variances are critical so that corrective action can be taken if warranted. The number of financial items related to a typical practice is significant, and every item cannot be continuously investigated. Practices might consider variances greater than 10 percent from budget as being significant enough to warrant further examination. A large dollar variance may also be considered to require further investigation.

One caution in performing variance analysis is to not rely solely on profit and loss as the most important metrics. The profit from the practice is a result of revenue minus expenses. Optimizing revenue and the utilization of costs optimizes the outcome in the form of increased profitability. Unless a careful examination of revenue and expense variances is undertaken, the opportunity for such optimization may be lost.

METRICS AND RATIOS

An endless number of metrics can be applied in medical practices. Regular maintenance of databases and the consistent measurement of those metrics deemed most important by the practice are important functions of practice managers and leaders. Certain metrics may require more focus from time to time, including those based on quality improvement activities or the identification of issues that need to be addressed. Appropriate metrics must be selected to achieve the desired managerial result.

Metrics fall into many categories. The most common include the following:

◆ Financial

◆ Operational

◆ Clinical

In this section, we focus on some key financial and operational areas.

Financial Metrics

A number of financial metrics should be monitored by the practice manager related to revenue, expenses, and productivity. Revenue is often expressed as a percentage of the billed charges that are collected, particularly in terms of the following time periods after billing:

◆ 0 to 30 days

◆ 31 to 60 days

◆ 61 to 90 days

◆ 91 to 120 days

◆ Greater than 120 days

◆ Percentage of total collections to charges

This division is important because the older an accounts receivable, the less likely it will be collected. Often receivables are uncollectible because the insurance information that was provided is inaccurate or the patient—whether insured, but with high deductibles and coinsurance, or self-pay, or uninsured—does not have the economic means to satisfy the bill.

Another important metric in the financial arena is the number of claims filed accurately with the payer the first time. This measure is usually expressed as a percentage of claims rejected due to inaccurate information. Careful management and quick review of denied claims is imperative to resubmit them as soon as possible. Modern practice management systems contain "scrubbers" to help ensure claims are properly prepared for filing.

At some point, outstanding accounts receivable need to be written off as bad debts or as uncollectible. This step helps the practice avoid having an unrealistic view of the number of collectible receivables. The practice should have a carefully crafted policy on how to manage older accounts receivable; some options are as follows:

◆   Write off as charity care.

◆   Send to a collections firm or continue internal collection activity.

◆   Write off as bad debt.

Bad debt is distinguished from charity care in that bad debt represents receivables that are collectible but the debtor is unwilling to pay, whereas in the case of charity care, the debtor is unable to pay or the practice had no expectation of payment at the outset of the encounter.

When the likelihood of collecting a debt is very small, the account should be written off to a special account so that a record is kept of the action but the account is no longer considered an active receivable. This way, the practice avoids creating a falsely inflated balance of viable receivables.

Operational Metrics

Dashboards can be very effective ways to express the operational health of the practice in a precise and timely way. Most practice stakeholders are busy and not well versed in financial matters; therefore, the use of dashboards, such as a heat map, may be an ideal way to keep everyone informed. Exhibit 7.9 shows an example of a practice heat map with four key metrics. Two of the indicators are in darker shades, indicating they are operating below expectation. The lighter-shaded indicator reflects higher-than-expected performance, and shades in between indicate performance as expected. Indicators with darker shading require investigation to improve. Notice that the positive indicator is productivity, which may indicate that the practice is producing well but lagging in other operational areas. Adjusted collection percentage is performing below expectations, which may be the primary source

EXHIBIT 7.9
Heat Map of Key
Metrics

Productivity 2000 wRVUs/provider	Adjusted Collection Percentage 60%
Expense Ratio 50%	Net Income

of concern and require additional attention from the practice manager. Colors may be substituted for shading, with green being positive, red being negative, and yellow being neutral, which is also referred to as a stoplight dashboard.

Performance Benchmarks and Important Financial Metrics

Performance benchmarks are numerous and varied. Some examples are shown in exhibit 7.10. Because so many potential metrics are available, the practice manager must carefully target those measures that are most meaningful to his or her concerns.

Organizations such as MGMA provide benchmarks that are useful in determining the ideal performance level of a practice. Without some understanding of what poor, average, or superior performance data are, the practice manager may have difficulty determining the areas that require more focus for improvement.

The financial systems maintained by medical groups are as follows:

Payroll

Billing systems
    Government third party

Employee benefits

Financial reporting
    Profit/loss statements (income
        statements)
    Variance analysis
    Financial control and audit functions
    External

Maintenance of fee schedules and
chargemasters

Accounts receivable
    Insurance
    Self-pay

Accounts payable
    Balance sheet
    Budgets
    Service and receipt (and its various
        forms)
    Internal

Compliance

Chart of accounts

PHYSICIAN AND OTHER PROVIDER COMPENSATION

Physician compensation is an important area of practice management that requires special attention and can be one of the most challenging aspects of the practice administration's compensation and benefits program. It is such an integral part of the financial management of the practice that it is discussed here rather than as part of the human resources chapter.

Physicians are compensated in a number of ways, ranging from a simple salary to a complex formula involving several components. How providers are compensated in the medical practice may depend on the ownership of the practice. In small, privately owned practices, the physician owners typically decide how they are paid.

In large, affiliated practices or practices owned by healthcare systems, compensation may be driven by market forces and by the human resource policies of the organization.

Formulas for Benchmark Equations and Metrics

$$\frac{\text{Bad debt}}{\text{Net collections}}$$

$$\frac{\text{Operating expenses}}{\text{Total revenue}}$$

$$\frac{\text{Staff FTEs}}{\text{Total revenue}}$$

$$\frac{\text{Current assets}}{\text{Current liabilities}}$$

$$\frac{\text{Cash, marketable securities, A/R (if on accrual system)}}{\text{Current liabilities}}$$

$$\frac{\text{Long-term debt}}{\text{Long-term debt and shareholder's equity}}$$

$$\frac{\text{Total liabilities}}{\text{Total liabilities and shareholder's equity}}$$

$$\frac{\text{Appointment no-shows}}{\text{Total schedule appointments}}$$

Gross Collection Rate

$$\frac{\text{Net collections}}{\text{Gross charges}}$$

$$\frac{\text{New-patient appointments}}{\text{Total scheduled appointments}}$$

$$\frac{\text{Floor space, expenses, bad debt, income}}{\text{FTEs}}$$

Average Daily Receivables

$$\frac{\text{Total receivables recorded in 60 days}}{\text{60 days}}$$

Days of Receivables Outstanding

$$\frac{\text{Total receivables}}{\text{Average daily receivables}}$$

Because of the private inurement rules discussed in chapter 4, compensation may be subject to certain limitations so that total provider income does not exceed the current market value for the services provided by the physician to the organization. The Office of Inspector General of the US Department of Health & Human Services recognizes certain standards for determining market-based compensation for providers and has devoted significant effort to informing the practice community of the rules and regulations regarding just compensation (OIG 2015, 2016). The practice must remain vigilant regarding compliance with all the rules and regulations pertaining to physician compensation. This requirement is especially relevant for not-for-profit organizations because of the potential to attribute compensation for referrals and other non-practice-related activities not provided at fair market value for the work performed by the practitioner.

DETERMINING PHYSICIAN COMPENSATION: ONE EXAMPLE

Here we examine one approach taken by a for-profit practice that is distributing the net proceeds of practice operations as income to the physicians (Darves 2011).

Establishing the compensation formula used by the practice requires significant input, analysis, and consideration by the stakeholders.

1. *Determine and clarify philosophy and objectives.* The philosophy and objectives of the practice help frame the mission, vision, values, and goals, which in turn inform the compensation. Examples of philosophy are the prevailing attitudes of practice staff toward productivity (often expressed as relative value units [RVUs]), the egalitarian nature of the practice, and the practice style differences among the physicians in the practice. For example, in a multispecialty practice, a pediatrician and a neurosurgeon would not be paid the same salary; however, the criteria for determining salary might be the same, such as productivity, patient satisfaction, physician citizenship, community benefit, credit for nonmedical care duties, research, quality indicators, longevity with the practice, and consideration for outreach activities.

2. *Determine what databases are needed as input for the compensation formula, and assess the quality of the information.* Practices often wish to include certain information and data in their compensation formulas without being able to accurately develop that information. This gap can lead to conflict if any questions arise about the validity of the data. Thus, the data must be valid, verifiable, reproducible, and timely.

3. *Select components to be used in the formula.* The philosophy of the practice regarding how complex to make the formula determines which components

and how many components are used. Some practices, particularly those in single specialties, may pay everyone in an equal manner. Other practices may differentiate compensation on the basis of the numerous characteristics previously discussed.

4. *Meet with stakeholders.* Stakeholders must be involved to determine whether the development of the compensation model is on track. At this stage of development, the practice manager must verify that the components being considered in the formula meet the expectations of the stakeholders and are consistent with the philosophy of the practice.

5. *Model the results.* Once consensus has been reached on the basic elements of the compensation formula, the results must be modeled or simulated, to project what would occur if adopted, using data that are as close to actual practice data as possible. The model should be shared with the stakeholders so none are surprised and so unintended outcomes are avoided.

6. *Gain approval.* Understandably, few issues are more sensitive to members of the practice than compensation. Therefore, the practice manager and other leaders must be sure the physicians understand how the compensation formula works and the probable outcomes of its implementation. One suggestion is to provide a carefully written explanation of how each step is derived and how the physician can use the methodology to calculate his or her personal income.

7. *Implement the compensation plan.* This step may take at least three different forms. The first is to launch the new compensation model with a transition phase, especially if the practice is using a formula that differs substantially from the proposed model. The transition could take one of a number of approaches, such as an incremental implementation whereby a portion of compensation is determined by the old formula and a portion is determined by the new formula. The second form of implementation is to maintain the old methodology while tracking compensation using the new formula so that a comparison can be made. This approach may help reassure members of the practice that their compensation will not change drastically, which is often a fear when new compensation models are adopted. The third implementation form is a straight switchover. This approach may be risky and produce unnecessary anxiety because the practitioner does not have the benefit of a pro forma view of the change. If the compensation model has been carefully constructed with adequate input from the stakeholders and carefully modeled to see if it will result in the desired outcome, delaying its implementation

serves little purpose and only focuses the individual practitioners on their self-interest.

8. *Review the outcomes.* Any compensation policy or method change in the practice should be reviewed on a regular basis to be sure it is functioning as intended. The sensitivity of compensation makes periodic review especially important. Often, this review is built into the implementation plan to reassure the practice members that any necessary adjustments will be made on a periodic basis. Compensation models change frequently in most medical practices in light of the dynamics of the medical care environment.

A general view of distributing income using a physician compensation formula for a practice is illustrated in exhibits 7.11 through 7.14. In this case, productivity, research, and quality metrics are factors in determining the final income of the physician.

Exhibits 7.12, 7.13, and 7.14 illustrate the income distribution process. In step 1, the compensation components are awarded to each of five physicians in the practice. Productivity is determined by the number of work RVUs produced by each physician, and points are awarded for quality metrics on the basis of a predetermined system, which may include a variety of outcome measures. The final measurement used in this formula awards points for clinical research. The totals are distributed to each physician as indicated in exhibit 7.12.

In step 2, relative percentages for each measure are determined as a straight-forward calculation. In step 3, the total available income of $500,000 is divided on

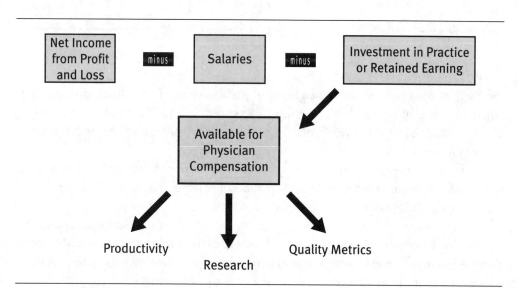

EXHIBIT 7.11
Basic Physician Compensation Framework

EXHIBIT 7.12

Example Physician
Compensation
Model, Part 1

In this example, there is a total of $500,000 in income to allocate to the physicians based on the formula.

Each physician—A, B, C, D, and E—will receive a share of the income based on work RVUs (wRVUs). The number of wRVUs for each physician is determined as a percentage of the total.

Quality metrics are expressed on a predetermined point system, where a total of 20 quality points is divided between the 5 physicians based on the metrics the practice has decided to measure. This could be patient satisfaction or engagement, core measures, complication rates, or a multitude of other possibilities. The points compiled for each physician are then converted to a percentage of total points.

In a similar way, research credit is determined by allocating a total of 20 points using a predetermined measure of research activity, such as number of studies, number of papers published or submitted, or number of projects funded. The points accumulated are then converted to a percentage of the total points.

Step 1: Determine measurements for the practice and each physician.

Measure	Physician A Measure	Physician B Measure	Physician C Measure	Physician D Measure	Physician E Measure	Total for the Practice
Productivity (number of wRVUs)	1,000	900	800	1,200	1,100	5,000 wRVUs
Quality metrics	3	5	5	3	4	20 points
Research	4	3	5	5	3	20 points

the basis of the predetermined weighting of each portion of the allocation measures, where in this case productivity represents 75 percent, or $375,000 of the total available for allocation; quality represents 15 percent, or $75,000; and research represents 10 percent, or $50,000.

In step 4, the distribution of dollars to each of the five physicians in the practice is transacted. Physician D received the highest allocation, largely due to his productivity and his research contribution.

This example is simple and straightforward, and in many practice situations, the income distribution formula is more complicated than the one illustrated here. Most practices use Microsoft Excel or other computer programs to calculate physician compensation, which allows for the easy incorporation of many factors and variables.

Exhibit 7.13
Example Physician
Compensation
Model, Part 2

Step 2: Determine relative percentage of measure for each physician.

Measure	Physician A Measure	Physician B Measure	Physician C Measure	Physician D Measure	Physician E Measure	Total for the Practice
Productivity (number of wRVUs)	20%	18%	16%	24%	22%	100%
Quality metrics	15%	25%	25%	15%	20%	100%
Research	20%	15%	25%	25%	15%	100%

Step 3: Determine the amount of income to be allocated in each category.

Productivity: $500,000 × .75 = $375,000
Quality: 500,000 × .15 =   75,000
Research: 500,000 × .10 =   50,000
Total to allocate: $500,000

Step 4: Determine the total dollar value for each physician by multiplying each category percentage by the dollar values available for allocation.

Exhibit 7.14
Allocation of
Income to the
Practice Physicians

Amount to Allocate $500,000	Physician A Measure	Physician B Measure	Physician C Measure	Physician D Measure	Physician E Measure	Total for the Practice
Productivity (number of wRVUs)	20%	18%	16%	24%	22%	100%
$375,000	$75,000	$67,500	$60,000	$90,000	$82,500	$375,000
Quality metrics	15%	25%	25%	15%	20%	100%
$75,000	$11,250	$18,750	$18,750	$11,250	$15,000	$75,000
Research	20%	15%	25%	25%	15%	100%
$50,000	$10,000	$7,500	$12,500	$12,500	$7,500	$50,000
Total allocation	$96,250	$93,750	$91,250	$113,750	$105,000	$500,000

Nonphysician Provider Compensation

Increasingly, nonphysician providers, including physician assistants and nurse practitioners, are compensated more like physician providers, using a formula containing a number of components. However, many nonphysician providers are still paid on an hourly or salaried basis, which may be supplemented by periodic bonuses for meeting standards in areas such as productivity, patient satisfaction, and quality.

THE FUTURE OF PRACTICE FINANCIAL MANAGEMENT

Financial management in medical practice is likely to see dramatic changes. Currently, practices focus much attention on volume and some operational aspects of financial management. In the future, that focus may move toward evaluation of outcomes in the context of new financial incentive systems where services are reimbursed much less on the basis of volume and much more for the outcomes of the services provided. Whereas now practice managers ask, "How many have we done?," in the future, payers may ask, "What good have your services done? And show us with data." This shift will have a dramatic impact on how physicians are compensated as value-based factors are increasingly incorporated into compensation models (Carr and Milliron 2014).

DISCUSSION QUESTIONS

1. Identify the three primary types of costs in the medical practice, and explain how they differ.
2. What is the main purpose of budgeting?
3. Describe the different components of the budgeting process.
4. What are the primary financial statements for the medical practice, and how is each used?
5. What are some benchmarks used in financial analysis for the medical practice?
6. Describe some of the factors used in physician compensation.

REFERENCES

Carr, J. D., and M. J. Milliron. 2014. "Integrating Value into Physician Employment Compensation Models." Published August 13. www.beckershospitalreview.com/compensation-issues/integrating-value-into-physician-employment-compensation-models.html.

Darves, B. 2011. "Physician Compensation Models: The Basics, the Pros, and the Cons." Published October 18. www.nejmcareercenter.org/article/physician-compensation-models-the-basics-the-pros-and-the-cons.

Gans, D. N., S. Andes, and R. J. Gold. 2014. *Chart of Accounts*, 6th ed. Englewood, CO: Medical Group Management Association.

Inmon, W. H. 2005. *Building the Data Warehouse*, 4th ed. New York: Wiley.

Office of Inspector General (OIG). 2016. "A Roadmap for New Physicians: Avoiding Medicare and Medicaid Fraud and Abuse." Accessed January 30. http://oig.hhs.gov/compliance/physician-education/roadmap_web_version.pdf.

———. 2015. "Fraud Alert: Physician Compensation Arrangements May Result in Significant Liability." Washington, DC: OIG.

CHAPTER 8

HUMAN RESOURCES MANAGEMENT

They're not employees, they're people.

—Peter Drucker

LEARNING OBJECTIVES

➤ Describe the range of human resource functions in the medical practice.

➤ Appreciate the range of professionals that are found in medical practices.

➤ Articulate the steps in the hiring function.

➤ Understand regulations that are specific to the employment process.

➤ Illustrate the steps in managing change.

➤ Describe why leading change is important to medical practice management.

INTRODUCTION

Healthcare employment constitutes about 9 percent of the American workforce, with about 3 percent being professionals (KFF 2016). Hiring and sustaining a high-caliber staff are two of the most important functions of managing a physician practice. Without a properly trained and motivated staff, providing high-quality services to the practice's patients is difficult. An old saying in human resources management, "Hire for attitude, and train for skill," is particularly applicable today, when in the highly competitive medical practice environment, patients have increasingly high expectations of their providers. Simply having technical skills is not adequate to build and maintain a successful practice. Staff must be able to engage patients in a positive and constructive way to earn their trust and satisfaction. Although data seem to conflict on this point, many researchers believe engaged and satisfied patients are more likely to comply with the instructions of their providers than are disengaged, unsatisfied patients, leading to better outcomes (e.g., Kane, Maciejewski, and Finch 1997). More recently, a study by Fenton, Jerant, and Bertaski (2012) found little connection between satisfaction and clinical outcome; in fact, the researchers found that mortality was higher, as were expenditures and utilization, among more satisfied groups. Other authors have observed this tenuous connection as well (Kennedy, Tevis, and Kent 2014). The controversy has intensified as more physician payment is tied to patient satisfaction. Some issues that complicate this concept are the lack of common definitions and measures of satisfaction and the complexity inherent in defining what produces satisfaction, which goes far beyond the clinical or office experience (Berkowitz 2016). Regardless of the evidence, satisfying and engaging patients is a desirable goal for any practice if for no other reason than it creates a pleasing practice atmosphere.

THE PEOPLE IN THE PRACTICE

A number of terms are used to describe medical practice employees in general, some of which are often used synonymously. They include *teammate*, *associate*, *colleague*, and *staff member*.

Furthermore, a variety of terms are used to describe the physicians and providers of the medical practice, with *medical staff* a common phrase. Interestingly, physicians often refer to each other as *partner*, even when the practice is not an actual legal partnership. The term *partner* in this sense denotes the collegial relationship among the physicians of the practice.

Practices may also employ many different nonphysician professionals. Exhibit 8.1 lists some of the numerous nonphysician practitioners who may be found in the medical practice.

The number and type of nonphysician practitioners vary dramatically from practice to practice, depending on size, specialties, and services provided by the practice. Small, single-specialty practices may have few on staff, whereas large, multispecialty practices likely employ several types of nonphysician practitioners.

THE EMPLOYMENT, RECRUITING, AND HIRING PROCESS

Hiring new staff requires careful planning and preparation. Depending on the size and complexity of the practice, recruiting may be the responsibility of the practice manager;

Nurse	Pharmacist	Physician assistant
Nurse practitioner	Allied health professional	Anesthesia technician
Art therapist/art psychotherapist	Athletic trainer	Audiologist
Cardiovascular technologist	Clinical laboratory scientist	Medical coder
Diagnostic sonographer	Dietitian/nutritionist	Electrocardiogram technician
Emergency medical technician	Environmental health officer	Exercise physiologist
Kinesiotherapist	Massage therapist	Medical assistant
Medical interpreter	Medical laboratory scientist	Medical radiation scientist
Music therapist	Neurophysiologist	Occupational therapist
Paramedic	Perfusionist	Phlebotomist
Practice manager	Public health epidemiologist	Physical therapist/ physiotherapist
Radiotherapist/ radiation therapist/ medical dosimetrist	Diagnostic radiographer	Recreational therapist
Rehabilitation counselor	Renal dialysis technologist	Respiratory therapist
Social worker	Speech and language pathologist	Surgical technologist

in large practices, that task likely is performed by a human resources department or hiring manager. The process should be similar to that described in this section regardless of who undertakes the endeavor. Physician recruiting may differ somewhat, and practice providers inevitably are involved in their hiring, whereas they may not be involved in nonphysician staffing. Often, physicians want to be involved in recruiting the members of the practice who will work directly with them.

Next, we discuss nine steps in the employment process, from identifying staffing needs to conducting interviews.

STEP 1. IDENTIFY NEEDS

Before any action is taken, the practice must determine its specific needs regarding a potential new employee. This step is especially important if the position is new and not simply a replacement for a departing member of the practice. Often, this determination is made through the use of a quality improvement process, which may help to determine how the position might change or whether the position continues to be necessary.

At the same time the job needs are being identified, the practice should be clear as to who will be responsible for overseeing the steps of the hiring process and who will conduct each step. Recruiting is a multistep process, and accountability for each step needs to be defined to ensure that no missteps or misunderstandings occur.

STEP 2. DEVELOP A POSITION DESCRIPTION

The position or job description is an essential document, for the hiring process and beyond, that articulates the responsibilities and requirements of the job and identifies tasks and accountabilities. In addition to recruiting a new member of the practice, the job description may serve as key evidence in any defense against discrimination claims in hiring should they arise.

Job descriptions should focus on the requirements of the job and the skills and education needed to fulfill the position's duties. Importantly, it should leave as little of the decision making to discretion as possible, as this could introduce bias. Therefore, the job description should be carefully worded to reduce the possibility of misunderstanding among all parties involved in hiring for the position.

The position description should contain information about the essential functions of the job, the purpose of the job, minimum requirements, and preferred requirements. Distinguishing between minimum and preferred requirements is important to assure applicants that only those individuals with the minimum requirements will be considered for the job. Targeted, specific language contained in the job description also improves search engine optimization when attracting candidates.

Beyond the hiring process for a candidate, the job description can be a valuable tool in career planning and training. Some practice employees may aspire to other jobs in the practice, and the job description for those positions helps the practice manager or human resources staff member guide the teammate in understanding the training and experience needed to achieve his or her goals. It is a blueprint for building one's career.

STEP 3. DEVELOP A RECRUITING PLAN

Once the job description has been created or updated, a recruiting plan for the position needs to be developed, which includes the following:

◆ Where will the job be posted to attract candidates? Recruiters have many options: Internet job boards, advertisements through professional societies, ads in local and national publications, word of mouth, and direct contact with training programs are a few. Asking current employees to refer qualified candidates is also an attractive option.

◆ How long will the posting appear? Although no specific standard is recommended for the optimal duration of a posting, it should be long enough to receive an adequate number of qualified candidates. In many cases, the position is posted until filled.

◆ How will resumes and applications be managed? In medical practices, this is an important consideration. Depending on the size and complexity of the practice, the practice manager or members of the practice dedicated to human resources management may be the primary people responsible for recruiting. In other cases, multiple individuals (e.g., a committee) may be involved if many stakeholders have a vested interest in the recruiting process. Hiring a new practice manager or administrator might be an activity for which a committee should be formed. In the case of hiring clinical staff, the physicians may wish to be involved, especially when, as noted earlier, the person being hired will work directly with them.

In some cases, the practice may use an outside recruiting agency if the internal capabilities of the practice are limited in the human resources area.

STEP 4. IMPLEMENT THE RECRUITING PLAN

During this step, the practice posts the position opening on job boards, career sites, and organizational job boards selected for appropriateness and reach to desired candidates. For example, the American College of Healthcare Executives and the Medical Group Management Association host extensive online job boards that are visited frequently by members of these organizations and are an excellent target audience for several practice positions. In some cases, newspapers and professional journals may be appropriate places for advertising the open position.

STEP 5. RECEIVE AND REVIEW APPLICATIONS

During this step, candidate applications should be compared against the criteria established in the job description. A spreadsheet or another tool that allows the recruiter to list the applicant's name followed by the job criteria he or she meets—or fails to meet—can be helpful in narrowing down the choices to the most qualified candidates for further review.

STEP 6. CONDUCT INTERVIEWS

The interview process may be divided into two phases. The first phase typically involves a telephone or Internet-based voice (e.g., Skype) interview with candidates who appear to meet the criteria established for the position. This phase is useful when several candidates meet the minimum qualifications or when some of the candidates would have to travel a long distance for a face-to-face interview. After this initial round of interviews is completed, face-to-face interviews with the top candidates are conducted.

Interviewing is an important skill set that should be developed by the members of the practice engaged in hiring. The sophistication of the interview is largely determined by the background and experience of the interviewer and the amount of recruiting the organization has performed (the main reason some organizations use recruiters).

Interviews can be undertaken by the recruiter along a spectrum of difficulty. Some interview approaches are considered light on substance or easy for the interviewee to perform well in, called softball interviews. On the surface, this tactic might sound appealing, but it is not recommended. The number one reason new members fail at a job is that they prove to be a poor fit with the organization. A rigorous but respectful and fair interview process helps to ensure a good fit. Few people set out to do a bad job in a new position; to help them succeed, the recruiter should articulate during the interview what is expected in the role and how the candidate's qualifications match up to these expectations.

A rigorous interview process does not involve treating candidates rudely or disrespectfully. The interview is likely the first opportunity the practice has to demonstrate to prospective employees or medical staff how it treats its employees, and it reflects on you as a manager.

Recruiting is a high-stakes undertaking for the practice to ensure that the "right" person is hired. One suggestion for gaining insight on how interviewees will fit with the practice is to watch how candidates interact with others. Are they courteous to everyone? Do they say hello to the receptionist and the housekeeping staff or any other practice members they meet? Do they smile? These are clues to the emotional intelligence (EQ) of the applicant. (EQ is discussed in more detail later in the chapter.) Applicants are likely on their best behavior, so negative signs about their interactions with other people may be an important indicator of future performance with patients and other employees.

Possible Candidate Interview Questions

A key aspect of effective interviewing is to have a prescribed process in place that is applied consistently so all candidates are posed questions that are similar in scope and specifics. Prescribed interviewing allows for a fair evaluation of candidates.

Interview questions vary significantly depending on the nature of the position and the skills required, but some recommended general questions to ask are as follows:

◆ Tell me about yourself.

◆ What are some of your personal and professional achievements?

◆ What are the critical factors for a satisfying practice for you?

◆ What factors will have the largest impact on your decision as to whether to join us?

The following additional questions can elicit insight on a candidate's strengths, weaknesses, and leadership abilities:

◆ Tell me about your interpersonal style.

◆ How do you get along with others?

◆ Do you like working as part of a team?

◆ How do you manage conflict?

◆ Tell me about a time you had to deal with a difficult situation with a colleague, someone you reported to, and someone who reported to you.

◆ What type of people do you have trouble working with?

◆ What type of patients do you have trouble dealing with? (This question is often specified on the basis of specialty.)

◆ How do you respond when you have problems with someone?

◆ What have you heard about our practice or organization that you have questions about or don't like?

◆ What interests you most about our practice/organization?

◆ Where do you see yourself in five to ten years?

◆   Why should I hire you?

◆   What kinds of situations or occurrences make you angry?

◆   How well do you work under pressure?

◆   Do you consider yourself a flexible person?

◆   What motivates you?

Questions You Should Never Ask

Personal questions that could form a basis for discrimination, such as questions about race, ethnicity, age, gender, sexual orientation, or marital status, should never be asked. Even questions about how the person will get to work can be interpreted as discriminatory and may lead to legal action if that person is not hired. The practice has a right to require staff to arrive on time for their scheduled shift, but how they get there is not the practice's concern. The best—and only—questions to ask are those that relate to the job and to the person's ability to perform the job functions.

Questions the Applicant Might Ask

Asking the applicant if she or he has any questions is an accepted and appropriate aspect of the interviewing process. Following are some common questions that may be asked by the applicant:

◆   What is the scope of the practice?

◆   What qualifications are you looking for in a candidate?

◆   Tell me about a typical workday or workweek.

◆   Why is the practice recruiting?

◆   What are the plans for the practice?

◆   Can you tell me more about the practice's community involvement?

◆   What hospital(s) does the practice use?

◆   Can I meet other members of my department?

◆   Does the practice plan to offer any new services in the near future?

STEP 7. DECIDE WHICH APPLICANT TO HIRE, AND MAKE THE JOB OFFER

The decision to hire an applicant may be made in a number of ways. In some organizations, the hiring manager or practice leader meets with practice members with whom the candidates will be working to hear their impressions of the candidates. Depending on the nature of the job and the size of the practice, physicians and other staff may also be involved. It is always a good idea to involve as many people as possible who will be in contact with the new hire. This is especially true of the smaller practice, since everyone will likely work in closer proximity to one another.

Making the job offer usually begins by contacting the successful applicant by telephone and offering him or her the job. Any verbal offers must be followed up with an offer letter that specifies the salary and benefits being offered, as well as other important details, such as the employment start date. The letter should also state that the offer is subject to the findings of a prehire health screening and background check (see step 8) and should request acknowledgment of the offer with the candidate's signature indicating formal acceptance of the job.

STEP 8. CONDUCT PREHIRE HEALTH SCREENING AND BACKGROUND CHECK

Medical practices engage in some of the most important human interactions people experience in life, and this role underscores the need for practices to employ dependable, honest teammates. One recommended hiring practice is to conduct a prehire health screening for drug use and a criminal background check for all new employees. Using a professional agency for screenings is advisable for smaller practices because of the special and sensitive nature of this task; the practice must avoid mistakes that could cause legal repercussions or the loss of a great employee.

STEP 9. WELCOME AND ONBOARD THE NEW EMPLOYEE

The practice should develop a thorough onboarding process for all new members. It should include activities as mundane as the location of their workspace, restrooms, and break facilities to those as specific as a detailed review and training regarding the specific job. See exhibit 8.2 for a sample onboarding checklist.

TALENT MANAGEMENT

Managing the human resources of the medical practice requires attention to a number of important elements, including performance management, compensation and benefits, and development of each person's potential.

EXHIBIT 8.2
Example Onboarding Checklist

What Needs to Be Done?	Who Will Do This Onboarding Work?	When Does It Need to Be Completed?	Status	Notes
Complete installation and acquisition for computer and software, new employee e-mail, etc.	Designate a team member			*Determine if there are any special requirements*
Select a location in building				*Indicate solution*
Supplies for office	Designate a team member	Before the employee begins		
Complete practice orientation	Team members		Give orientation checklist	
Talk with new employee's leader about her expectations of the role			Schedule	
Assign a team "buddy"	Designate team members	Immediately on arrival		*Who will be the go-to person to answer questions and check on how things are going?*
Introduce to all team members and provide opportunity to become familiar with current work	Designate team members	By the end of the first 2 weeks		
Meet other leaders	Department buddy/ leadership	Within the first 30–60 days		
Use Departmental Orientation Checklist to provide information on specific issues and topics	All listed on the attached orientation document	Ongoing	Bring to new hire's attention on the first day and give them a copy; a lot of whom to go to for what items and resources they may need	
First 30 Days Schedule—includes orientation, lunches, training, regular meetings, first 30-day check-in				
View facilitator's guide	New employee should review			

Sources: Fallon and McConnel (2013); Fried and Fottler (2011).

PERFORMANCE MANAGEMENT

Each practice makes its own determination of what factors are most important in setting goals, measuring performance, and assessing and reviewing employees. Although many organizations consider performance management to be a perfunctory activity to be conducted once a year, high-performing practices recognize the importance of these functions. Performance, or talent, management activities should be ongoing throughout the year and form the basis for many of the interactions that employees, managers, and supervisors have with each other.

Some important components of the talent management process include the following:

◆   *Goal setting.* Goals should be framed in terms of the SMART method: specific, measurable, achievable, realistic, and timely. The manager and the employee should work together to construct meaningful SMART goals and base performance measurement on them. Exhibit 8.3 shares a defining question to help clarify each element of the SMART goal design.

◆   *Performance measurement.* Measurement should be based on predetermined indicators of success in achieving the goals established for the employee. Measurement should be credible and easy to observe or document, and the manager and employee should be in agreement that they are reasonable expectations for the job. The employee should be able to check his or her

EXHIBIT 8.3
SMART Goals

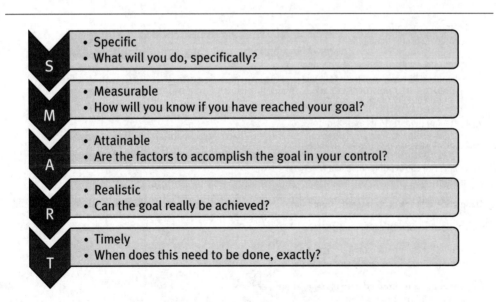

- Specific
- What will you do, specifically?

- Measurable
- How will you know if you have reached your goal?

- Attainable
- Are the factors to accomplish the goal in your control?

- Realistic
- Can the goal really be achieved?

- Timely
- When does this need to be done, exactly?

Source: Doran (1981).

progress at any time so that when a formal review is undertaken, no or few surprises are encountered.

◆ *Assessment and review.* Many processes are available for conducting performance reviews, either manually or electronically. Managers typically think of performance assessments in terms of nonprovider employees, and certainly tools for reviewing the performance of providers are less common, but conducting provider assessments is an essential element of effective practice management. Exhibit 8.4 is an example of a provider assessment tool.

Whether for a nonprovider or a provider, assessments and reviews should be based on the practice's values, the important competencies required for the job, and achievement of the goals established by the employee and his or her manager. Reviews are an opportunity for staff development; ideally, assessment and review should not be tied to compensation adjustments. This is not the common approach, but in the experience of the author, it is a recommended strategy, as it increases employee satisfaction, enhances employee

EXHIBIT 8.4
Provider
Assessment Tool

	Physician Assessment				
	Always	Often	Sometimes	Occasionally	Never
1. I communicate effectively with patients.					
2. I communicate effectively with patients' families.					
3. I communicate effectively with other healthcare professionals.					
4. Within the range of services I provide, I perform technical procedures skillfully.					
5. I maintain quality medical records.					
6. I select diagnostic tests appropriately.					
7. I critically assess diagnostic information.					
8. I make the correct diagnosis in a timely fashion.					
9. In general, I select appropriate treatments.					
10. I handle transfer of care appropriately.					
11. I provide a clear understanding about who is responsible for continuing care of the patient.					
12. I communicate information to patients about rationale for treatment.					
13. I recognize psychosocial aspects of illness.					

Physician Assessment					
	Always	**Often**	**Sometimes**	**Occasionally**	**Never**
14. I maintain confidentiality of patients and their families.					
15. I coordinate care effectively for patients with other healthcare professionals.					
16. I coordinate the management of care for patients with complex problems.					
17. I respect the rights of patients.					
18. I collaborate with medical colleagues.					
19. I am involved with professional development.					
20. I accept responsibility for my professional actions.					
21. I manage healthcare resources efficiently.					
22. I manage stress effectively.					
23. I participate in a system of call to provide care for my patients when unavailable.					
24. I recognize my own limitations.					
25. I handle requests for consultation in a timely manner.					
26. I advise referring physicians if referral request is outside of scope of my practice.					
27. I assume appropriate responsibility for patients.					
28. I provide timely information to referring physicians about mutual patients.					
29. I critically evaluate the medical literature to optimize clinical decision making.					
30. I facilitate the learning of medical colleagues and coworkers.					
31. I contribute to the development of quality improvement programs and practice guidelines.					
32. I participate effectively as a member of the healthcare team.					
33. I exhibit professional and ethical behavior toward my physician colleagues.					
34. I show compassion for patients and their families.					

EXHIBIT 8.4
Provider
Assessment Tool
(continued)

development, and increases employee aspiration attainment. Everyone wants to feel he or she is appreciated, cared about, and encouraged to grow.

COMPENSATION AND BENEFITS

The way physicians are compensated in practices is often different than for other employees of the practice. Therefore, for purposes of this discussion, we consider physician compensation separately in chapter 7. Here, we focus on the compensation of the other members of the practice.

Exempt and Nonexempt Employees

Nonprovider employees are usually divided into two categories—exempt and nonexempt—and are governed by the Fair Labor Standards Act (FLSA). With few exceptions, to be exempt, an employee must meet the following guidelines:

◆ Be paid at least $23,600 per year ($455 per week).

◆ Be paid on a salary basis.

◆ Perform exempt job duties.

These requirements are set by the US Department of Labor (2016) and outlined in the FLSA regulations. Most employees must meet all three of the above-listed tests to be exempt.

PROFESSIONAL DEVELOPMENT

Each person working in the medical practice should have an individual development and aspirational plan. The steps for establishing this plan are as follows:

1. Determine goals and the reason for development.

2. Identify what skill area the person would like to learn or improve on.

3. Pinpoint what actions the person needs to take to address this need.

4. Define the ways in which the practice can help the person make advances on the plan.

Frequent follow-up meetings should be held to check in on progress and a tracking mechanism developed to reflect what has been learned and achieved.

EMPLOYMENT POLICIES AND PROCEDURES

Every physician practice must have in place carefully crafted and maintained policies and procedures regarding employment. Employment policy establishes the standards for performance and conduct for all employees and provides employees with information about the terms of their employment. Common areas addressed in a set of employee policies include the following:

- A welcome for new employees

- Background information on the practice

- Statements regarding antidiscrimination

- Business ethics and conduct

- The employment process

- Disciplinary action and processes

- Any prohibitions on outside work or hiring of relatives

- Privacy and security

- Terms of employment

- Performance evaluations

- Payroll functions

- Working conditions and working hours, which may include permissible conditions of computer usage or e-mail usage

- Corporate compliance

- Patient care

- Occupational Safety and Health Administration issues

- Emergency procedures

Employee benefit programs, as part of an employee's compensation, are another area to be formalized and documented. These programs vary greatly among practices, but they typically include some or all of the following:

- Paid time off
- Bereavement leave

◆ Jury duty

◆ Health insurance

◆ Disability insurance

◆ Dental insurance

◆ Retirement benefits

◆ Military leave

Employment policy should be updated on a regular basis and refresher sessions given to the practice members to avoid misunderstandings and to ensure that employees have the opportunity to receive the benefits they are entitled to. The practice leader should request acknowledgment by all staff members, with their signature indicating that they have read and understand the policies and procedures and will abide by them.

ORGANIZATION DEVELOPMENT

According to Warren Bennis (1969), organization development is concerned with the effectiveness of the organization in carrying out its mission. It focuses on strategies and interventions intended to influence the mission, beliefs, values, and behaviors that affect the performance of the practice. In many ways, the modern medical practice should rethink the way it accomplishes its work and how it structures and manages its relationships with other entities. As healthcare becomes more of a collaborative effort and more team based, building good relationships becomes increasingly important.

Communication is a cornerstone of high-quality care and of employee development and interaction. It is also essential to organization development. Effective communication leads to understanding and trust, which can result in improved compliance, outcomes, and satisfaction for patients and employees. The results of effective communication are illustrated in exhibit 8.5.

EMPLOYEE DEVELOPMENT

We cannot develop our organizations if we do not develop our employees. Early in this chapter, we discussed a performance management strategy that focuses on fairness and encouraging employees to nurture their own aspirations. This is a major part of employee development. Fair compensation is also an important part of this development.

Other important aspects of employee development include coaching and mentoring. These two terms are often used interchangeably, although coaching often involves a supervisor–employee relationship in which one-on-one discussions take place to enhance

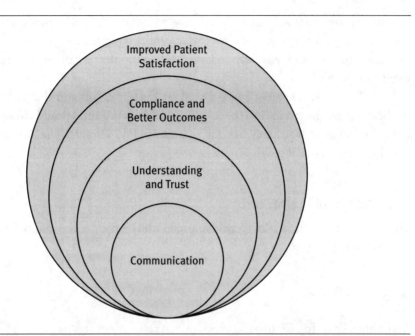

Exhibit 8.5
Communication Is
the Cornerstone of
Good Care

the performance of the individual or resolve problems, while mentors are often not in direct contact with the employee on a day-to-day basis. Mentorships are mutual and entered into voluntarily, they may be more aspirational in nature than coaching relationships are, and they involve one-on-one discussions about the mentee's future and steps to take toward achieving personal goals (Reitman and Benatti 2014). A practice manager can serve as both coach and mentor.

CHANGE MANAGEMENT

US society has seen more change in the past 100 years than the rest of human history. One of the great challenges in medical practices today is dealing with the rapid rate of change (Kurzweil 2001). As discussed in chapter 1, the medical practice is faced with a perfect storm of change. However, people are not well equipped to deal with change; in fact, humans' neurobiological makeup is designed to resist change.

Change involves the shifting of paradigms and requires people to adjust their mind-set about how they think things should be. A paradigm is a powerful force that resists change and anchors people to the status quo, dictating how they make decisions.

Some of the great developments of the twentieth and twenty-first centuries include the automobile, Swiss watches, personal computers, the Internet, smartphones, the advent of online education, and the evolution of medical practice. All these developments and many others required paradigm shifts to be successful, and in almost every situation, prominent naysayers did not believe in the paradigm shift. The first cars were met with bemusement and ridicule. The Swiss watch industry, itself calling for an adjustment to portable time keeping, virtually collapsed following the paradigm shift to quartz movement timepieces.

Change management is a key skill set for leadership and the management of the medical practice now and into the future. To address **organizational change**, we consider the use of an effective change model such as the PAST model, illustrated in exhibit 8.6 and discussed in detail next.

Organizational change
A process by which the organization evolves to help it adapt to a new set of environmental and competitive factors.

THE PAST CHANGE MODEL

The components of the PAST change model (developed by the author) are prepare, act, sustain, and transform.

Prepare

Make the Case for Change

Members of the practice must be educated about the factors surrounding the need to change and come to understand why change is necessary. Members of the practice who

EXHIBIT 8.6
The PAST Change
Model

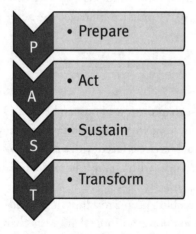

P • Prepare
A • Act
S • Sustain
T • Transform

Prepare the case for change
• The emotions of change
• Assess gaps in readiness

Act
• Assess current state
• Design and develop
• Implement and measure

Sustain
• Reinforce change
• PDSA cycle
• New standard work

Sustain
• Reinforce change
• PDSA cycle
• New standard work

Transform
• Define standards, not rules
• Set expectations
• Feedback and accountability

do not believe change is required will be resistant, and any efforts to change will likely be unsuccessful. Stated another way, this understanding creates the foundation for meaningful and effective change management.

Anticipate the Emotions of Change

Change is an emotional process. Negative emotions often arise from the perception that change is dangerous. Staff often wonder whether they will be needed in the future or if they will be able to learn the new procedures or processes. The easy position to take is, "I am comfortable with the way things are."

The practice manager needs to recognize that these emotions are natural. Furthermore, they will evolve during the change process, progressing through stages that are similar to the stages of dealing with loss popularized by Elisabeth Kubler-Ross (1969) in her seminal work, *On Death and Dying*:

1. *Shock and denial.* Change is sometimes difficult to acknowledge.

2. *Anger and blame.* Once people come to believe change must happen or is already happening, they tend to express anger about it. This anger needs to be expressed and acknowledged so that it can be processed and allowed to dissipate.

3. *Bargaining.* Individuals facing change next turn to bargaining by offering a trade-off to avoid the change, which by now is recognized as inevitable. The trade-off typically takes the form of a promise to behave differently if the change isn't implemented.

4. *Depression.* Like death, change can feel bleak. Practice members should be encouraged to support each other through the sadness and seeming hopelessness of change.

5. *Acceptance.* Eventually, people experiencing change begin to accept it as reality. Those who face it proactively and support others throughout the process tend to adapt in due time, grow comfortable with it, and see its positive attributes.

Not everyone moves through each stage in a sequential fashion; some may regress and pass through stages more than once. How long does this process take? The answer depends on how significant the impact of the change is on the individual, how well he or she prepared for change, and how effectively the leadership guides him or her through the change process. One way to help people through the emotions of change is to have them answer questions about the change. This idea is rooted in the neuroscience of change: In an emotional state, people do not process information; by asking themselves questions, they reengage their forebrain (thinking brain), which allows rational thought to occur about the change. The practice manager should also be available to answer questions and to reassure staff, as appropriate, about the change. In the absence of knowledge, people tell themselves stories about a change, and those stories are usually more dire than the actual change.

Individual differences in how people process change need to be considered in this process. Managers who have heightened awareness of individual practice members' emotions engage them differently depending on how they are dealing with change. Open dialogue helps the practice members through the emotions of change as well. Conversations around how staff are feeling can bring issues to light that can then be addressed.

Assess Gaps in Readiness

In managing change, consider the readiness for change. Readiness can be evaluated in formal as well as informal ways.

Virtually all the formal assessment tools assess readiness at the leadership, organizational, personal, and technological levels. These tools are available from commercial vendors and consultants. Informal assessments are also useful in change management. In some cases, readiness can be determined simply by asking people the following questions (HRSA 2016):

◆ How do you feel about this change?

◆ What are your fears and concerns?

◆ What information do you need to feel comfortable with the change?

Act

Assess the Current State

Assessing the current state of the process to be changed or of the organization as a whole is important in change management and should be the first step in the action phase of managing change. One approach to this assessment is to flow-chart current activities to validate the proposed change in consideration of enhancing patient flow, productivity, stakeholder satisfaction, or other needed areas of improvement.

Design and Develop

What will this change look like once it is implemented? This is one of the key questions to consider in the design and development phase of change. A clear pathway from the current state to the new state needs to be established, with signposts to mark progress and assignments of responsibility shown along the way. Before changes are implemented, it is important to consider how the practice will determine if the change is successful. Predetermined measures are essential. So often we implement a change and then retrospectively evaluate success without clear standards for measuring that success. Because we all want to be successful, it is natural that we tend to look for measures that may have little impact on the success of the practice as a way of measuring the success of the change. Practice managers need to exercise rigor when evaluating change because not all change will produce the desired results.

Implement and Measure

At this stage of change management, implementation begins with sharing the vision for the change. Then, the following steps are taken:

◆ Define roles. Who will do what? How will their role or job change?

◆ What are the goals of the change, in the short and longer term? This needs to be shared clearly and repeatedly.

◆ Determine milestones for the progress of the change.

◆ Share progress with all concerned.

◆ Celebrate successes and milestones.

◆ Evaluate and adjust as needed. Things do not always work as planned, so accept suggestions and be open to additional ideas.

Sustain

Implement the Plan-Do-Study-Act Cycle

A mechanism for continuous process improvement must be in place to continue positive changes into the future. The Plan-Do-Study-Act (PDSA) cycle is an effective tool to help sustain and continue improvement. Rarely does a change produce all the desired results when first implemented; therefore, continuous improvement is a desirable aspect of change management.

The PDSA cycle is easy to understand and apply to process improvement efforts. Exhibit 8.7 shows a graphical representation of PDSA, and its components are delineated in exhibit 8.8.

Reinforce Change by Adopting New Standard Work Processes

Among the most difficult aspects of undertaking a change process is sustaining that change. Returning to the old methods or procedures over time is not unusual and, in fact, can occur quickly. To prevent reversion, change must be reinforced through the development of new standard work. New standard work documents the new way of doing things and comes with the expectation that everyone uses the new process. The manager needs to verify that

EXHIBIT 8.7
The PDSA Cycle

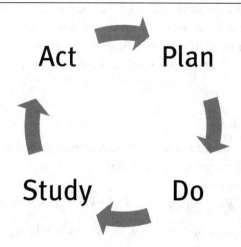

the new standard work process is consistently used; otherwise, he or she will have no way to determine with certainty whether the change works as intended.

Consider this simple example. I want to stop eating cookies, and I adopt a new standard work to not purchase them and bring them home, because no matter how much willpower I have, if those cookies are easily available, I will eventually succumb to the temptation and eat them. In the same way, a new standard work replaces the old standard, making reversion to the old way of doing things difficult and increasing the likelihood that the change will be successful.

Additional tools, ideas, and suggested methods for improvement are available from the Institute for Healthcare Improvement (2017) and the Deming Institute (2017).

Transform

Changes in practice management are intended to be transformative, meaning they significantly affect the practice. To hardwire transformative change, the following guidelines should be followed:

- *Define standards, not rules.* Everyone involved needs to be clear about the expected outcomes so the change is not just a rote process.

- *Set expectations.* Simply stated, you get what you ask for. A practice manager should never assume people know what they are expected to do; he or she must let them know.

- *Establish feedback and accountability mechanisms.* Accountability cannot occur without feedback. Absent feedback, a practice cannot improve or achieve a high level of performance.

Step 1. Plan

Assemble a team that has knowledge of the problem or opportunity for improvement.
- Identify roles and responsibilities.
- Establish timelines.
- Develop a meeting schedule.

Develop an aim statement.
- Try to answer these three fundamental questions:
  - What are we trying to accomplish?
  - How will we measure improvement?
  - What change will result in improvement?

Describe the current process.
- What is the practice doing now?
- What are the major steps in the process?
- Who is involved?
- What do they do?
- What is done well?
- What could be done better?

Possible tools to consider in this step:
- Check sheets
- Control charts
- Strengths, weaknesses, opportunity, and threats (SWOT) analysis
- Run charts
- Fishbone diagrams
- Scatterplots
- Nodes of influence analysis
- Affinity diagrams
- Brainstorming
- Flow diagrams
- Focus groups and focused conversations
- Prioritization matrix

Describe the problem.
Using the aim statement, indicate what the practice wants to accomplish. Use data that are available. For example, if your objective is improving patient satisfaction, you might look for data in the patient engagement survey about items such as waiting time.

Write a problem statement.
Write a problem statement to summarize the consensus of the problem. For example, "Waiting times are too long because there are not enough doctors in the office at one time." Do not suggest a solution at this step.

EXHIBIT 8.8
Detailed Steps in
the PDSA Cycle

(continued on next page)

Exhibit 8.8
Detailed Steps in
the PDSA Cycle
(continued)

Identify causes and alternatives.
• Consider the cause
• Work to identify causes of the problem using tools such as
  – Process control charts
  – Fishbone diagrams
  – Flowcharts
  Examine the practice process and ask questions about the efficiency, cost, and variation in how the process is done. The PDSA team can then consider alternatives that they believe will address the objective. This can often be done by filling in the blanks of the simple statement, "If we do _____, then _____ will happen."
• Select an option to try from the alternatives identified.
Develop an action plan that outlines all resources that are needed, including people, materials, and the time involved.

Step 2. Do
Implement the selected alternative. It is important to collect data to determine if the improvement is successful. For example, if waiting time was selected as the problem, then measuring waiting time after the intervention is implemented would provide evidence of improvement.

Step 3. Study
Did the team's actions result in an improvement? Was the improvement worth the cost? Consider, for example, if waiting times only improved a small amount, it might not be perceived as an improvement by the patients and, therefore, not worth the cost of implementing the change. Alternatively, it may be worthwhile to consider other actions that might have a larger impact on waiting times.

Ask more questions: Are there any trends, any new insights or findings that the PDSA cycle uncovered? Were there unintended consequences of the action that were unexpected and potentially created additional problems?

Use process improvement tools to study your results. This could include flowcharts, process control charts, Pareto charts, and many others.

Step 4. Act
It is important to reflect on the actions taken and see if additional improvement can be made by additional PDSA cycles. The new process needs to be standardized and incorporated into daily practice.

Finally, it is always important to celebrate improvements and share lessons learned. This includes the following:
• Communicate to all stakeholders what is being done
• Sustain your accomplishments through new standard work
• Plan for additional improvements

THE INFLUENCER MODEL FOR CHANGE

Another effective model for addressing change in a medical practice is the influencer model, developed by VitalSmarts (2016) and described in the book *Influencer: The Power to Change Anything* (Patterson et al. 2008). As shown in exhibit 8.9, the influencer model focuses on what motivates people to change, or wish to change, and their ability to make required changes. The ability to change involves the availability of necessary resources, the permission to act, and the knowledge to act.

Further, the influencer model suggests that change occurs at three levels: structural, social, and personal. Finally, the model is underpinned by the fundamental concept of vital behaviors that are demanded of all members of the practice to ensure accountability. Being accountable is a necessary element of professionalism in the medical practice; those who lack it must change to make professionalism a reality.

CONFLICT MANAGEMENT

The modern medical practice is home to an increasingly diverse set of interests among its many stakeholders. This diversity inevitably produces conflicts. To address issues of discord, conflict management has become an important skill set for practice managers. Among the most useful tools for managing conflict is the Thomas-Kilmann Conflict Mode Instrument (TKI). As with many organization development tools, the TKI allows the individual and the group to self-assess their preferred conflict resolution style and, importantly, to understand the importance of using the five different styles in different situations (Kilmann Diagnostics 2016):

- Competing
- Compromising
- Collaborating
- Accommodating
- Avoiding

Self-assessment leading to self-awareness is critical to conflict management. Leaders must create awareness of their tendencies, preferences, and behaviors. A number of commercial products are available that measure aspects of temperament, personality, and behaviors. They include the following:

- The Management by Strengths Survey (Management by Strengths 2016)
- DiSC (DiscProfile 2016)
- The Predictive Index (PI 2017)

EXHIBIT 8.9
Influencer Model for Change

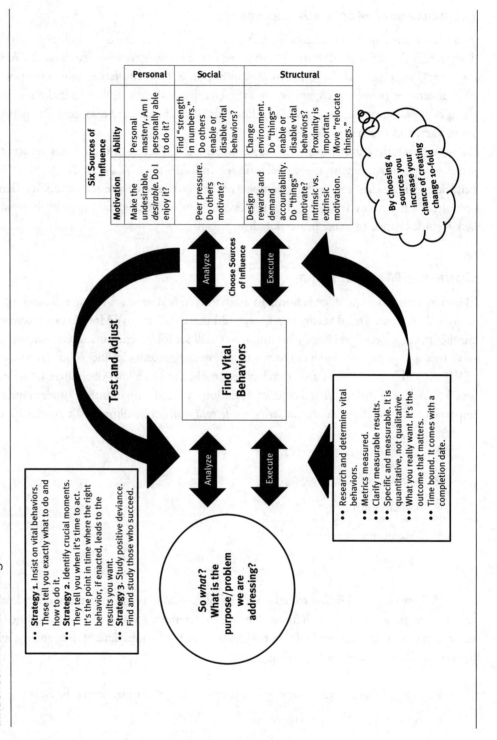

A complementary concept to awareness is emotional intelligence (EQ). It was popularized by Daniel Goleman (1995) in his seminal work, *Emotional Intelligence: Why It Can Matter More Than IQ*. Goleman discusses four critical attributes of emotional intelligence:

◆ *Self-awareness*, which includes developing emotional self-awareness and self-confidence and having an accurate assessment of oneself and how one responds to others

◆ *Social awareness*, which involves having organizational awareness, being service oriented, and having empathy for others

◆ *Self-management*, which revolves around self-control, being trustworthy, being conscientious, being adaptable, being achievement-oriented, being driven to succeed, and having initiative

◆ *Relationship management*, which is composed of a group of traits relating to being influential, being an inspirational leader, developing others, having influence with others, building lasting bonds with stakeholders, and having an orientation toward teamwork and collaboration

Underestimating the importance of EQ is difficult when one considers its emerging role in evaluating and compensating practices to assess the quality of their care. The Medicare Access and CHIP Reauthorization Act and other pay-for-performance programs place a high premium on EQ. For example, the patient satisfaction metric, which is tracked by virtually all healthcare organizations, relies heavily on the EQ of physicians and other practice members to effectively deal with patients and their families.

DIVERSITY AND INCLUSION

US society has become increasingly diverse, a trend that will continue in the coming years. Issues of diversity and lack of inclusion have been shown to limit the ability of diverse populations to access and receive appropriate medical care (Betancourt et al. 2003). Some of the many dimensions of diversity are included in the box titled "Dimensions of Diversity."

Dimensions of Diversity

Age	Income and insurance status
Beliefs about healthcare	Parental status
Disabilities	Prior experience with the healthcare system
Education	Race
Ethnicity	Religious beliefs
Gender and gender identity	Sexual orientation
Geography	Work background
Health literacy	

At the heart of diversity and inclusion is the ability to effectively communicate with patients and their families. Communication is an essential element in so many aspects of human interaction, particularly in the healthcare delivery environment. Communication leads to understanding, which leads to trust, which then increases the likelihood that patients will be activated and adhere to the instructions of the provider. Enhanced communication results in improved patient satisfaction, which, as noted previously, is becoming increasingly important in the new outcomes-based reimbursement system.

Everyone in the medical practice must be aware of and actively defend against conscious and unconscious bias. Bias is a fact of the human condition; to pretend that one has no bias or to allow another's ignorance and bias go unchallenged is unacceptable in the modern medical practice. Practice managers should engage the members of the practice in education related to diversity and addressing bias. Policies should clearly state the practice's intention to promote diversity and inclusion.

REWARD AND RECOGNITION

An essential aspect of practice management is the reward and recognition of practice members. Although economic rewards are important, they are not the only way to demonstrate appreciation. Sometimes a simple "thank you" or another considerate gesture is an ideal acknowledgment.

The practice should design reward and recognition strategies that increase employee satisfaction and engagement, leading to improved performance. Many successful practices recognize birthdays and major events in the lives of practice members while respecting their privacy. Celebrating successes such as reaching important milestones or completing a difficult set of tasks can build morale for the team.

One strategy takes acknowledgment a step further by asking employees how *they* wish to be recognized. Some people do not enjoy or feel comfortable with public recognition; they prefer receiving accolades in a private setting. We all have preferences about what makes us feel special and appreciated, and the wise practice manager finds out what those preferences are for his or her staff (Fried and Fottler 2015; MGMA 2015).

THE FUTURE WORKFORCE

According to a Pew Research Center study, two thirds of Americans believe that in the next 50 years, robots will be performing much of the work humans do now (Smith 2016). A key implication of this prediction is that the future medical practice workforce should learn to excel at those activities that robots and computers cannot. Fundamental among these activities is human interaction.

Shifting demographic patterns and technological change toward economic globalization will have a significant impact on the future workforce. A study released by the RAND Corporation (2004) found four significant implications related to these trends:

Employees will work in more decentralized, specialized firms, and employer-employee relationships will become less standardized and more individualized.

Slower labor force growth will encourage employers to adopt approaches to facilitate greater labor force participation among women, the elderly, and people with disabilities.

Greater emphasis will be placed on retraining and lifelong learning as the U.S. workforce tries to stay competitive in the global marketplace and respond to technological changes.

Future productivity growth will support rising wages and may affect the wage distribution; the tie between employment, and access to fringe benefits will be weakened.

All these implications will have an impact on the future of the medical practice. In terms of telemedicine, telehealth, and other trends toward electronic intermediaries between the practice and the patient, many employees can now work from home performing billing and other office work. It is only a matter of time before clinicians routinely conduct remote patient care. With the overall US workforce aging (e.g., the average age of urologists in the United States is 50), the healthcare delivery system is likely headed toward shortages in several medical specialties as well as other highly trained workforce members in the medical field.

BURNOUT

According to a recent study published in the *Journal of the American Medical Association*, 45.8 percent of physicians report at least one symptom of burnout, and the range of burnout incidence among medical specialties is significant, with emergency management positions reporting the highest level of burnout (Shanafelt et al. 2012). Thus, healthcare worker burnout is becoming a major issue facing every medical practice (Shin, Gandhi, and Herzig 2016).

Just one reason among many for burnout is the dramatic change taking place in medical practices and for physicians. From the Affordable Care Act reforms to new payment mechanisms to increasingly sophisticated and complex electronic records systems to pressures to do more work (see more patients, process more claims, and so on) with fewer resources to the increasing scrutiny on medical care delivery by the media and regulators, medical practice is a shifting landscape, and some practitioners are clearly feeling exhausted.

PROVIDER HEALTH

The health of medical practice members should be of great concern to practice managers and leaders. Without a healthy workforce, the practice cannot provide the best possible care to its patients or operate at an optimal level.

Attention to members' well-being actually begins with the hiring process, which is the first step in the employment management function, and continues with the establishment of effective lines of communication and the monitoring of practice activities to increase the likelihood that any health issues can be identified early.

One step toward helping providers and others in the practice avoid burnout is to make available the abbreviated Maslach Burnout Inventory (Maslach, Jackson, and Leiter 1996; Maslach and Goldberg 1998). This straightforward self-administered assessment is illustrated in exhibit 8.10.

The person taking the self-assessment simply checks the appropriate column in response to each question. The columns are totaled, and the proper weighting is applied. The interpretation of the assessment is shown in exhibit 8.11.

If the practice uses the burnout inventory, it should also consider how it will respond to those who have high burnout scores. If the practice does not intend to address these issues, it should not consider using this tool.

SIMPLE WAYS TO DECREASE BURNOUT

The practice can suggest a few simple approaches to help people deal with burnout. Uncertainty is a major source of stress, especially in these times of rapid change, so an initial recommendation might be to avoid overthinking the situation—you cannot predict the future, no matter how smart you are.

Second, suggest that the individual "own what you can own." This phrase means paying attention to one's work and the issues that are in one's control. People often worry so much about things beyond our control that we lose sight of what we can affect or influence.

How often:	Not at All	Rarely	Sometimes	Often	Very Often
Do you feel run down and drained of physical or emotional energy?					
Do you find that you are prone to negative thinking about your job?					
Do you find that you are harder and less sympathetic with people than perhaps they deserve?					
Do you find yourself getting easily irritated by small problems, or by your co-workers and team?					
Do you feel misunderstood or unappreciated by your co-workers?					
Do you feel that you have no one to talk to?					
Do you feel that you are achieving less than you should?					
Do you feel under an unpleasant level of pressure to succeed?					
Do you feel that you are not getting what you want out of your job?					
Do you feel that you are in the wrong organization or the wrong profession?					
Are you becoming frustrated with parts of your job?					
Do you feel that organizational politics or bureaucracy frustrate your ability to do a good job?					

EXHIBIT 8.10
Maslach Burnout Inventory (Abbreviated)

(continued on next page)

How often:	Not at All	Rarely	Sometimes	Often	Very Often
Do you feel that there is more work to do than you practically have the ability to do?					
Do you feel that you do not have time to do many of the things that are important to doing a good quality job?					
Do you find that you do not have time to plan as much as you would like to?					
Sub Totals: Count number of checks in each column, and multiply total by appointed number	×1	×2	×3	×4	×5
Column Totals					
Add column totals to get Total Burnout Score _____					

Source: Maslach, Jackson, and Leiter (1996).

Score	Comment
15–18	Little sign of burnout.
19–32	Little risk of burnout, unless some factors are severe.
33–49	Caution: You may be at risk of burnout, especially if several of your items were rated high.
50–59	You may be at severe risk for burnout. Do something about this soon.
60–75	You may be at very severe risk for burnout. Do something about this now!

Third, take positive action to move an aspect of life forward. This suggestion may involve creating new routines that eliminate triggers for stress; learning new stress-relieving techniques, such as mindfulness meditation; or taking a moment to relax and reflect on one's gratitude for the positive aspects of one's life.

A final bit of advice is to engage in healthful behaviors. This means getting enough sleep, eating correctly, and getting regular exercise. Studies have shown that a brisk walk can be as effective in combating mild depression as antidepressant pharmaceuticals (Mead et al. 2009).

As a medical practice leader, your most important asset is the people. Hire and manage with care, and encourage healthful behaviors to ensure an optimum workforce to take care of patients.

DISCUSSION QUESTIONS

1. List the steps in the hiring process, and explain why each is important.

2. Write a brief outline of the employee onboarding process.

3. What are some nonphysician practitioner categories often found in the medical practice?

4. What are the components of a SMART goal?

5. Often physicians are not assessed on a regular basis. Do you think regular assessments should be required for physicians? Why or why not?

6. What options does the practice manager have in addressing professional burnout?

REFERENCES

Bennis, W. 1969. *Organization Development: Its Nature, Origins and Prospects*. Reading, MA: Addison-Wesley.

Berkowitz, B. 2016. "The Patient Experience and Patient Satisfaction: Measurement of a Complex Dynamic." *OJIN: The Online Journal of Issues in Nursing* 21 (1): manuscript 1.

Betancourt, J., A. Green, J. Carrillo, and O. Anaaeh-Firempong. 2003. "Defining Cultural Competence: A Practical Framework for Addressing Racial/Ethnic Disparities in Health and Healthcare." *Public Health Reports* 118 (4): 293–302.

Deming Institute. 2017. "Management System." Accessed June 2. https://deming.org/management-system.

DiscProfile. 2016. "DiSC Overview." Accessed March 25. www.discprofile.com/what-is-disc/overview.

Doran, G. T. 1981. "There's a S.M.A.R.T. Way to Write Management's Goals and Objectives." *Management Review* 70 (11): 35–36.

Fallon, F. L., and C. McConnel. 2013. *Human Resource Management in Health Care: Principles and Practices*. New York: Jones & Bartlett Learning.

Fenton, J., A. Jerant, and K. Bertaski. 2012. "The Cost of Satisfaction: A National Study of Patient Satisfaction, Healthcare Utilization, Expenditures and Mortality." *Archives of Internal Medicine* 172 (5): 405–11.

Fried, B. J., and M. D. Fottler. 2015. *Human Resources in Healthcare: Managing for Success*, 4th ed. Chicago: Health Administration Press.

———. 2011. *Fundamentals of Human Resources in Healthcare*. Chicago: Health Administration Press.

Goleman, D. 1995. *Emotional Intelligence: Why It Can Matter More Than IQ*. New York: Bantam.

Health Resources and Services Administration (HRSA). 2016. "Readiness Assessment & Developing Project Aims." Accessed July 28. www.hrsa.gov/quality/toolbox/methodology/readinessassessment.

Institute for Healthcare Improvement. 2017. "How to Improve." Accessed May 10. www.ihi.org/resources/Pages/HowtoImprove/default.aspx.

Kaiser Family Foundation (KFF). 2016. "State Health Facts/Healthcare Employment." Menlo Park, CA: KFF.

Kane, R., M. Maciejewski, and M. Finch. 1997. "The Relationship of Patient Satisfaction with Care and Clinical Outcomes." *Medical Care* 35 (7): 714–30.

Kennedy, G., S. Tevis, and C. Kent. 2014. "Is There a Relationship Between Patient Satisfaction and Favorable Outcomes?" *Annals of Surgery* 260 (4): 592–600.

Kilmann Diagnostics. 2016. "Thomas-Kilmann Conflict Mode Instrument." Accessed March 25. www.kilmanndiagnostics.com/catalog/thomas-kilmann-conflict-mode-instrument.

Kubler-Ross, E. 1969. *On Death and Dying: What Dying Has to Teach Doctors, Nurses, Clergy and Their Own Families*. New York: Simon & Schuster.

Kurzweil, R. 2001. "The Law of Accelerating Returns." Published March 7. www.kurzweilai.net/the-law-of-accelerating-returns.

Management by Strengths. 2016. "The MBS Survey." Accessed March 25. www.strengths.com/MBS_Survey_Page.html.

Maslach, C., and J. Goldberg. 1998. "Prevention of Burnout: New Perspectives." *Journal of Applied and Preventive Psychology* 7 (1): 63–74.

Maslach, C., S. E. Jackson, and M. P. Leiter. 1996. *The Maslach Burnout Inventory*, 3rd ed. Palo Alto, CA: Consulting Psychologists Press.

Mead, G., W. Morley, P. Campbell, C. Greig, M. McMurdo, and D. Lawlor. 2009. "Exercise for Depression." London: Cochrane Collaboration.

Medical Group Management Association (MGMA). 2015. "Human Resources." In *Body of Knowledge Review Series*, 3rd ed. Englewood, CO: MGMA.

Patterson, K., J. Grenny, D. Maxfield, and R. McMillan. 2008. *Influencers: The Power to Change Anything*. New York: McGraw-Hill.

Predictive Index (PI). 2017. Home page. Accessed May 12. www.predictiveindex.com.

RAND Corporation. 2004. "The Future at Work—Trends and Implications." Santa Monica, CA: RAND.

Reitman, A., and S. R. Benatti. 2014. "Mentoring Versus Coaching: What's the Difference?" Published August 8. www.td.org/Publications/Blogs/Human-Capital-Blog/2014/08/Mentoring-Versus-Coaching-Whats-the-Difference.

Shanafelt, T., S. Boone, L. Tan, L. Dyrbye, W. Sotile, D. Satele, C. West, J. Sloan, and M. Oreskovich. 2012. "Burnout and Satisfaction with Work-Life Balance Among US Physicians Relative to the General US Population." *Journal of the American Medical Association* 172 (18): 1377–85.

Shin, A., T. Gandhi, and S. Herzig. 2016. "Make the Clinician Burnout Epidemic a National Priority." Published April 21. http://healthaffairs.org/blog/2016/04/21/make-the-clinician-burnout-epidemic-a-national-priority.

Smith, A. 2016. "Public Predictions for the Future of Workforce Automation." Published March 10. www.pewinternet.org/2016/03/10/public-predictions-for-the-future-of-workforce-automation.

US Department of Labor (DOL). 2016. "Compliance Assistance—Wages and the Fair Labor Standards Act (FLSA)." Accessed April 21. www.dol.gov/whd/flsa.

VitalSmarts. 2016. "Influencing Organizational Change." Accessed June 18. www.vitalsmarts.com/products-solutions/influencer.

CHAPTER 9

LEADING, MANAGING, AND GOVERNING WITHIN ORGANIZATIONAL DYNAMICS

Treat people as if they were what they ought to be, and you help them become what they are capable of being.

—Johann Wolfgang von Goethe

LEARNING OBJECTIVES

➤ Appreciate the types of leaders and leadership styles.

➤ Understand the difference between leadership and management.

➤ Describe the dyad management model.

➤ Appreciate the importance of managing disruptive behavior in the medical practice.

INTRODUCTION

Many definitions and descriptions of management and leadership have been offered by numerous observers. In essence, and for purposes of this discussion, leadership is the process of social influence in which one person can enlist the aid and support of others in the accomplishment of a common task or goal. This definition is captured by a quote from former

First Lady Rosalynn Carter: "A leader takes people where they want to go. A great leader takes people where they don't necessarily want to go, but ought to be" (Goodreads 2017).

Leaders also need to know themselves, and they need to know their followers. They are good teachers and help their followers understand the nature of the medical practice's mission. Good leaders explain the "why," and not simply the "what." People need to know why they carry out activities to be fully invested in them. They often become so busy focusing on the what that they forget the why. Staff cannot demonstrate passion for what they do not understand or support, and they cannot support something they do not understand. If practice members do not support and understand the mission and respect the values it espouses, the practice cannot prosper. Leading a divided practice is difficult, if not impossible. To avoid such divisions, leaders must focus attention on aligning practice members with the mission and vision of the practice (Wagner 2003).

Much of leadership and management (later in the chapter, we consider the differences between leadership and management) relates to how the leader interacts with his or her team. Does she delegate or collaborate? Does he direct, dictate, or facilitate? Readers may consider this question as they proceed through the chapter, with the understanding that people do not need to limit their approach to leadership to their natural tendencies. All styles have their place, and each can be learned. Think about the surgeon in the operating room. We expect and desire that surgeon to be directive and dictate what needs to be done. The operating suite is no place for a lengthy discussion or collaboration on solutions if the patient faces an imminent threat. Now place the same surgeon in a practice meeting that requires a collaborative solution and the input of all stakeholders to arrive at an optimal outcome for the patient. In this case, a direct or dictating style of leadership is counterproductive. This scenario represents one of the challenges for medical practice managers and leaders: the need to help people develop the flexibility to use the proper leadership style in the appropriate situation. This skill comes with awareness and with practice, and the modern medical practice is charged with developing leaders who appropriately use multiple leadership and management styles in the operation of the practice.

THE BASICS AND THEORIES OF LEADERSHIP

While a detailed description of each is beyond the scope of this text, some of the most prominent leadership theories are listed here for review. Many of the following focus on the behaviors and characteristics of leadership to explain performance and organizational impact (Northouse 2015; Nohrina and Khurna 2010):

◆ Great man theory

◆ Role theory

◆ Participative leadership

- Lewin's leadership styles

- Situational leadership

- Hersey and Blanchard's situational leadership

- Trait theory

- Behavioral theory

- Contingency theory

Regardless of the theory one subscribes to in terms of leadership styles and development, leadership and its proper application are essential elements of a viable medical practice. As in many types of organizations, medical practice leadership is in increasingly short supply (Hay Group 2006).

Exhibit 9.1 summarizes an important aspect of the most prominent theories of leadership: the need to either serve their stakeholders or be more self-centered in perspective.

In general, we see two kinds of leaders: those who are focused on power, economic reward, and authority (will to power) and those who are oriented toward service (will to serve). Those possessing the will to serve tend to be more transformational, and those with the will to power tend to work in organizations that are transactional in nature. **Transformational leadership** is intended to create change in individuals and in the medical practice. The goal of transformational leadership is to encourage valuable and positive change in the followers and promote growth in both followers and leaders. Transactional leadership, sometimes called managerial leadership, focuses on supervising followers and managing group performance; leaders employing this style of leadership promote compliance through rewards and punishments. Transformational leadership is the style most needed in today's practice environment.

Transformational leadership
A form of leadership intended to create change in individuals and the medical practice by encouraging valuable and positive change in followers and promoting growth in both followers and leaders.

EXHIBIT 9.1
Transactional Power Versus Transformational Power

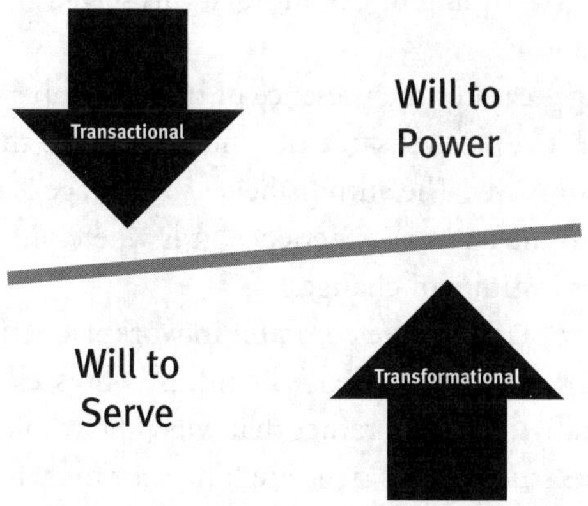

Transactional — Will to Power

Will to Serve — Transformational

In his book *Good to Great*, Jim Collins (2001) proposes five levels of leadership, which are applicable to the medical practice:

Level 1: The highly capable person is able to give to the practice thorough knowledge, skills, and other good work habits.

Level 2: The contributing team member is a person who begins to use her talents to give to the practice.

Level 3: The competent manager understands basic organization of employees and resources and how to use them to meet objectives and goals of the practice.

Level 4: The effective leader stimulates a higher performance standard for the practice.

Level 5: A leader who builds enduring greatness through humility and professional will.

Level 5 leaders find their success through the success of others and of the practice; they do not put their own ambitions first. The level 5 leader is rare, so it is true that other levels of leadership can be successful; however, leaders can, and should, all strive to become level 5 leaders (Collins 2001).

In the medical practice, trust is essential, and that trust must be built between the practice manager, its leaders, and the other stakeholders in the organization. Perhaps because of this need for trust, the concept of tribal leadership, developed by David Logan, John King, and Halee Fischer-Wright in their book, *Trial Leadership: Leveraging Natural Groups to Build a Thriving Organization*, also may be particularly applicable to the medical practice. This theory identifies five stages of tribal culture and demonstrates how managers and leaders can help the entire "tribe" move from one stage to the next. These stages are as follows (Logan, King, and Fischer-Wright 2008):

Stage 1: Members of the tribe are hostile to one another and to the company or practice. According to the authors, this stage is not commonly seen in organizations.

Stage 2: This stage features the presence of tribal members who are negative, antagonistic, passive, sarcastic, and resistant to the positive initiatives of the company. The authors believe this stage is commonly seen, and from the author's experience, it is where one often finds medical practices in times of change.

Stage 3: This stage is even more common in workplace tribes and can be characterized by "knowledge hoarders" who seek to outwit competitors on an individual level rather than view the whole as a tribe. Tribal members stuck in this stage are lone warriors who primarily care about being seen as the best individual in the tribe. This stage, too, describes many medical practices.

Stage 4: The tribe begins to move from "I'm great" to "we're great." Members become motivated to work together for the benefit of the whole organization. Leaders, managers, and practice members must work very hard to achieve this stage, as the practice of medicine is heavily focused on the individual, and the natural inclination is for the individual to see the success of the practice primarily as a result of his or her own personal efforts.

Stage 5: Innovative members use their talents to make an impact on the community for the greater good. According to the authors, less than 2 percent of workplace tribal cultures achieves this stage. Although the medical practice must always focus on its primary mission—the excellent care of individual patients—the emerging interest in and reimbursement for population health management and community health require the medical practice culture to look outward to the communities it serves.

LEADERSHIP VERSUS MANAGEMENT

Another debate that often occurs regarding leadership and management is whether leadership and management are different. In his article "Are Leadership and Management Different? A Review," Algahtani (2014) provides an overview of the scholarship on leadership and management. People often use the terms *leadership* and *management* synonymously; however, generally speaking, leadership and management are not the same concept. The two disciplines share a number of overlapping skill sets, especially when applied in smaller practices. That said, leaders tend to be externally focused on the environment, with particular concern for the mission and the future direction of the practice. They are typically visionary, seeking the ideal levels of operational performance, service, and concern for the well-being of their stakeholders. Managers focus on internal issues and the tasks that must be accomplished to achieve an effective degree of operation. They translate goals into action. Successful organizations find a collaborative balance between leaders and managers and the role each brings to the practice (Algahtani 2014).

Some medical practices may be structured in a way that requires practice managers or clinical leaders to serve both leader and manager functions, but even in these situations understanding the difference is helpful so that the leader-manager is capable of assuming the appropriate role for the situation at the correct time and in the context of the individual practice.

In a discussion of leadership versus management, defining what each term means is important. Leaders need followers, and therefore the number one responsibility of a leader is to paint a compelling vision of the future. Otherwise, why would anyone follow? Exhibit 9.2 provides a list of leadership characteristics compiled from a review of many leading researchers in the field.

The simplest definition of *management* is the process of controlling things and people. As is often said of healthcare in general, practice management is both art and science. This notion can be seen in exhibit 9.3, which lists management characteristics as described by several leading researchers (see, e.g., Bass, Bennis, Covey, Kotterman, and others listed in the Additional Reading section at the end of this chapter).

THE DYAD LEADERSHIP MODEL IN PRACTICE MANAGEMENT

Modern medical practices often employ the dyad leadership model for running the practice, as practices can have difficulty finding a staff member with the expertise needed to run both the clinical and nonclinical parts of the practice. The typical arrangement is such that a nonphysician executive is in charge of administrative issues and a physician or another

EXHIBIT 9.2 Leadership Characteristics	Is adaptable to situations
	Is ambitious and achievement oriented

EXHIBIT 9.2

Leadership Characteristics

Is adaptable to situations	Is alert to social environments
Is ambitious and achievement oriented	Is assertive
Is cooperative	Is decisive
Is dependable	Focuses on people
Has a high-activity level	Is persistent
Has self-confidence and takes risks	Tolerates stress
Is willing to assume responsibility	Is trustworthy and inspires trust
Is inspiring	Is influential
Has followers	Uses influence
Empowers others	Does the right thing
Originates	Challenges the status quo
Has a long-range perspective	Has eyes on the horizon
Is transformational	Follows personal values
Asks what and why	Is innovative
Sets strategies and vision	Facilitates decision making

EXHIBIT 9.3
Management
Characteristics

Has subordinates	Establishes agendas
Is the classic good soldier	Asks how and when
Relies on control	Accepts responsibility
Focuses on doing things right	Has a short-range perspective
Holds formal authority	Is a problem solver
Is tough-minded	Budgets
Is analytical	Plans
Maintains stasis	Focuses on systems
Uses power cautiously	Delegates cautiously
Minimizes risk	Is a stabilizing force
Administers	Has eyes on the end result
Takes a structured approach	Is deliberate
Coaches	Manages
Decides on action plan	Monitors activities against plans
Sets timetables	Organizes staff

clinician is responsible for the clinical aspects of the practice. Numerous duties require cooperation where clinical and nonclinical functions overlap; the interdependent nature of administrative and clinical functions is particularly evident in patient care.

In a study by the Medical Group Management Association (MGMA 2016), 58 percent of respondents indicated they used a physician–administrator dyad leadership model, and 75 percent of those dyads were said to meet at least monthly.

DEVELOPING A DYAD MANAGEMENT STRUCTURE

The first step in developing a dyad leadership model in a medical practice is to establish an agreement, sometimes called a covenant, between the nonclinical and clinical leaders. This agreement answers the questions shown in exhibit 9.4 and records the answers in the form of the covenant framework.

As physician practices continue to consolidate and become part of larger integrated organizations, the need for practice physicians to increase their management and executive skill set is becoming prevalent. However, in the past practices have often erred in assuming that medical expertise alone confers on physicians the ability to manage

1. What does dyad leadership look like to us?
2. What is your perception of why we need dyad leadership in our practice?
3. What is our agreement vision for group/practice? Is it different than what is currently recorded?
4. What are our goals for group/practice?
5. Our goals for the group/practice aligned?
6. What schedule will we commit to for routinely discussing issues affecting the operations of the practice? Options are daily/weekly/monthly/quarterly and as needed.
7. How do we convey our commitment and support to the dyad leadership process to the members of the practice?
8. How will we handle conflicts between nonclinical staff and clinical staff?
9. How will we resolve our differences of opinion about issues?
10. What decisions do we make together? Examples:
    a. Strategic decisions
    b. Recruiting
    c. On-boarding
    d. Mentoring
    e. Team development
11. What decisions do we make independently?
    a. Daily operating decisions
    b. Giving feedback
12. How will we develop agendas?
13. Who will chair and coordinate meetings?
14. Other items that may be unique to the practice.

Signed: _____
Date: _____

Signed: _____
Date: _____

and lead. Management and leadership are unique skills, separate from clinical skills. Good doctors do not necessarily make good leaders or managers. The assumption that a good clinician can be a good leader or manager often leads to the fulfillment of the Peter Principle, whereby individuals are selected for promotion to their highest level of incompetence on the basis of their current role, only to fail (Asghar 2014). Therefore, physician managers and leaders must receive the education and training needed to fulfill the responsibilities of their new roles (Zismer and Bruggemann 2010; Zismer and Person 2008).

Training may be developed internally; sought through external resources, such as the American College of Healthcare Executives (ACHE), MGMA, the American Association for Physician Leadership, the American Medical Group Practice Association, the American Academy of Family Physicians, the American College of Surgeons, the American College of Physicians, the American College of Cardiology, or any of the numerous other professional organizations; or by using a hybrid internal–external training approach.

Medical practices, especially large ones, can offer significant training themselves. Regardless of which approach the practice chooses, management and leadership training should focus on the following:

◆ What must leaders know as professionals in this practice?

◆ What must individual leaders know to be able to achieve personal, practice, and professional goals?

◆ What do leaders require of the practice to enable them to succeed in their new role?

In addition, training specific to dyad-managed practices should cover the following areas:

◆ Leadership and the mission, vision, and strategy

Objective: Clarity about the co-leadership role.

— Discuss models of dyad leadership.

— Discuss and describe the evolution of dyad leadership in the practice (purpose, history, roles, etc.).

— Create and share a dyad leadership agreement.

◆ Communication styles

Objective: Understand your communication style and how you can best work with your co-leader.

— Take the Management by Strengths, DiSC, or Predictive Index profile and discuss the results to understand yourself and others.

◆ Quality and process improvement

Objective: Attain a firm grasp of quality and process improvement. Understand the practice's initiatives and the tools and resources available to support them.

    — Plan

    — Do

    — Study

    — Act

◆ Recruiting, onboarding, mentoring, and developing

    Objective: Understand how best to recruit, onboard, and develop staff.

    — Discuss the role of physicians in recruiting other physicians.

    — Discuss the purpose and benefits of staff development.

    — Review tools to help recruit, mentor, and develop staff.

◆ Managing disruption

    Objective: Learn best practices for managing disruption.

    — Understand your style of conflict management using the Thomas-Kilmann Instrument or a similar tool.

    — Review best practices for managing disruption.

◆ Business decision making

    Objective: Understand how to run the practice together while balancing service and profitability.

    — Explore the decision-making process.

    — Identify and understand the key performance metrics.

The importance of training in these areas is highlighted in the sections that follow.

LEADERSHIP: MISSION, VISION, AND VALUES

Peter Drucker once said that above all else, "leaders must have followers," and to ensure followership, those leaders must establish the mission, vision, and values of the organization. In fact, one defining characteristic of the trusted leader is his or her ability to paint a compelling vision of the future.

    The mission statement provides the reason the organization exists and the intentions of the organization. The vision statement provides the aspirations of the organization and what the future state of the organization will be when it is successful. The values statement indicates what the organization believes and how it will behave, often declaring how its members will behave as individuals and how they will interact with their stakeholders.

The statements should be clear, concise, and simple. They should leave little room for interpretation, and they should be known and acknowledged by all members of the organization. If anyone in the practice cannot articulate the why, what, and how represented by the mission, vision, and values statements, they need further training. If additional training and support fail to improve the individual's understanding of the statements, he or she may not be a good fit for the practice. These statements are the framework for all decision making; they should guide all actions of the practice and should have a profound impact on how it operates, what services it provides, and how the work will be performed.

Developing the mission, vision, and values statements is an important function of the governing body because it sets the tone and standard for all that the organization does. Of course, the first question is whether the practice should develop a mission, vision, and values statement at all, considering this activity is more than a simple exercise.

For example, a practice's mission, vision, and values statements might be as follows:

Mission: To be the leading provider of medical services in the community.

Vision: We will be the community's preferred provider of high-quality care at an affordable price.

Values: We provide service to all members of our community regardless of their ability to pay.

Many variations are possible, but they should always be true to the practice's intentions: what the practice hopes to achieve and how it expects to achieve those aims. These documents must be carefully developed and taken seriously, or they should not be developed at all.

Many practices expand the concept of the values statement by providing a list of their values and the commitment they have made to the patients of their practice. Some examples of values that might be articulated and posted or given to the patient as a commitment to them include the following:

- ◆ Putting the patients' needs first

- ◆ Treating the patient and his or her family with courtesy, respect, and compassion

- ◆ Communicating information clearly and thoroughly

- ◆ Always using integrity and sound judgment in all decisions

- ◆ Working collaboratively with the patients, staff, and other colleagues (patient-centered care)

- ◆ Using evidence-based care and best business practices

- ◆ Having a high-performing culture that attracts and keeps the most talented individuals

- ◆ Delivering the highest-caliber care possible

- ◆ Earning trust through action, service, and behavior

- ◆ Maintaining an atmosphere of quality improvement and continuous learning

PROFESSIONALISM

In today's modern practice environment, professionalism and ethics are paramount considerations. What is professionalism?

- ◆ It is a vocation or calling and implies service to others.

- ◆ It involves knowledge of a distinctive base of expertise that is kept up-to-date.

- ◆ It is determined by a set of standards and examination of achievement in those standards.

- ◆ It involves developing a special relationship with those the individual serves.

- ◆ It involves the adoption and demonstration of particular ethical principles.

All the above points apply to professionalism in medical practice. In addition, professionals exhibit the following attributes:

- ◆ Honesty

- ◆ Altruism

- ◆ Service

- ◆ Commitment

- ◆ Communication

- ◆ Commitment to excellence

- ◆ Accountability

- ◆ Lifelong learning

Dr. Gerald Hickson and his colleagues at Vanderbilt University have worked for many years to perfect a system for improving professionalism in medical practice. As shown in exhibit 9.5, professionalism and ethical behavior require the right balance of intentional system design and professional accountability. To put it another way, the practice must develop rules of acceptable conduct and make its expectations for that conduct known while relying on the individual professionals to be accountable to ensure that the highest standards of professionalism and ethical behavior are maintained.

Hickson and colleagues (2007) have also found a strong connection between negative behaviors by members of the practice and malpractice litigation. By progressively addressing negative disruptive behaviors, in almost all cases behaviors are decreased, with a resulting significant decrease in malpractice claims and other negative consequences in the practice. Exhibit 9.6 shows the spectrum of disruptive behaviors seen in medical practices, ranging from the most common to the most severe.

PROFESSIONALISM AND SUBSTANCE ABUSE

Medical practice leaders need to be in tune with potential causes of disruptive behavior that hinder professionalism; in some cases, it may be due to substance abuse or mental illness. In these situations, many barriers can impede early diagnosis and intervention with professionals, including the following:

◆   The "conspiracy of silence"

◆   Denial on the part of family, friends, colleagues, and even patients

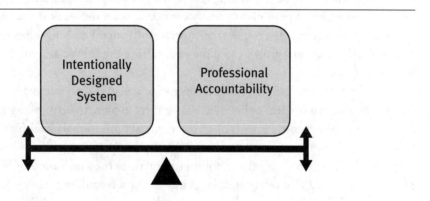

EXHIBIT 9.5
Balancing System Design and Professionalism

Source: Hickson et al. (2007). Used with permission of Gerald Hickson.

EXHIBIT 9.6

Spectrum of
Disruptive
Behaviors

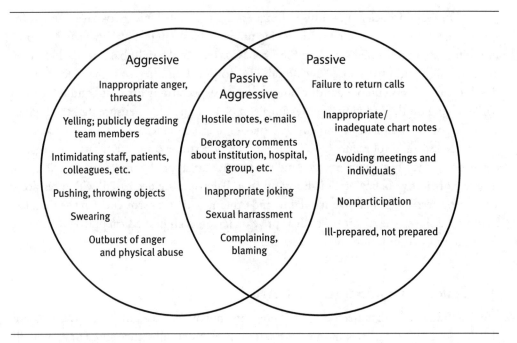

Source: Swiggart et al. (2009).

These barriers are the products of a lack of education concerning the true nature of addiction as a primary biogenetic and psychosocial disease. Tenacious denial is the common feature of alcoholic or addicted physicians, as knowledge of the effects of drugs and alcohol create the delusion that special insight provides immunity from addiction. Alcoholic or addicted physicians usually cannot see themselves as sick and often do not accept dependency as a disease. Furthermore, family members and colleagues contribute to the denial by covering up or making excuses for the physician and do not demand he or she seek help.

However, signs and symptoms emerge in professional life, family life, and social life. The practice must have clear policies and procedures in place to help colleagues in this area. In most states, the medical boards operate a medical professionals' health program, which is designed to provide assistance to the individual while protecting him or her from actions that would permanently affect the ability to practice. The Federation of State Physician Health Programs (2016) offers additional information regarding these programs. Practice managers and leaders should be familiar with these resources should the need arise to tap into them.

LEADERSHIP STYLES

A brief discussion of leadership styles may be useful for leaders of medical practices. Weber (1958) categorized leadership styles as bureaucratic, charismatic, or traditional. More important for our purposes, Burns (1978) and Bass (1999) added to this perspective by proposing the categories of transactional and transformational leadership. With transformational style being the preferred approach over transactional leadership, exhibit 9.7 illustrates some key attributes of the transformational leader and shows how they vary from transactional leadership (Bass 1990; Bass and Avolio 1994).

Burns (1978) noted the attachment of morality to leadership, proposing that moral leaders are sensitive to the needs, beliefs, and values of their followers, whereas immoral leaders disregard the beliefs of followers. Furthermore, he suggested that amoral leaders rule followers through coercion and fear, an approach that is generally discounted as ineffective.

Rather, transformational leaders use internal, or intrinsic, motivating factors to influence, and they provide individualized consideration, inspirational motivation, and intellectual stimulation to achieve outcomes. Transactional leaders use external, or extrinsic, motivating factors and manage by exception and contingency.

Transformational leaders and managers are able to articulate their attitudes and demonstrate their behaviors in a way that is inspiring and motivating to their followers. This cycle is illustrated in exhibit 9.8.

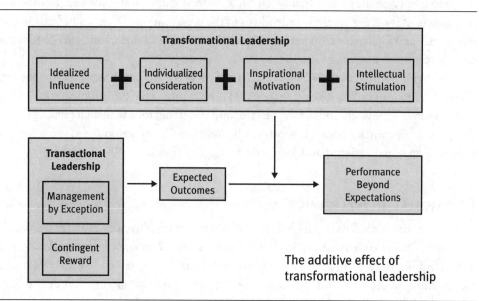

EXHIBIT 9.7
Results of Transformational Leadership

Source: Adapted from Bass and Avolio (1994).

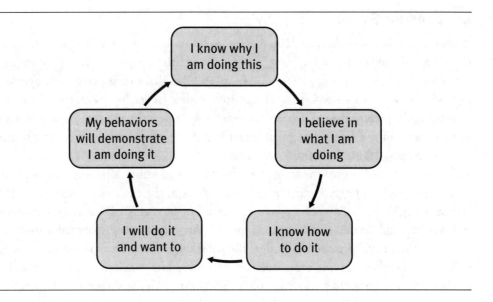

ORGANIZATIONAL CONSCIENTIOUSNESS

Most people recognize conscientiousness as the personality trait of being careful and vigilant. In an organizational sense, we add the notions of efficiency, orderliness, and the general desire to complete the task at hand well. In a sense, organizational conscientiousness is a summation of the traits of all the individuals in the organization. When considered in those terms, care and vigilance in operations require leadership to set the tone and demonstrate conscientiousness as an organizational value.

Organizational conscientiousness has often been expressed as, "First do the right thing; then do it right." Practice managers and leaders must take this simple phrase to heart as they examine the operations of the practice and its interactions with all its stakeholders in the spirit of the conscientious relationship. Organizational conscientiousness is fundamental to having an organization that demonstrates integrity (Becker 1998).

EMOTIONAL INTELLIGENCE

Most successful leaders have a high degree of emotional intelligence (EQ). As discussed in chapter 8, Daniel Goleman's (1995) book *Emotional Intelligence: Why It Can Matter More Than IQ* brought EQ to the forefront of theories in the management world. His insights and application are based on the work of Mayer and Salovey (1997), who define EQ as "the ability to perceive emotions, to access and generate emotions so as to assist thought, to understand emotions and emotional knowledge, and to reflectively regulate emotions so as to promote emotional and intellectual growth."

EQ involves the recognition and regulation of ourselves and our relationships. According to Goleman (1995), EQ traits can be described as follows:

- Self-awareness
    - emotional self-awareness
    - accurate self-assessment
    - self-confidence
- Social awareness
    - empathy
    - organizational awareness
    - service orientation
- Self-management
    - self-control
    - transparency
    - adaptability
    - achievement driven
    - initiative
- Relationship management
    - inspirational leadership
    - developing others
    - influence
    - change catalyst
    - conflict management
    - building bonds
    - teamwork and collaboration

A 2009 literature review found an important connection between highly successful nursing practice and EQ, a relationship that also applies to other providers in the medical practice (Smith, Profetto-McGrath, and Cummings 2009).

One exercise for developing EQ in the organization is to ask your team, or an individual team member, to close their eyes and think about a person on whom they really rely and whom they trust—someone they consider the ideal team member. Then ask them to think about someone who would be in the opposite camp: difficult, untrustworthy, and hard to get along with—someone they generally dread dealing with. Now ask, at the most basic level, what is the difference between these two people? The answer is probably their EQ. One lacks self-awareness when he disregards his effect on the people he interacts with. He is not service oriented, he lacks self-control, and he responds poorly when changes are necessary. The individual lacking EQ cares little about developing others and seems to enjoy conflict instead of building bonds and collaboration.

Although task-oriented competencies are important in determining success, the critical factor is EQ. The practice manager should strive to help practice members develop this intelligence.

GENERATIONAL ISSUES IN THE MEDICAL PRACTICE

Generational issues are emerging in the medical practice as never before. According to a report released by the Pew Research Center, 10,000 people turn 65 every day in the United States, and that trend is expected to continue to at least 2029 (Heimlich 2010). This shift toward an aging population has a profound impact on the medical practice in a number of ways. As people age, in general they need more medical care, and practices need to be adept at caring for older people.

Although some physicians and practices specialize in the care of older individuals, most seniors receive care from practices that see a wide range of ages. Consider that older individuals may need more time, not only for navigating the practice but also to explain their medical needs. In addition, those medical needs are often for treating multiple diseases (Shi and Singh 2015). As of 2009, 56 percent of people over age 65 had at least one of five serious chronic conditions, and many had three or more (Lee, Cigolle, and Blaum 2009). These factors present a resource challenge for the practice in determining ways to provide care to a population that is getting increasingly older while the practice is simultaneously experiencing restrictions on reimbursement.

Our workforce is also aging, and individuals are choosing, for many reasons, to delay retirement. As stated in chapter 1, for the first time in history, five generations are present in the workplace, a situation that offers both opportunities and challenges for medical practices. The two largest groups are the baby boomers and the millennials. On the one hand, boomers bring experience and a long-term perspective, place work as a high priority, and are comfortable with hierarchy. On the other hand, millennials generally enjoy collaborative working relationships, technology, and a desire for greater work–life balance (Smola and Sutton 2002).

Furthermore, millennials tend to be less oriented toward planning than members of the baby boom generation are. Consider a little story about going to dinner. A group of boomers decide to go to dinner. They will plan for this event and even make a reservation at the restaurant. They go to a place they are familiar with. They may recall their favorite dish and look forward to having it again. In addition, they have planned what they will do after dinner. The millennial group going to dinner decides to get something to eat and tweets or texts that information among themselves and with other friends. "Getting something to eat. Join us?" They look online for a place to get the type of food they are in the mood for; the location and number of people to dine are not determined ahead of dinner. They drive by the first choice and notice that the parking lot is too full, so they tweet that they are proceeding to the next possible location. In the meantime, more and more of their friends join in and plan to meet with them. Finally, they come to a place where they all are satisfied and they get something to eat.

The point is that the goal of getting something to eat was accomplished by both parties; the difference was in the process. Which is right? Which is wrong? The answer, of course, is neither, but recognizing the approach that each group took in getting the goal accomplished is helpful. Planning has its place, and so do flexibility and spontaneity. Extending the example to the medical practice, leaders and managers must be open to incorporating new ideas and processes into the workplace by taking into account the aptitudes and values each generational group brings.

Furthermore, they must work to effectively develop teams that take advantage of the many positive attributes of each group. Open dialogue regarding their differences in which they are acknowledged is key because each brings its own set of strengths and weaknesses. The more practice leaders recognize the value of each group, the more effectively they can manage the practice. For example, a practice converting its records system to an electronic health record is wise to consider the points of view of all the generations working in the practice. Younger team members may have a solid grasp on the use of new technologies, and older workers see the limitations of the technology that balance the team's deliberations.

DIVERSITY AND INCLUSION ISSUES FOR LEADERSHIP

We have now seen how age and generations can have a great impact on the operations of the medical practice. And age is only one aspect of diversity. Next, we explore other diversity elements and how we can effectively manage them to improve the practice.

The process starts with the recognition that "We don't know what we don't know." Practice managers and leaders are charged with helping practice members become aware of diversity and inclusion issues.

The following steps are involved in improving diversity and inclusion in the medical practice (Holvino, Bernardo, and Merrill-Sands 2004):

1. Establish clear expectations in the policies and the values expressed by the practice that it supports a diverse and inclusive environment. These expectations should apply to employment issues, educational activities, patient care activities, and community outreach efforts.

2. Shape attitudes and policies toward diversity and inclusion through training and education, recruiting, onboarding, and development. When possible, practices should strive to be representative of the communities they serve.

3. Measure and evaluate the practice's current status regarding diversity. Have conversations with community leaders and activists to gain feedback on their perspective of the practice in terms of diversity and inclusion issues.

4. Take corrective action when necessary, such as making operational changes, addressing performance issues, and curbing any activity that will affect the practice and its stakeholders. Such action might be taken by members of the practice toward each other and the patients or by patients toward practice members.

Following are two illustrative stories.

ONE DAY, Mr. Jones calls the practice administrator of Happy Practice USA. He complains that he did not want to be cared for by a doctor because of his race. Does the administrator accommodate the patient and assure him that he will not have to see a physician because of his race? The ideal conversation might go like this: "Mr. Jones, I assure you that all of the physicians in our practice are highly qualified and that they work as a team. In our efforts to make sure you receive timely and appropriate care, we would be irresponsible if we guaranteed you would not see a particular physician in the practice. In fact, you may need to see this physician when you are in the most difficult of circumstances, as in the emergency department when our physicians are on call. For these reasons, it is not possible, nor is it our policy, to have patients change caregivers solely on the basis of what you have described. We would certainly like to have you as our patient, and we want you to feel comfortable and confident in the care that we provide. Mr. Jones, please consider what I've said, and if you feel you cannot have the confidence in all our caregivers to provide the care you need, it might be best for you to find another practice to care for you. Of course, we will give you adequate time to make your decision and find a different practitioner if that is your desire. We will do everything we can to make that a smooth transition." This dialogue should be followed up with a letter indicating the essence of the conversation to prevent complications and the potential for an allegation of abandonment. (All states and medical societies have standards on appropriate ways to dismiss a patient. Failure to follow these rules can result in an abandonment complaint, which can lead to sanctions from the state medical examining board.)

ONE DAY, a supervisor frantically enters the administrator's office and says, "I have a serious employment question that I need to discuss with you." The administrator listens carefully to the story. "I just had a person with a disability apply for a position in my department. I don't know why human resources would send me an applicant like this. What should I do?" An appropriate discussion could proceed as follows: "Is the person qualified to do the job? Is she the best applicant to perform the job that we have posted to fill?" The supervisor replies, "Yes on both counts." The administrator asks, "Can we make reasonable accommodations so that she can do the work?" The supervisor replies, "It will not take a lot to do that." The administrator replies, "Then you should hire her."

These conversations are also great opportunities to coach supervisors on diversity and inclusion practices. They should be treated as a learning opportunity rather than in a punitive manner. The supervisor's contact with people with disabilities may be limited, and his or her reaction in this situation may have arisen from a lack of understanding rather than due to malicious intent. Remember, "We don't know what we don't know"; effective practice managers and leaders help develop people in all respects, including diversity and inclusion.

They should never miss an opportunity to provide leadership on diversity and inclusion and, when necessary, coach on the values that the practice espouses. Although in some cases, legal issues may be involved, such as discrimination on the basis of age, race, ethnicity, gender, national origin, and disability (EEOC 2016), in all cases, hiring for inclusion is the right thing to do.

One final thought on diversity and inclusion goes to an issue that is not often included in this category, and that is the way individuals think. Practices must allow some diversity of thought; failing to do so means they miss opportunities to include innovative ideas in practice operations. Encourage members of the practice to provide ideas and speak up with innovative thoughts. Diversity and inclusion can be a strength for any medical practice.

GIVING AND RECEIVING FEEDBACK

Among the most difficult tasks of managers and leaders is providing feedback to subordinates; receiving feedback is fraught with difficulty as well. Successful practices master the art of giving and receiving feedback to all members of the practice.

Why is feedback so difficult? Many people have had poor experiences in receiving and giving feedback. Because it is a skill that requires time and attention to develop, much of the feedback people have received in the past may have been given in an inappropriate way, resulting in negative feelings about feedback in general—even about accepting positive feedback.

Effective medical practices see giving and receiving feedback as essential skills, and they seek to cultivate those skills in everyone in the practice. To begin, establish a clear understanding that the practice engages in providing feedback to one another and that feedback is a gift (Stone and Heen 2014). If managers and leaders are unaware of behaviors, performance issues, or other opportunities for improvement, they cannot address those issues. Likewise, failing to provide reinforcement for constructive behaviors and excellent performance is a missed opportunity to institutionalize the behaviors the practice seeks and the performance it desires. We all want recognition for what we do, and much of the time, that can be in the form of constructive feedback.

When giving feedback, always consider what your intentions are and what you hope to achieve from the session. When receiving feedback, consider what the intentions of the person giving feedback might be, and listen to that feedback carefully.

GUIDANCE ON PROVIDING POSITIVE FEEDBACK

Following are tips for providing positive feedback:

- ◆ Express your positive intent, and describe the behavior your feedback is intended to address.

  - Describe the behavior in a specific manner.

  - Avoid generalizing about the behavior. Generalizations are always less effective than concrete, specific comments, and they are less meaningful to the recipient.

  - Be sincere in your presentation.

  - Do not mix criticism with praise.

- ◆ Describe the impact of the behavior in terms of the goals of the practice or department.

- ◆ Always thank the recipient for his or her contributions to the practice or department.

GUIDANCE ON PROVIDING NEGATIVE FEEDBACK

Considerations when giving negative feedback are as follows:

- ◆ Giving feedback when it is not positive but constructive in nature is often challenging. Prepare for the feedback session carefully by determining the desired outcome. Make the feedback useful and actionable.

- ◆ Be sure you have observed the behavior directly. Do not rely solely on hearsay before conducting the feedback session.

- Always choose a private location and allow adequate time for the session.

- Always show that your intent is positive. Be objective with your wording and approach, and discuss what you have observed, not what others have told you.

- Describe the behavior and its impact on the work group, department, or practice. Focus on the behavior, not the person, and express your desire for a mutual solution. Avoid being accusatory or creating a confrontational environment.

- Encourage the person to respond, and listen carefully to that response. The dialogue is an opportunity to demonstrate active listening by summarizing the speaker's key points and clarifying any statements that may be unclear.

- Ask the person for solutions, and, if appropriate, suggest a specific change.

- Summarize the discussion.

- Agree on next steps. Express encouragement, show confidence in the person, and be sure that the steps are clear and that a follow-up date is established.

GUIDANCE ON RECEIVING NEGATIVE, CONSTRUCTIVE FEEDBACK

None of us is perfect, and in a high-performing practice, every member should expect to receive constructive or negative feedback on occasion. In fact, an absence of the occasional constructive feedback is a sign that the organization is not committed to being open and honest with its members.

Following are considerations for receiving negative or constructive feedback:

- Think about how you react to feedback of a constructive nature. Is your manner defensive? Do you quickly apologize, or do you react in a positive way by seeking to learn and understand what the feedback is meant to tell you?

- When possible, think about your responses before the session takes place. Often, people have a sense that a constructive feedback session may occur, especially in a practice that is open and honest about feedback.

- Listen actively and calmly. Be sure you understand the points being made and acknowledge the concerns.

- Discuss a mutually appropriate solution, and develop an action plan.

- Always reflect on any feedback session to learn not only about the specific behaviors and situations discussed but also how to improve your management and leadership skills in the future. Self-reflection is a powerful tool for growth.

GUIDANCE ON RECEIVING POSITIVE FEEDBACK

Who doesn't like positive feedback? Surprisingly, many people feel uneasy when receiving positive feedback, and such feedback sessions can become awkward. To avoid difficult positive feedback situations, first, understand that the feedback is a reflection not only of your performance but also of what the practice values. More than a simple expression of appreciation, it is an indication of activities and behaviors you should continue to do to support the practice. Next, seek advice on learning to be gracious and appreciative of positive feedback.

Learning to give and receive feedback of all types is essential for the high-performing medical practice. A culture that respects and engages in consistent, fair, and well-executed feedback does not develop by accident; it requires the organization to establish an environment conducive to open and honest feedback (Stone and Heen 2014; Patterson et al. 2011).

GOVERNANCE AND ORGANIZATIONAL DYNAMICS

Organizational dynamics
The script for the organization's human capital, or the ways in which individuals and processes interact in the company.

The governance and **organizational dynamics** of a medical practice cover a wide range of issues, many of which have been discussed in other parts of the text. For our purposes in this discussion, we cover the key aspects of governance and the manner in which these functions influence organizational culture.

The governance of a medical practice involves numerous areas of responsibility, including the following.

◆ *The appropriate legal structure for the organization.* This function includes considering and balancing the framework of governing bodies with attention to these elements:

— The size of the board and committees. Board size varies greatly among organizations on the basis of the size and diversity of the practice, as an inverse relationship exists between the size of a governing body and its ability to act, so careful consideration must be given to size. In addition, think about the time frame in which action is needed. Often, operational and strategic issues may be separated, with consideration for the need to act more quickly on operational issues and more deliberatively on strategic ones.

— How members are chosen. If members are elected, how? By majority? Or by a specified percentage greater than 50 percent (called a super majority)? By appointment? In some cases, individuals are simply appointed by the practice. For example, the board may appoint members of a quality management committee. By rotation? In this structure, an individual may rotate into a position of authority on the basis of an agreed-on schedule or process.

— Extent of authority held by members. Most practices, like most other types of organizations, place limits on the authority of any one person or group of individuals. Authority typically is limited in terms of the amount of money that can be spent, what contracts and obligations can be entered into by the group or individual, and so on. It also includes changes in the bylaws or voting rules, legal changes to the practices, or merger and acquisition activity. The practice should avoid an overly complicated oversight process, for example by giving responsibility to a committee or an individual only to require their decisions to be reviewed or revised at one or more additional levels of governance.

— What committees to establish. Committees, such as an executive committee, a compensation committee, a quality management committee, a safety committee, a medical records committee, or a research committee, may be ad hoc or permanent committees. An ad hoc committee is formed for a particular purpose or task and disbanded once that task is completed. An example is an ad hoc committee seated for the selection and purchase of a medical records system (a permanent IT committee may also be in place, which would have responsibility for system oversight going forward).

◆ *Record-keeping of the activities of the governing bodies.* Accurate minutes and other documents related to meetings must be kept and distributed as appropriate. One area related to record-keeping is ensuring proper follow-up occurs on action items. Failures to establish and execute follow-up procedures result in forgotten items resurfacing as even more problematic or urgent concerns.

◆ *If incorporated, development and maintenance of the corporate mission, vision, and values statements and the organization's culture.* This area of responsibility should be visited yearly or when appropriate depending on current events. For example, a practice merger or acquisition should prompt this action.

◆ *Development and maintenance of the practice's strategic plan and its implementation.* This area should also be visited yearly or when appropriate depending on current events. For example, the possible repeal and replacement of the Affordable Care Act may compel the practice to consider changes to its strategic plan.

◆ *Setting compensation standards for physicians, other professionals, and staff.* Compensation standards may be established with the help of the compensation committee, survey data from MGMA, and benchmark information from other physician practice organizations. A compensation consultant may be needed in some cases, as when the issues are particularly problematic, are complex, or involve legal questions.

◆ *Approving expectations or programs for the practice.* Expanding the scope or geographic reach of the practice represents major commitments that require careful planning and support, so thorough vetting by the governance structure is essential.

◆ *Facilitating and encouraging physician leaders to become knowledgeable, participative stakeholders.* The practice's management and leadership must devote time and resources to educating the members of the governing bodies. Retreats devoted to reflection and renewal of the practice are opportunities for education on good governance.

◆ *Ensuring the quality of the medical care provided by the practice.* The governing bodies of the practice must ensure that the practice delivers high-quality care. This responsibility is accomplished through the following steps:

— Establish quality goals, and educate everyone in the practice on those goals.

— Develop and monitor appropriate quality benchmarks using data analysis and surveys, such as patient satisfaction surveys.

— Take action when quality measures are not met by engaging in quality improvement projects.

— Take action when serious or recurring complaints arise.

— Take all patient and provider complaints seriously.

— Review individual quality data with all providers, and establish an action plan for improvement when necessary. Schedule regular follow-up sessions for reviewing progress.

◆ *Participating in advocacy endeavors at local, state, and federal levels.* Efforts include the following:

— Membership in local civic organizations, such as the Rotary Club. These organizations are often unaware of or uninformed on important healthcare issues.

— Participation in local business organizations, such as the area's business roundtable or others that may be unique to the community.

— Engaging with state legislators. Be available to help and inform when issues affecting patients and practices arise.

— Engaging with members of the US Congress and their committees.

— Involvement in professional organizations, such as ACHE, MGMA, and other specialty-specific organizations.

On a regular basis, the governance process should be reviewed and the governing body educated on its responsibilities and obligations to the practice and to the patients it serves. Unlike many other organizations, the governing body of a medical practice may have a limited knowledge of business and governance. Because the governing body is often composed of the practice's physicians and providers, this makeup presents challenges whereby decisions can be influenced by personal preference or interest. An important step is to remind members of the governing body that they should act in the best interest of the practice.

Governance and organizational dynamics have taken on additional importance for all organizations in recent years. The modern medical practice is no exception, and in a sense, it is in greater need for focused attention to this topic as healthcare comes under ever-increasing scrutiny. Rising costs, medical errors and other quality concerns, potential conflicts of interest, and spiraling technology costs all lead to the need for much more attention to governance and organizational dynamics than has been required in the past.

In a practical sense, however, governance and organizational dynamics can be summed up as *a need to change and to protect the new status quo in a cycle of continuous improvement.* Effective governance and the management of organizational dynamics are essential to a successful medical practice. Governance and organizational dynamics must have a higher priority for practices in the future. Above all else, leaders must develop their followers in the standards and expectations of governance to facilitate the flow of new ideas in the changing healthcare environment.

CONDUCTING MEETINGS

An important skill for practice leaders is the ability to conduct an effective meeting. This task may sound simple, but in reality, it requires a great deal of thought, preparation, and execution to have meetings that produce results.

An effective meeting is divided into three sets of activities:

1. Before the meeting:

    a. Determine the structure of and purpose for the meeting. Ask yourself if the meeting is necessary. Can the issue be handled in some other way?

   b.   Carefully consider who is being asked to attend the meeting and why they are there.

   c.   Determine the objective and desired outcome of the meeting.

   d.   Compile and distribute (well in advance) any prior communication, documents, or other information that will help the attendees prepare for the meeting.

   e.   Develop and distribute an agenda that includes the items to be discussed, the time allotted for discussion, and the actions needed. Meeting items that may be listed as "information only" often can be handled by memo or other means of communication.

   f.   Establish rules for the conduct of the meeting.

2.   Conducting the meeting:

   a.   Always start the meeting on time.

   b.   Remind participants to limit discussion to the items on the agenda to make sure all are addressed.

   c.   Go over the rules of the meeting and ask if any participants have changes or objections. Obtain agreement that the meeting will be conducted under these rules.

   d.   Any important items that arise that are not on the agenda may be placed in the "parking lot," a device for recording and deferring critical but unplanned issues for later consideration.

   e.   Manage the discussion. Medical practice meetings involve people who often have strong personalities and opinions. The facilitator of the meeting should manage the discussion in a way that provides for all attendees to have input, such as allowing each attendee to comment in turn in "round robin" style.

   f.   Limit discussion to the time allotted for each agenda item. Time management of meetings is important to maintain interest and credibility for future participation.

   g.   Stay on topic. The facilitator can bring the discussion back to the topic at hand should the conversation drift to other areas.

   h.   Follow-up actions should be decided by the group. The group should also decide who is responsible for completing each action.

    i.   Minutes of the meeting should be recorded, including required follow-up activities.

    j.   Set follow-up meetings if appropriate. In medical groups, one strategy is to establish standing meeting times that account for provider schedules. That said, beware of standing meetings that have no purpose. Meetings can always be canceled, and should be when no useful purpose is apparent.

    k.   Always end the meeting on time.

3. After the meeting:

    a.   Thank the participants for their attendance and contribution.

    b.   Prepare and distribute minutes.

    c.   Develop an action list of the items requiring follow-up. Distribute those action items to the responsible parties, and establish a time frame for their action.

    d.   Inform stakeholders of important actions that resulted from the meeting, including follow-up activities and timelines.

    e.   Monitor progress on follow-up activity.

ASSESSING LEADERSHIP SUCCESS

The professional practice manager goes through career stages from competent to expert, from studious to intuitive. When others ask for her opinion and not for the facts, it might be said that she "has arrived." Opinions are based on the integration of knowledge and facts, of skills and insights—and above all, trust. The trust that we speak of is authentic trust, not naive trust. Authentic trust is built over time and, unlike naive trust, does not require that we always be right, only that we always be worthy of the trust we have been given.

Authentic trust is a close ally of integrity. Think about someone you really trust. What makes that person trustworthy? Is he or she infallible? Probably not, but that individual has done all he or she could to make appropriate decisions given the information available. This person recognizes when he or she is wrong and takes actions to correct mistakes (Wagner 2003).

When one's judgment is valued and one's professionalism is respected, that individual has achieved success.

Discussion Questions

1. In your own words, explain the difference between leaders who have a will to power and those who have a will to serve.

2. Compare the transformational and transactional leadership styles.

3. What is meant by a dyad leadership system?

4. What are some leadership characteristics?

5. What are some management characteristics, and how do they differ from those of leadership?

6. Describe some examples of disruptive behavior, and discuss their implications.

7. What choices does the practice manager have in dealing with disruptive behavior?

References

Algahtani, A. 2014. "Are Leadership and Management Different? A Review." *Journal of Management Policies and Practices* 2 (3): 71–82.

Asghar, R. 2014. "Incompetence Rains, Er, Reigns: What the Peter Principle Means Today." Published August 14. www.forbes.com/sites/robasghar/2014/08/14/incompetence-rains-er-reigns-what-the-peter-principle-means-today/#458768b7631b.

Bass, B. 1999. "Two Decades of Research and Development and Transformational Leadership." *European Journal of Work and Organizational Psychology* 8 (1): 9–32.

———. 1990. *Bass and Stogdill's Handbook of Leadership*. New York: Free Press.

Bass, B., and B. Avolio. 1994. *Improving Organizational Effectiveness Through Transformational Leadership*. Thousand Oaks, CA: Sage.

Becker, T. E. 1998. "Integrity in Organizations: Beyond Honesty and Conscientiousness." *Academy of Management Review* 23 (1): 154–161.

Burns, J. 1978. *Leadership*. New York: Harper & Row.

Collins, J. 2001. *Good to Great: Why Some Companies Make the Leap . . . and Others Don't*. New York: Harper Business.

Federation of State Physician Health Programs. 2016. "State Programs." Accessed June 18. www.fsphp.org/state-programs.

Goleman, D. 1995. *Emotional Intelligence: Why It Can Matter More Than IQ.* New York: Bantam.

Goodreads. 2017. "Quotable Quote: Rosalynn Carter." Accessed May 10. www.goodreads.com/author/show/96533.Rosalynn_Carter.

Hay Group. 2006. *Confronting the Leadership Crisis: What Works, What Doesn' t, What Lies Ahead.* Stamford, CT: Chief Executive Group.

Heimlich, R. 2010. "Baby Boomers Retire." Published December 29. www.pewresearch.org/daily-number/baby-boomers-retire.

Hickson, G. B., J. W. Pichert, L. E. Webb, and S. G. Gabbe. 2007. "A Complementary Approach to Promoting Professionalism: Identifying, Measuring, and Addressing Unprofessional Behaviors." *Academic Medicine* 82 (11): 1040–48.

Holvino, E., M. F. Bernardo, and D. Merrill-Sands. 2004. "Creating and Sustaining Diversity and Inclusion in Organizations: Strategies and Approaches." In *The Psychology and Management of Workplace Diversity*, edited by M. S. Stockdale and F. J. Crosby, 245–76. Malden, MA: Blackwell.

Lee, P., C. Cigolle, and C. Blaum. 2009. "The Co-occurrence of Chronic Diseases and Geriatric Syndromes: The Health and Retirement Study." *Journal of the American Geriatrics Society* 57 (3): 511–16.

Logan, D., J. King, and H. Fischer-Wright. 2008. *Tribal Leadership: Leveraging Natural Groups to Build a Thriving Organization*. New York: HarperCollins.

Mayer, J. D., and P. Salovey. 1997. "What Is Emotional Intelligence?" In *Emotional Development and Emotional Intelligence: Implications for Educators*, edited by P. Salovey and D. Sluyter. New York: Basic.

Medical Group Management Association (MGMA). 2016. "Do You Currently Utilize a Physician Administrator (Dyad) Leadership Team Model?" Published March 8. www.mgma.com/industry-data/polling/mgma-stat-archives/do-you-currently-utilize-a-dyad-leadership-team-model.

Nohrina, N., and R. Khurna (eds.). 2010. *Handbook of Leadership Theory and Practice*. Boston: Harvard Business Review Press.

Northouse, P. 2015. *Leadership: Theories and Practice*, 7th ed. Thousand Oaks, CA: Sage.

Patterson, K., J. Grenny, R. McMillan, and A. Switzler. 2011. *Crucial Conversations: Tools for Talking When Stakes Are High*, 2nd ed. New York: McGraw-Hill Education.

Shi, L., and D. Singh. 2015. *Delivering Health Care in America: A Systems Approach*, 6th ed. New York: Jones & Bartlett Learning.

Smith, K. B., J. Profetto-McGrath, and G. G. Cummings. 2009. "Emotional Intelligence and Nursing: An Integrative Literature Review." *International Journal of Nursing Studies* 46 (12): 1624–36.

Smola, K. W., and C. D. Sutton. 2002. "Generational Differences: Revisiting Generational Work Values for the New Millennium." *Journal of Organizational Behavior* 23 (4): 363–82.

Stone, D., and S. Heen. 2014. *Thanks for the Feedback: The Science and Art of Receiving Feedback Well*. New York: Penguin.

Swiggart, W. H., C. M. Dewey, G. B. Hickson, A. J. R. Finlayson, and W. A. Spickard. 2009. "A Plan for Identification, Treatment, and Remediation of Disruptive Behaviors in Physicians." *Frontiers of Health Services Management* 25 (4): 3–11.

US Equal Employment Opportunity Commission (EEOC). 2016. "Discrimination by Type." Accessed January 2. www.eeoc.gov/laws/types.

Wagner, S. L. 2003. "Integrity, Trust, Leadership and Professionalism: Defining the ACMPE Fellow." *College Review* (Fall): 27–30.

Weber, M. (H. Gerth, trans.) 1958. "The Three Types of Legitimate Rule." *Berkeley Publications in Society and Institutions* 4 (1): 1–11.

Zismer, D., and J. Bruggemann. 2010. "Examining the 'Dyad' as a Management Model in Integrated Health Systems." *Physician Executive* 36 (1): 14–19.

Zismer, D., and P. Person. 2008. "The Future of Management Education and Training for Physician Leaders." *Physician Executive* 34 (6): 44–46.

ADDITIONAL READING

Bass, B. 2010. *The Bass Handbook of Leadership: Theory, Research, and Managerial Applications*. New York: Simon & Schuster.

———. 1985. *Leadership and Performance Beyond Expectations*. New York: Free Press.

Bennis, W. G. 1989. "Managing the Dream: Leadership in the 21st Century." *Journal of Organizational Change Management* 2 (1): 6–10.

Bennis, W. G., and B. Nanus. 2007. *Leaders: The Strategies for Taking Charge*. New York: HarperCollins.

Capowski, G. 1994. "Anatomy of a Leader: Where Is the Leader of Tomorrow?" *Management Review* 83 (3): 10–18.

Covey, S. R. 1991. *Principle-Centered Leadership*. New York: Simon & Schuster.

Drucker, P. F. 1999. "Knowledge-Worker Productivity: The Biggest Challenge." *California Management Review* 41 (2): 79.

House, R. J. 1977. "A 1976 Theory of Charismatic Leadership." In *Leadership: The Cutting Edge*, edited by J. G. Hunt and L. L. Larson, 189–205. Carbondale: Southern Illinois University Press.

Kotter, J. P. 2001. "What Leaders Really Do." *Harvard Business Review* 79 (11): 85–96.

Kotterman, J. 2006. "Leadership Versus Management: What's the Difference?" *Journal for Quality & Participation* 29 (2): 13–17.

Lunenburg, F. C. 2011. "Leadership Versus Management: A Key Distinction—At Least in Theory." *International Journal of Management, Business, and Administration* 14 (1): 1–4.

Maxwell, J. C. 1998. *21 Irrefutable Laws of Leadership*. Nashville, TN: Thomas Nelson.

Mullins, L. J. 2010. *Management & Organisational Behaviour*. London: Pearson Education.

Zaleznik, A. 1977. "Managers and Leaders: Are They Different?" *Harvard Business Review* (May/June): 67–78.

CHAPTER 10

QUALITY MANAGEMENT IN THE PHYSICIAN PRACTICE

Quality and reliability are system properties.

—W. Edwards Deming

LEARNING OBJECTIVES

➤ Articulate the nature of performance management.

➤ Describe the approaches to performance improvement.

➤ Appreciate the impact of variation on performance.

➤ Discuss the components of the Triple Aim.

➤ Describe process improvement.

INTRODUCTION

One of the most important issues to address in the medical practice is the quality and safety of the care provided to patients. The Institute of Medicine (IOM 2001), a prestigious branch of the National Institutes of Health, stated in its landmark report *Crossing the Quality Chasm: A New Health System for the 21st Century*, "In its current form, habits, and environment, American health care is incapable of providing the public with the quality health care it expects and deserves."

Another historic IOM (2000) report, *To Err Is Human: Building a Safer Health System*, indicated that a shocking number of people—an estimated 44,000 to 98,000 per year—are harmed by the healthcare system. A more recent study found that this number has increased since publication of the 2000 IOM report despite substantial efforts to improve. Medical errors have now become the third leading cause of death in the United States (Makary and Daniel 2016).

The complexity of medical service and the inconsistency with which these services are delivered, not to mention the fragmented nature of the system, have led to a number of quality concerns (Mosadeghrad 2014), including a lack of systematic approaches to care delivery and quality improvement. Efforts to improve quality in the medical profession have a long tradition of focusing on individual performance versus system performance. Exhibit 10.1 illustrates the potential flaw in this thinking. The bell-shaped curve, P-1, represents the overall performance of any given system. Curve P-2 illustrates an improved system of performance where the median performance is moved from M-1 to M-2. If an organization seeks to improve by only focusing on the low performers, it experiences only a small improvement, shown as I-1. By improving the system as a whole, a much larger improvement is seen, as demonstrated by I-2. Although focusing on removing bad behavior and poor performance is necessary, it will not produce the optimum level of improvement being sought in the US healthcare system.

QUALITY AND SAFETY IMPROVEMENT

Much of the work in quality improvement has focused on healthcare institutions such as hospitals; however, the findings of the IOM research are applicable to the medical practice as well. A common denominator in all healthcare environments is the healthcare provider.

EXHIBIT 10.1
Performance
Improvement

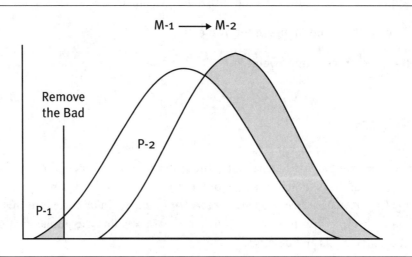

In a landmark study published by RAND Corporation in 2006, quality was found to be lacking in the services offered by medical practices. Overall, adults received about half of the recommended care; furthermore, that finding did not vary significantly across metropolitan areas. In addition, wide variability in the quality of care received was noted across communities for the same disease state. All social and demographic groups were affected. One conclusion of the study is that the lack of care received by patients was caused by the absence of investment in systemwide information technology, performance tracking, and incentives for improving care (RAND 2006).

For the most part, practices still are not reimbursed for services by third-party payers on the basis of the quality of care delivered, but on volume (McKesson 2016). Although no practice wishes to provide care in a way that produces poor quality, the focus on volume and the lack of focus on outcomes create distortions in the way leaders manage their practices. In fact, this reimbursement methodology is a major contributing factor to misaligned incentives (Network for Regional Health Improvement 2008; Miller 2009). These ideas are not new, but progress toward moving to value from a volume-based system has been slow, painstaking, and resisted by stakeholders. As discussed in the "Change Management" section of chapter 8, healthcare is plagued by high resistance to change.

The National Committee for Quality Assurance (NCQA) has also made striking observations about the US healthcare system. A report published in 2007 states, "Research shows that the quality of health care in America is, at best, imperfect, and, at worst, deeply flawed" (NCQA 2007).

In *Crossing the Quality Chasm*, IOM (2001) recommends that private and public purchasers, healthcare organizations, clinicians, and patients work together to redesign healthcare processes in accordance with the rules that follow:

1. **Care should be based on continuous healing relationships.** Patients should receive care whenever they need it and in many forms, not just through face-to-face visits. The health care system should be responsive at all times (24 hours a day, every day), and access to care should be provided over the Internet, by telephone, and by other means in addition to face-to-face visits.
2. **Care should be customized based on the patient's needs and values.** The system of care should be designed to meet the most common needs but should have the flexibility to respond to an individual patient's choices and preferences.
3. **The patient should be in control.** Patients should be given necessary information and the opportunity to exercise as much control as they choose over health care decisions that affect them. The health system should be able to accommodate differences in patient preferences and should encourage shared decision making.
4. **The system should encourage shared knowledge and the free flow of information.** Patients should have unfettered access to their own medical

information and to clinical information. Clinicians and patients should communicate effectively and share information.

5. **Decision making should be evidence-based.** Patients should receive care based on the best available scientific knowledge. Care should not vary illogically from clinician to clinician or from place to place.

6. **Safety should be a property of the system.** Patients should be safe from injury caused by the care system. Reducing risk and ensuring safety will require systems that help prevent and mitigate errors.

7. **The system should be transparent.** The health care system should make information available to patients and their families that allows them to make informed decisions when selecting a health plan, a hospital, or a clinical practice or when choosing among alternative treatments. Patients should be informed of the system's performance on safety, evidence-based practice, and patient satisfaction.

8. **The system should anticipate patients' needs.** The health system should be proactive in anticipating a patient's needs, rather than simply reacting to events.

9. **The system should constantly strive to decrease waste.** The health system should not waste resources or patients' time.

10. **The system should encourage cooperation among clinicians.** Clinicians and institutions should actively collaborate and communicate with each other to ensure that patients receive appropriate care.

The prevailing mind-set and attitude about quality and safety should be in alignment with the sentiment from this quote from *Antigone*, by Sophocles (2005): "All men make mistakes, but a good man yields when he knows his course is wrong, and repairs the evil. The only crime is pride." Errors of commission, errors of omission, errors of communication, errors of context, and diagnostic errors are all to blame. Furthermore, the human desire to be perfect contributes to the problem, not the solution (James 2013). The illusion of perfection is a point of view that is unrealistically held by the public. In the face of all these issues and variables surrounding patient safety and quality, leaders and managers of medical practices can no longer cling to the status quo.

THE TRIPLE AIM

Medical practices are at the forefront of population health management, as the medical practice is often the first contact patients have with the healthcare system. The Triple Aim is a cornerstone population health concept developed by Donald M. Berwick, MD, founder, president emeritus, and senior fellow of the Institute for Healthcare Improvement (IHI). In a sense, the approach has become national health policy in terms of the way many healthcare providers are beginning to think about healthcare. As shown in exhibit 10.2, the Triple Aim is focused on the following intersecting elements (IHI 2017):

EXHIBIT 10.2
The IHI Triple Aim

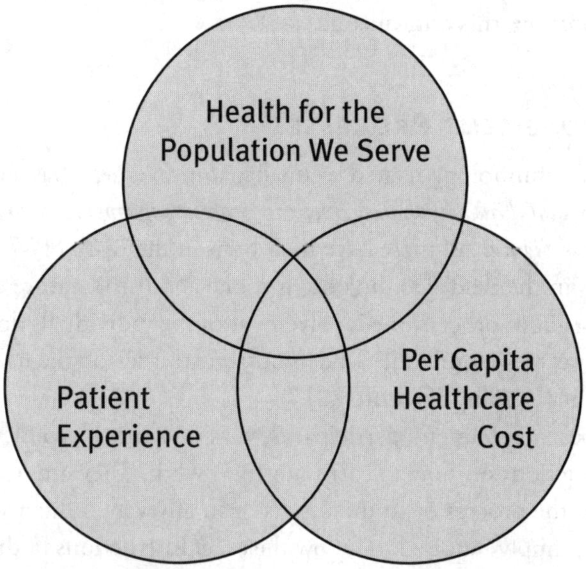

Source: Adapted from IHI (2017).

◆ *Per capita cost.* This component of the Triple Aim intends to lower the cost of care per person (not cost in aggregate, because as population increases, costs should naturally rise).

◆ *Patient experience.* The Triple Aim is concerned with patient experience because it has a huge impact on whether patients adhere to the treatment prescribed by providers. Evidence shows that patients who are satisfied with the care they receive and consider the care experience to be "good" are more likely to comply with the recommendations of their providers than are those who perceive their experience as unsatisfactory. Another benefit of consistently positive patient experiences is that it provides for an overall pleasant environment in the practice (Manary et al. 2013).

◆ *Better health for the population as well as the individual.* Considering the care of individual patients is no longer sufficient; to improve patient care, medical practices must take a broad look at the communities and populations served and develop strategies that improve the overall health of those groups.

Naturally, medical practices are focused on individuals and individual care. They want to achieve the best outcome for each patient. However, attending to the health of the entire population is important because small segments of that population use enormous amounts of healthcare resources, and society is asking the medical practice to take a substantial role in addressing this critical issue.

QUALITY IMPROVEMENT PROCESSES

Over the years, the terminology related to quality improvement has shifted from *quality improvement* (QI) to *total quality management* to *process improvement, Lean,* and *Six Sigma,* and now to *Lean Six Sigma.* All these have their basis in the work of W. Edwards Deming and other pioneers in the field. Deming often spoke about the nature of the process and outcomes, teaching about process, the involvement of the individuals doing the work, and how important it was to the outcome. To demonstrate this lesson, he used a tool called the red bead experiment (Deming Institute 2017).

In the red bead experiment, participants work on a mock production line. They are given specific instructions on how to carry out their work. They are not allowed to make any adjustments to the process or to the inputs or in any way influence how the result is produced. They are simply required to follow the exact instructions of their supervisor and "work hard."

The objective is to make white beads, not red beads. Some participants are given paddles containing small holes to accommodate the beads. They dip the paddle in a container full of red and white beads, shake off the excess, and take the paddle to an inspector, who counts the number of white beads the producer has made. Importantly, the inspector's role adds no value to the process. The process is repeated, and frustration mounts as the participants realize achieving the best outcome (producing all white beads) is impossible because the input of red and white beads into the paddle is random.

This simple but extremely effective experiential activity demonstrates the fact that the process is fundamental to the outcome of any activity. For example, over-reliance on incentives to deliver performance is misguided; instead, practices must rely on providers' internal motivation to do the right thing while having an environment and processes in place that create trust and allow employees to flourish. No one ever comes to work on any given day intending to do a poor job. When medical practices rely only on incentives to motivate members, they may accomplish their metrics, but as research has shown, they do not necessarily see improvement (Heidenreich et al. 2016). Metrics often are set too low to ensure success, and any failures to meet the metrics are easily explained. Practices must help all members of the practice evolve in terms of process improvement to contribute to and produce the outcomes desired by engaging teammates' greatest asset—their mind. In this section, we discuss a variety of tools for process improvement. All these tools should be used with discretion and judgment and with a skill base that develops over time.

VARIATION AND QI

Another important issue in quality and safety are the standards established for the work performed. Medical practices are now expected to create standard work processes that allow activities to be completed in the best way each time to reduce variation. Consider a practice that sees many patients each day. Several of those patients have similar attributes: the same diagnosis, the same gender, the same age, and so on. Why does one patient leave the practice pleased and praising the experience and another leave upset and threatening to never return? They saw the same provider, may even have been in the same corridor, and were seen in adjacent and presumably similar rooms. How could their experiences be so different? The answer is variation. Variation is the enemy of quality and of standard processes. In the absence of standards, tremendous variation emerges in all activities, producing a wide range of experiences and outcomes.

To illustrate this point further, conduct the "draw a pig" exercise, related to visual cues and carefully crafted instructions, known as standard work. The complete exercise can be found in the Minnesota Office of Continuous Improvement Toolkit (MNCI 2016). Briefly, participants are asked to perform four sequential stages of this exercise.

Stage 1:   Each participant is given a sheet of paper with nine equal squares on it. They are asked to draw a pig. Each participant is given two minutes to complete the activity. The facilitator collects all the papers, and the group views the outcomes. The results vary tremendously in the appearance of the pig (the outcome). Each person has applied his or her creativity in producing the pig, which is limited by each person's expertise in drawing. Significantly, many participants tend not to finish the exercise in the time allowed.

Stage 2:   Each participant is given a sheet of paper with nine equal squares on it, as in the first stage. The difference this time is the facilitator also provides a carefully written set of instructions on how to draw the pig. The participants are again given two minutes to draw the pig. Each person reads and interprets the instructions according to his or her own frame of reference. The facilitator again collects all the papers, and again the group sees a great deal of variation, albeit less than in stage 1. As in the first stage of the exercise, a number of the participants typically are unable to finish the activity in the time allowed.

Stage 3:   Each participant is again given a sheet of paper with nine equal squares on it. This time, the facilitator provides the group with instructions for drawing the pig as well as an image of what the final result should look like. The participants are given one minute to complete the task.

At the end of the time, the facilitator collects the drawings and finds that virtually everyone was able to complete the task, with a striking reduction in the variation of the drawings (see exhibit 10.3).

Stage 4: The participants review the group's drawings from each stage, further illustrating the points of the exercise.

The overall lesson from this exercise may be obvious, but it is a dramatic demonstration in an experiential learning framework that allows the participants to see the nature of variation as well as how important standard work is in reducing that variation. It also emphasizes the importance of experience in the work performed. The more learning opportunities of this nature that practice members experience, the more able they are to understand why similar patients may have very different experiences and perceive a difference in service in a practice.

The red bead experiment and the "draw a pig" exercise might be seen as contradictory. The red bead experiment implies that work should not be standardized and that workers should be involved in how the work is done, whereas the "draw a pig" exercise seems to support the notion that standardization improves quality by reducing variation. Both implications are true. Practices must standardize effective processes and continually

EXHIBIT 10.3
The Standard Pig

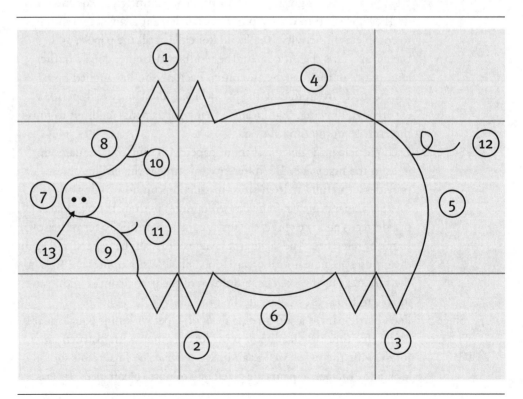

improve them through worker involvement. In that way, they provide the best methods of performing the work at any given time to all their patients.

Direct contact with the patient requires that professional judgment and variation be applied, but these direct contact processes, including front- and back-office operations and how patients flow through the practice, can all benefit from standardization.

LEAN

Regardless of a practice's size or the services it provides, a fundamental knowledge of the quality improvement process is essential. We can always do better, and we should always consider that opportunity in everything we do. The minute a practice stops improving or looking for opportunities to improve, it begins to stagnate. Staying the same in a medical practice is not an option.

Lean is a quality improvement process created by the Toyota Motor Company that focuses on the elimination of waste (Liker 2004). Waste is defined from the perspective of the customer—for medical practices, the patient—as unnecessary steps in a process or procedure that create no value for the customer.

The eight commonly identified types of waste in Lean are as follows:

◆ *Overproduction*, or doing more than is required or doing it earlier than needed.

◆ *Waiting*, for people, supplies, or activities, at any step in a process. Waiting to see the clinician, standing in line to register, or being on hold during a phone call are examples.

◆ *Transportation*, or getting people or things to their required locations. Moving mobile equipment from place to place is an example.

◆ *Inventory*, such as records, supplies, and unfinished work. Having unfinished charts or keeping more supplies at the work station than needed are examples.

◆ *Motion*, or extra steps taken because of inefficient layouts of the workplace. Having a work station far away from the examining rooms is an example.

◆ *Defects*, or rework that must be done because of an error. A lost lab test or record is an example; another is repeat phone calls to the practice due to slow follow-up.

◆ *Underutilization of people*, or having people work beneath their skill level and not listening to their ideas.

The time a patient waits to see a provider in a medical practice provides no value to the patient and, in fact, provides no value to the practice. In the author's experience, the number one complaint for many medical practices is waiting time: Of the more than 5,000 complaints reviewed, roughly 4,000 were related to complaints about wait times or delays in receiving test results. A typical Lean project in a medical practice undertaken to address patient wait times is demonstrated by the following story. The CEO of a well-known healthcare organization was showing a Lean master from Japan around the organization. With much pride, the CEO guided the master from place to place and gave a careful explanation of the services and aspects of each location. When they entered a waiting room, the Lean master asked, "What space is this?" The CEO replied, "It's a waiting room." The Lean master responded, "What waits here?" And the CEO, now startled, replied, "Patients, of course!" The Lean master said, "Didn't you know they were coming?" The CEO said, "Of course. Some of them have had appointments for almost a year." At that, the Lean master looked the CEO in the eye and said, "Aren't you ashamed?" He meant, shouldn't the practice be ashamed that it was not better prepared to receive patients even though it had ample time to do so? The CEO gained a new perspective following this visit (Virginia Mason Medical Center, personal communication, 2013).

The Lean master only asked questions up until the final statement. He was helping the CEO understand the nature of the situation, not simply telling him what it was. In addition, the story helps us see that we are often too interested in explaining why something is wrong or why it cannot be changed, rather than thinking deeply about how we might improve the situation. This excuse making may be particularly evident in healthcare because of the industry's reluctance to admit its shortcomings.

Another important aspect of Lean is visual management. Lean relies on visual management to be effective; this means going to see what is happening in the work area, not simply reading a report or reviewing second-hand information. Leaders must be present in the *gemba*, the place where the work occurs, and determine for themselves what is taking place. Reports and accounts by others have a biased frame of reference, are subject to misinterpretation, and in the rare case are intentionally deceptive. Visual management is an essential skill for the effective practice manager; it can even be practiced at some level in the largest provider practices.

The Five Whys

One Lean tool used for root cause analysis is known as "the five whys." If you ask why in response to each statement when looking at a situation, the root cause of the issue will emerge if "why" is asked enough times. Take the following example:

1. Why do patients have to wait? Because we do not allow enough time for each visit.

2.   Why? Because we have routinely scheduled patients at 15-minute intervals.

3.   Why? Because that's the way we have always done it, and we need to see a certain number of patients each day.

4.   Why? The providers often do not stay on schedule.

5.   Why? Because they're too busy.

All these answers hold the possibility for change. One can begin to see the nature of the five whys and its usefulness as a technique in root cause analysis. Implicit in the technique is the idea of helping others discover solutions and the causes of problems rather than relying on management to tell them what to do. A fundamental aspect of Lean leadership and management is to create problem solvers.

The Six Ss

Another easy-to-apply Lean tool is the six Ss. This technique is useful in helping practice members organize their work area. The steps include the following:

1.   *Sort*. Remove all unnecessary supplies and items from the work area. In essence, reduce the clutter.

2.   *Set*. Organize the remaining items in the work area in a way that is logical and useful.

3.   *Shine*. Clean the work area and inspect it for needed repairs.

4.   *Standardize*. Prepare written standards for how the workspace is to be organized, which may include labels or even outlines of where particular items are to be located.

5.   *Sustain*. Ensure that the standards are applied on a regular basis by inspecting the work area.

6.   *Safety*. Ensure that the work area is safe and free of visible hazards, such as electrical cords that create a trip hazard or medicines that are not stored properly and pose a poison hazard.

Success is achieved when waste created by a poorly organized work area is eliminated, thereby removing the need to look for supplies or equipment. This strategy can also eliminate the largest waste of all: an injury caused by unsafe working conditions (Jackson 2009).

CONDUCTING A LEAN PROJECT

The philosophy of continuous improvement is often referred to as *kaizen*, a Japanese business term, and can be used interchangeably with "Lean project." After a six S is completed, a more ambitious undertaking in the medical practice is a Lean process improvement project. Some additional training in Lean is advisable for those who wish to become proficient practitioners of the technique (Martin and Osterling 2007). A Lean process improvement project involves seven important steps:

Step 1: Introduce the Project

Introduction of the project is a critical first step in the process. All members of the team must understand the nature of and the desired outcome for the project. Also important is to gain commitment to the project from each team member.

Most practices have several issues that require attention and could benefit from an improvement project. On the basis of input from different areas of the practice, the leadership should select projects and prioritize them according to the greatest benefit to patients in the practice. Examples include reducing waiting time, reducing the time patients are left on hold when they call, reducing billing cycle time, reducing medical record error rates, and increasing immunization rates for children in the practice.

Practices need not undertake and complete one project at a time. In fact, multiple simultaneous projects may be considered, depending on the capacity of the practice.

Step 2: Define the Problem

Projects often fail because participants lack clarity about the nature of the project and, more specifically, a clear definition of the problem being addressed. Problem statements need to be concise, measurable, and within the power of the team to manage. For example, addressing Medicare regulations would be unrealistic for a process improvement team as they are beyond the power of the team to change them. Of course, a process that helps the practice comply with a particular regulation might be a worthy project.

Process improvement projects are always data driven. The process being examined must have measurable features that can be tracked over time as a way of measuring improvement. The adage, "You can't manage what you can't measure" is true for process improvement. The team must determine what metrics (measurements) will be collected for the project. Existing data are helpful for establishing a baseline measurement for the process.

A simple charter for the team can be used that indicates the purpose of the team, the problem it is addressing, and the desired outcome. Such a document helps prevent "scope creep," when the purpose and focus of the project begin to drift and the team loses sight of its original purpose. Certainly, revising the problem statement is necessary if the team discovers new information that better addresses the original concern. However, this decision should be made in a deliberate and orderly fashion.

Step 3: Introduce the Project, Form a Team

Unlike some approaches to problem solving in which the leadership or the manager makes the decision about what to do, effective QI procedure takes a team approach, such that the stakeholders of the process take part in improving the process. This notion stems from the understanding that those who perform the work have the greatest insight into how to improve any work process. The team should be multidisciplinary, as attention should always be paid to how the work comes to the practice, what the practice does with it, and who encounters the results of the work. These teams should be relatively small; five to seven members is often deemed an appropriate number, depending on the size of the practice.

One essential member of the team is a physician champion. This individual is a physician who has demonstrated an interest in the project, works well on teams, and has the time and inclination to serve on the team. A physician champion not only provides expertise but also represents the clinicians and can help explain and garner support for the project, which will be necessary for its acceptance and success.

Another valuable idea for beginning a process improvement activity is to start with a small issue first. This approach allows the group to develop expertise, experience some success, and gain a thorough knowledge of the concepts before beginning large, complex projects.

Step 4: Determine the Present Circumstances

Defining the current situation is crucial in process improvement. A process flowchart, also known as a value stream map, may be helpful in identifying all the parts of the process, particularly those areas that are of the greatest concern. Exhibit 10.4 illustrates a simple flowchart.

A flowchart defines an overall process, such as patient flow through the practice, or a subset of that operation, for example, the check-in process.

The critical points in the process flowchart include the input, which is the starting point of the process; the tasks performed using the input; and the production of an output, which can be further utilized in the operation.

The input should be carefully identified, as should each task and the desired output from the process. The pace of the process, or the time taken to perform each task, is called *takt time*. Takt time is often used as a metric in process improvement, especially in processes that seem to get bogged down and produce substantial waiting times or other unnecessary delays.

EXHIBIT 10.4
Simple Process
Flowchart

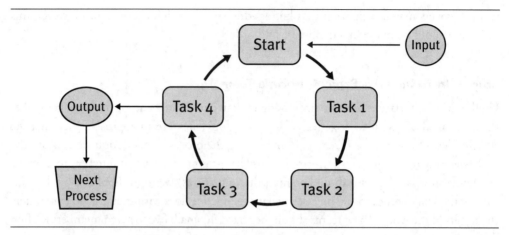

With a well-designed flowchart, the team should be able to identify areas that require improvement (Jackson 2013).

Step 5: Launch the Plan-Do-Study-Act Cycle

At this point in the Lean process, the team must determine what possible solutions may improve the process being examined, and a pilot of the solution should be tested. The Plan-Do-Study-Act (PDSA) cycle, discussed in chapter 8, allows the team to experiment with a proposed solution to determine its effectiveness in improving outcomes. As shown in exhibit 10.5, the PDSA cycle can be repeated with new ideas and solutions until an optimum outcome is achieved. At that point, new standard work is created to sustain the improvement over time. If new standard work is not documented and communicated to those involved in doing the work, the process quickly reverts to its old methodology. As the illustration shows, the new standard work becomes the wedge that prevents the improvement from going back in time.

Step 6: Implement the Improvement

Once the team is satisfied with the results of the pilot study, widespread implementation of the new standard work is deployed. This implementation requires careful communication, changes in job aides or procedure manuals, and any training to adopt the new process. The importance of this step must not be underestimated. Adequate time and attention must be taken to ensure acceptance and understanding of the new procedure. Variation is the enemy of quality, and implementing new standard work around important processes in the medical practice is essential to improving the outcome of practice activities.

Exhibit 10.5
Standard Work

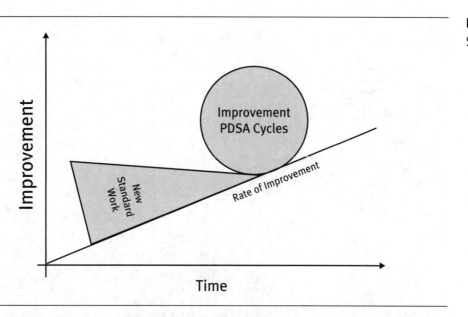

Step 7: Reflect on the Process

Every learning activity must be followed by reflection. This step provides an opportunity to ask what went well and what did not go as well as expected. What should the practice do differently next time to improve the process of quality improvement? It is also a good time to celebrate the success of the project. In this step, the three Rs are essential (ASQ 1996; Bicheno and Holweg 2008):

1. *Reflection.* What have you learned from this experience, not only in terms of the process being examined but of carrying out a Lean project?

2. *Reward.* The success and sometimes the simple completion of the project should be celebrated. Rewards can be simple recognitions of the efforts that individuals made in the learning.

3. *Renewal.* This is a good time for renewal and thinking about refocusing on the mission of the practice and on each member's role in producing the outcomes the practice wishes to achieve. That sense of renewal and refocus is instrumental in helping motivate and maintain the commitment necessary for optimal practice performance.

The IHI developed an informative and practical tip sheet, titled "The Seven Spreadly Sins," for successfully sharing the results of process improvement work to increase adoption and utilization of the new standard work (exhibit 10.6).

Exhibit 10.6
Tips for Sharing
Results from
Improvement Work

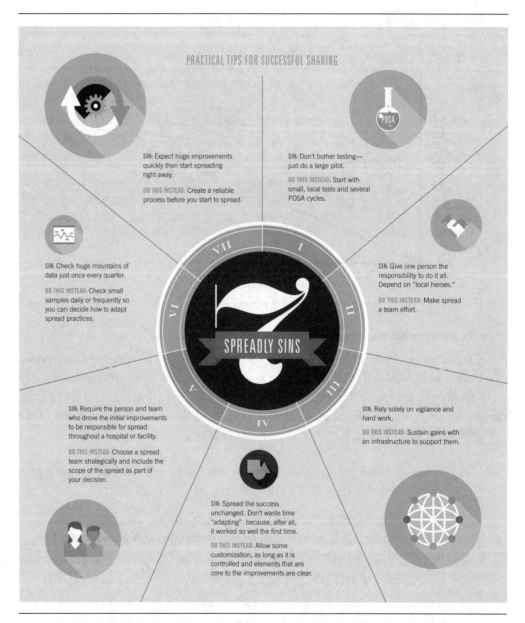

PRACTICAL TIPS FOR SUCCESSFUL SHARING

SIN: Expect huge improvements
quickly then start spreading
right away.

DO THIS INSTEAD: Create a reliable
process before you start to spread.

SIN: Don't bother testing—
just do a large pilot.

DO THIS INSTEAD: Start with
small, local tests and several
PDSA cycles.

SIN: Check huge mountains of
data just once every quarter.

DO THIS INSTEAD: Check small
samples daily or frequently so
you can decide how to adapt
spread practices.

SIN: Give one person the
responsibility to do it all.
Depend on "local heroes."

DO THIS INSTEAD: Make spread
a team effort.

SIN: Require the person and team
who drove the initial improvements
to be responsible for spread
throughout a hospital or facility.

DO THIS INSTEAD: Choose a spread
team strategically and include the
scope of the spread as part of
your decision.

SIN: Rely solely on vigilance and
hard work.

DO THIS INSTEAD: Sustain gains with
an infrastructure to support them.

SIN: Spread the success
unchanged. Don't waste time
"adapting" because, after all,
it worked so well the first time.

DO THIS INSTEAD: Allow some
customization, as long as it is
controlled and elements that are
core to the improvements are clear.

SPREADLY SINS

Source: IHI (2015). Used with permission.

Quality Improvement Tools

The art and science of quality improvement are not limited to Lean, and often many additional tools can be used in a Lean project or independently to help the manager and leaders of the practice address improvement issues. QI is a continuous process, and the following list of tools can be used to assist in identifying and managing quality issues (HRSA 2017):

◆   *Checklist or check sheet.* These simple tables or lists enumerate all the necessary steps or processes needed to complete a function. They are designed to assist the team or the individual performer and prevent him or her from forgetting any of the important steps in a process or procedure.

Atul Gawande brought new attention to using checklists as a way of reducing errors and increasing quality in surgery. The concept stems from the fact that human beings can only focus on so much at one time and cannot always remember to do everything in a complex sequence of activities (Gawande 2011). Reason (1990) adds that unaided recall is only about 90 percent accurate, which, for activities as important as healthcare delivery, is simply not good enough. In the Six Sigma methodology (discussed later in this chapter), "good enough" is represented by an error rate of 3.4 defects per million opportunities, of six standard deviations (6σ) from the mean, or 99.997 percent error free, as shown in exhibit 10.7.

Relying on human accuracy only, one might expect ten defects per hundred opportunities, or 100,000 errors per million opportunities, versus 3.4 if 6σ is achieved (Total defects ÷ Total opportunities × 1,000,000).

◆   *Control chart.* A control chart is used to measure the variation in a process over time. It records the activity of a process as a single line plot and indicates the upper and lower limits the process has produced. The wider the limits, the more variation is in the process, and this kind of chart allows the user to determine when the process is out of control and if the cause of the variation is due to special causes or normal variation.

◆   *Strengths, weaknesses, opportunities, and threats (SWOT) analysis.* As discussed in chapter 5, SWOT analysis is a way to capture the strengths, weaknesses, opportunities, and threats of the practice as part of a strategic planning or evaluation process.

◆   *Run chart.* Similar to a control chart, a run chart measures a process over time as a single line measure. It is the simplest form of plotting activity. Unlike the control chart, it does not contain upper and lower limits.

◆   *Fishbone diagram.* These diagrams are also known as Ishikawa diagrams or cause-and-effect diagrams, which is more descriptive of their use. The fishbone diagram is a visual way of capturing possible root causes of a problem.

◆   *Scatterplot.* These plots are simple graphs depicting two variables as discrete events on two axes as a way to determine a potential correlation.

◆   *Nodes of influence analysis.* This is an analytical tool for determining who in any group of people has influence on the other members of the group.

EXHIBIT 10.7

Graphic
Representation of
Six Sigma

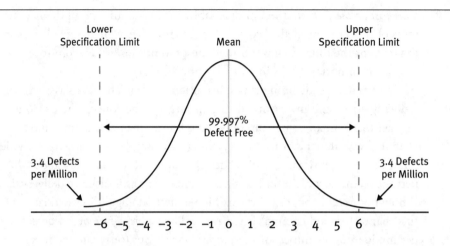

This technique is useful when determining the key individuals to enlist in introducing change to a practice.

◆ *Brainstorming*. Usually conducted with facilitation, brainstorming is a technique for obtaining input from a group without placing undue influence on the individual members of the group, thereby obtaining many ideas from the maximum number of people.

◆ *Affinity chart*. This tool provides a method for organizing key themes from a brainstorming activity.

◆ *Focus group*. For this type of information gathering, members of a target group are convened to obtain facilitated input on issues or questions important to the practice.

◆ *Focused conversation*. Similar to the focus group, a focused conversation usually involves a facilitator and the issues or questions are related to particular issues or questions. However, focused conversations typically are conducted with only one or two individuals.

◆ *Appreciative inquiry*. This method seeks input from stakeholders by asking for examples of when they have had a positive experience. For example, a medical practice might ask a patient an appreciative inquiry question similar to this: "Tell me about a time when you received excellent care." With this approach, the facilitator is able to glean important information about what made the visit a positive experience. It also focuses on the positive rather than simply looking for the counterfactual in reviewing complaints, and it does not presume an understanding of what patients expect. We often like to think we know, but we usually don't.

◆ *Histogram.* This tool is a simple graph consisting of rectangular bars that represent proportional frequency of the process or activity being measured. It provides a means to convey information quickly and in a way that illustrates variation.

◆ *Pie chart.* This simple graph illustrates a group of data where each section of a circle represents a proportion of the whole. Pie charting is one of the simplest ways to present information.

◆ *Prioritization matrix.* A prioritization matrix is a simple tool to sort a diverse group of items by order of priority. The priority is determined by the criteria of the user.

Six Sigma

Six Sigma was developed by Bill Smith at Motorola Corporation (Aveta Business Institute 2016) and was based in part on the work of Walter Shewhart, a statistical process control engineer and mathematician (Shewhart and Deming 2011) and on the concept of the normal curve, which dates back to the research of Carl Gauss in the eighteenth century (Tent 2006).

As with all work that relies on statistical analysis, Six Sigma looks at inputs as a function of their output. This relationship can be expressed as

$$Y = f(x),$$

where Y is the inputs, and the outcome is a function (f) of the individual components (x) that drive outcome.

Six Sigma uses the DMAIC methodology to work through improvement processes as follows:

1. *Define* what is critical to the patient, and map those processes at a high level.

2. *Measure* the inputs by planning the data collection to validate that the measurements are accurate. Establishing baseline measures for the processes

being studied is a key activity in DMAIC. This step also includes identifying the variables that are most responsible for producing the desired outcome.

3.   *Analyze* by using statistical methodology to test which inputs have the greatest influence on the outcome.

4.   *Improve* by designing solutions and selecting one to pursue and then determining the controls and type of culture needed to prove its effectiveness and sustain it.

5.   *Control* by developing feedback loops, creating a process control plan to sustain the gains implemented, and then replicating the cycle.

Six Sigma allows organizations to convert a practical issue into statistical terms and then find a statistical solution that is then implemented in practice. For example, when looking at wait times, a medical practice measures them to identify the components that affect the wait time, performs statistical analysis to determine those components that are most important, creates a solution that should address them, and implements the suggested solution. Say the overall wait time from check-in to leaving the practice following the visit is 15 minutes on average. The practice notes that the check-in portion of this wait creates a significant increase in the patient's overall waiting time at the office and institutes a solution—routine preregistration—that is expected to reduce check-in time. By reducing check-in time, the practice reduces overall wait time.

As with Lean, most Six Sigma practitioners receive training on the tools and techniques involved (Barry, Brubaker, and Murcko 2002; Pyzdek and Keller 2014).

One debate that surfaces from time to time in QI circles is whether to use Six Sigma or Lean strategies. On the one hand, achieving an error rate of 6σ, the "namesake" goal of the Six Sigma methodology, or 3.4 defects per million opportunities, is such a daunting prospect that people feel demoralized and unable to commit to the QI process. Lean, on the other hand, focuses on improvement without placing a value judgment on the magnitude of that improvement. Although the ideal aim is to maximize the opportunities to improve the care provided to patients and the processes that serve the practice, the Lean process tends to be more palatable in practice than Six Sigma is.

That said, Six Sigma is often very effective in the hands of skilled quality improvement practitioners. The primary differences between Lean and Six Sigma are illustrated in exhibit 10.8.

As a rule of thumb, use Lean when streamlining any process and reducing process waste; use Six Sigma when process metrics are more difficult to collect or understand and project success requires analysis of multiple inputs. These are often chronic problems. Regardless of the strategy chosen, success hinges on applying the right tools.

EXHIBIT 10.8
Comparison of
Lean and Six
Sigma

Lean = Improvement focused on improving patient flow and eliminating the eight deadly wastes.	Six Sigma = Process breakthroughs, design, or improvement. Teams focused on eliminating chronic problems and reducing variation in processes.
• Define value • Measure • Analyze process (flow) • Improve process (pull) • Create new standard work (for the improvement)	• Define • Measure • Analyze • Improve • Control

DATA ANALYTICS

Data analytics is discussed in detail in chapter 12 because it plays a big role in the future of healthcare. In this section, we introduce data analytics in the context of QI.

Data are useless unless they can be turned into information that can be acted on. The lack of utility of the enormous amounts of data generated by the healthcare system has been a significant issue in the field. Paper records, multiple sources of records, and the general inability to bring information together to make sense of it are just some of the barriers to using data effectively.

Consider this story: As a population health strategy, a large multispecialty practice aims to determine if A1c levels—an important measurement of diabetic control in patients—are recorded not only for all diabetic patients but also for patients diagnosed with a heart condition. Despite the meaningful use mandates, the practice has not yet converted its paper-based charts to an electronic health record system. In the absence of digital retrieval capabilities, the practice manager begins the data collection process by asking for a list, by chart number, of the records for all relevant patients. Next, he asks the medical records department to pull each of the charts on the list to check if an A1c level was recorded. When he receives the first hundred charts, he looks at the first chart and notes that the A1c level is not recorded, even though this chart is for a diabetic patient. He walks back to the medical records department to see if the laboratory record was simply not placed in the chart. Receiving an inconclusive answer, he seeks out the provider to verify that the A1c level was ordered. Ultimately, he cannot find any A1c data for this patient. He cannot be sure if the test was performed; the only verifiable information he obtained is that the level was not recorded.

How does a practice in this situation collect the data necessary to conduct population health activities and monitor the effectiveness of the practice without an efficient data collection process? The conclusion is obvious: Practices must develop digital systems to collect and manage patient information to improve the health of a patient population. Payers and patients alike are demanding such capabilities.

Making decisions on the basis of large sets of data without the use of powerful analytical tools is beyond the capacity of the human mind and any manual capability. However, the use of these tools is still fragmented and uneven in healthcare, especially in small medical practices. Without data analytics, the practice can be distracted by its paradigms and beliefs, which may obscure reality. We must use data to drive decisions, reduce bias, and effect improvements in the delivery of care.

DISCUSSION QUESTIONS

1. Describe the difference between "removing the bad" and "moving mean performance" for improving practice quality.

2. Describe each component of the Triple Aim and its importance to the US healthcare delivery system.

3. Identify and discuss the principles of Lean process improvement.

4. Write a brief outline of the steps in the Lean process.

5. How do Lean and Six Sigma differ?

6. Identify the components of the PDSA cycle, and discuss how each component is used in quality improvement.

7. Discuss the "seven spreadly sins." Why are they important to quality improvement?

REFERENCES

American Society for Quality (ASQ). 1996. *Handbook for Basic Process Improvement*. Published May. http://rube.asq.org/gov/handbook-for-basic-process-improvement.pdf.

Aveta Business Institute. 2016. "The History and Development of Six Sigma." Accessed July 7. www.sixsigmaonline.org/six-sigma-training-certification-information/the-history-and-development-of-six-sigma.

Barry, R., C. Brubaker, and A. Murcko. 2002. *The Six Sigma Book for Healthcare: Improving Outcomes by Reducing Errors*. Chicago: Health Administration Press.

Bicheno, J., and M. Holweg. 2008. *The Lean Toolbox: The Essential Guide to Lean Transformation*, 4th ed. Johannesburg, South Africa: Picsee.

Deming Institute. 2017. "Red Bead Experiment." Accessed May 22. https://deming.org/management-system/red-bead-experiment.

Gawande, A. 2011. *The Checklist Manifesto: How to Get Things Right*. New York: Picador.

Health Resources and Services Administration (HRSA). 2017. "Quality Improvement." Accessed May 23. www.hrsa.gov/quality/toolbox/methodology/qualityimprovement.

Heidenreich, P., P. Solis, M. Estes, G. Fonarow, C. Jurgens, J. Marine, D. McManus, and R. McNamara. 2016. "2016 AHA Clinical Performance and Quality Measures for Adults with Atrial Fibrillation or Atrial Flutter." *Circulation: Cardiovascular Quality and Outcomes* 9: 443–88.

Institute for Healthcare Improvement (IHI). 2017. "Triple Aim for Populations." Accessed May 22. www.ihi.org/Topics/TripleAim/Pages/default.aspx.

———. 2015. "Seven Spreadly Sins." Cambridge, MA: IHI.

Institute of Medicine (IOM). 2001. *Crossing the Quality Chasm: A New Health System for the 21st Century*. Washington, DC: National Academies Press.

———. 2000. *To Err Is Human: Building a Safer Health System*. Washington, DC: National Academies Press.

Jackson, T. 2013. *Mapping Clinical Value Streams*. Washington, DC: Rona Consulting Group and Productivity Press.

———. 2009. *5S for Healthcare*. Washington, DC: Productivity Press.

James, J. 2013. "A New, Evidence-Based Estimate of Patient Harms Associated with Hospital Care." *Journal of Patient Safety* 9 (3): 122–28.

Liker, J. 2004. *The Toyota Way*. New York: McGraw-Hill Education.

Makary, M. A., and M. Daniel. 2016. "Medical Error—the Third Leading Cause of Death in the US." Published May 3. www.bmj.com/content/bmj/353/bmj.i2139.full.pdf.

Manary, M. P., W. Boulding, R. Staelin, and S. W. Glickman. 2013. "The Patient Experience and Health Outcomes." *New England Journal of Medicine* 368: 201–3.

Martin, K., and M. Osterling. 2007. *The Kaizen Event Planner: Achieving Rapid Improvement in Office, Service, and Technical Environments*. Washington, DC: Productivity Press.

McKesson Corporation. 2016. "Value-Based Reimbursement vs. Volume-Based Care." Accessed July 1. www.mckesson.com/population-health-management/population-health/know-the-challenges.

Miller, H. 2009. "From Volume to Value: Better Ways to Pay for Health Care." *Health Affairs* 28 (5): 1418–28.

Minnesota Office of Continuous Improvement (MNCI). 2016. "CI Toolbox." Accessed July 4. https://mn.gov/admin/continuous-improvement/resources/projects/toolbox.

Mosadeghrad, A. M. 2014. "Factors Influencing Healthcare Service Quality." *International Journal of Health Policy and Management* 3 (2): 77–89.

National Committee for Quality Assurance (NCQA). 2007. *The Essential Guide to Health Care Quality*. Washington, DC: NCQA.

Network for Regional Health Improvement. 2008. *From Volume to Value: Transforming Health Care Payment and Delivery Systems to Improve Quality and Reduce Costs*. New York: Robert Wood Johnson Foundation.

Pyzdek, T., and P. Keller. 2014. *The Six Sigma Handbook*, 4th ed. New York: McGraw-Hill Education.

RAND Corporation. 2006. "The First National Report Card on Quality of Health Care in America." Santa Monica, CA: RAND.

Reason, J. 1990. *Human Error*. Cambridge, UK: Cambridge University Press.

Shewhart, W., and W. E. Deming. 2011. *Statistical Method from the Viewpoint of Quality Control*. Mineola, NY: Dover.

Sophocles. 2005 (441 B.C.). *Antigone*. Clayton, DE: Prestwick House.

Tent, M. B. W. 2006. *The Prince of Mathematics: Carl Friedrich Gauss*. Natick, MA: A K Peters/CRC Press.

CHAPTER 11

EMERGENCY MANAGEMENT AND THE MEDICAL PRACTICE

An investment in knowledge pays the best interest.

—Benjamin Franklin

LEARNING OBJECTIVES

➤ Appreciate the need for emergency planning and management in the medical practice.

➤ Understand the connection between the medical practice and the community in the context of emergency planning and management.

➤ Identify the key resources typically available in the community for managing an emergency.

➤ Recognize the steps of an emergency plan and their functions.

➤ Be able to develop an emergency plan for a medical practice.

INTRODUCTION

In 1990, the administrator for a medical practice at a health system in Louisville, Kentucky, left his downtown office to visit one of the medical clinics he helped manage. Something about how his day was progressing drew him to that office. Upon entering the practice, he approached the appointment desk, where he saw Dr. Patrick Casey, a young family practitioner. He said, "Dr. Casey, how's it going today?"

Dr. Casey replied, "Well, it's actually my day off, but I have a very difficult patient who needs to go to the hospital. I just came in to try and convince him to get the services he needs."

A few other pleasantries were exchanged, and the two walked toward the examination room. Upon arriving outside the exam room, the administrator placed his arm around Dr. Casey and told him to take care and enjoy the rest of his day off. He then turned the corner, leaving Dr. Casey to enter the exam room to see his patient.

In a matter of seconds, a gun shot rang out, and then another. It was hard to fathom at first what the sound was, but it soon became apparent that someone was shooting in the building. The administrator immediately asked people to leave the building or hide as quickly as possible. He told them that shots had been fired and that the situation was unclear. A 911 call was placed immediately, and the administrator headed to the pharmacy on the other side of the building while ushering people along the way to the safest possible locations, either sheltering in place or exiting the building. Reaching the pharmacy, he informed the staff of the situation; they sheltered in place and waited as law enforcement officers secured the building.

In the aftermath of the emergency, the administrator learned that Dr. Casey had been shot when he entered the exam room by the patient waiting to see him. The patient then turned the gun on himself. Dr. Casey died almost immediately, as did the patient. (*Courier-Journal* staff 1990).

This is a true story, and the administrator was the author of this text. This event was a defining moment of my career because it helped me realize the unthinkable can happen and we must be prepared for that possibility. It brought into focus what it means to lead in a difficult time, during unfamiliar events. I also knew I had to do more to prepare as an administrator to deal with emergencies.

In the past, the need for emergency preparedness and emergency management in the medical practice was limited. In general emergency or disaster situations, medical offices could close the practice if needed, allowing emergency matters to be dealt with by community agencies and the local hospitals. As in many small businesses, the threat of active shooters and other similar emergencies was rare and not a high priority in terms of preparedness for the practice.

THE NEW NATURE OF EMERGENCIES

That thinking is beginning to change. It has become clear that the nature and types of emergencies playing out in a wide range of communities pose threats to the safety and protection of the patients and employees of the practice. In addition, as we have learned from disasters such as 9/11, Hurricane Katrina, incidents such as Dr. Casey's death, and other catastrophic situations, emergencies do affect medical practices, and their scope can be virtually unimaginable. The need to marshal all the community's medical resources, in conjunction with community, state, regional, and federal agencies in emergency preparedness and management, has become clear.

The Medical Group Management Association defines a practice emergency as any incident or activity that disrupts the practice for more than 24 hours (Gans 2016). Medical practices may be exposed to several categories of emergency, including the following:

◆ Natural events, such as weather conditions

◆ Acts of violence, such as an active shooter or a violent patient

◆ Building-related emergencies, such as a fire

◆ Public health outbreaks, such as Ebola or Zika, or even influenza

Medical practices have become sophisticated in their understanding that the scope of an emergency may be such that it requires all available resources be brought to bear to resolve or survive it. Every practice manager and leader must have a basic knowledge of emergency preparedness and management. In addition, each practice needs to have an emergency preparedness plan in place—and review it routinely—should the need arise to enact it.

Emergency planning must focus on protecting the human resources of the practice; safeguarding the practice's assets; and managing patients in terms of capacity, flow, and degree of injury or illness in a wide-scale emergency scenario. Practices have numerous options for the type and format of plan they adopt, and these options need to be examined and procedures developed in accordance with the other existing policies of the practice. These plans and procedures must also be communicated to all stakeholders, including the providers, nonclinical staff, community members, and patients.

Options for medical practices during an emergency include the following:

◆ Close the practice and refer all patients to the nearest hospital emergency department or urgent care center.

◆ Close the office to face-to-face encounters and perform telephone triage only, such as assisting patients in refilling prescriptions and providing guidance to patients seeking an alternative channel of care.

◆ Remain open and care for those needing urgent attention.

◆ Assign the clinical staff and critical support staff to work with local emergency facilities to address the care needs of the community.

◆ Join the Medical Reserve Corps (MRC) and perform duties in accordance with the community's needs. The MRC operates under the purview of the US Department of Homeland Security; local groups are formed that are primarily made up of both retired and practicing clinicians (Ready.gov 2017).

This list reflects progressive levels of involvement in emergency management, but all require substantial consideration and planning, from how alternative operating procedures work to what contribution the practice is willing to make to community preparedness and response.

Effective emergency planning depends on the ability to anticipate and play out multiple scenarios (scenario development) and the potential responses to those scenarios. Often, practice personnel must think in terms of the unimaginable—events that were once a far-fetched thought but now are not unrealistic. In the case of Hurricane Hugo in 1990, no hurricane of that magnitude had ever reached Charlotte, North Carolina, in recorded history. Charlotte-based medical providers were unable to reach many facilities because the roadways were completely obstructed by trees and other debris (Lyttle 2014). It was the unimaginable scenario that is now possible.

Questions that practices need to consider as they select and develop an emergency plan are as follows:

◆ What are the patients' expectations of the practice in an emergency scenario?

◆ Do patients expect the practice to be open and available for their care in a widespread emergency?

◆ Will you treat patients who present without records? If so, how?

◆ What resources and personnel is the practice willing and able to provide in case of a local, regional, or national emergency?

◆ What alternative operating plans do you have for the practice?

— What if the Internet is down and other communication methods (e.g., landline, cell phone) are unavailable?

— What contingencies are in place for emergencies that damage the office building or limit access to medical records and other information?

To address the last question, for example, off-site storage and ready availability of records are essential. Next to its people, a medical practice's records are its most important asset. Without the medical, billing, and other records, you are literally and figuratively out of business.

Prior to events such as 9/11 in 2001; Hurricane Katrina in 2005; and the devastating EF-5 tornado in Joplin, Missouri, in 2011, medical practices did not always think about the scope of disasters. Years ago, practices commonly stored records in a nearby location, but Katrina taught us a lesson: A disaster of regional proportions may destroy any local storage locations, giving the term *off-site* new meaning.

In the electronic age, of course, the US healthcare system has become dependent on all manner of electronic systems. Planning, policies, procedures, and drills for "downtime"—regardless of the cause—are essential for all medical practices so that they may meet the expectation of the practice to operate during outages or emergencies.

The expectations of patients in these unusual circumstances need to be understood by the practice, and the intentions of the practice to meet those expectations must be understood by the patients. Of course, the type of practice has an important bearing on this determination. Practices that routinely see life-threatening emergencies and acute situations may find locating alternative channels of care difficult and thus may be likely to remain open under disaster-related circumstances even if it is with a small staff dealing only with the most urgent needs.

THE KEY DILEMMA

One dilemma that any medical practice faces with emergency preparedness and management is whether the practice expends valuable resources to prepare for an event that has a low probability of occurrence but that, once it occurs, brings devastation, making the failure to prepare for it costly.

An important aspect of this dilemma is the ongoing nature of emergency preparedness. Although some organizations do a good job in the planning process, they often fail to keep those plans current and engage in activities to keep staff aware and prepared. If the staff of a practice is unfamiliar with and poorly trained in emergency preparedness plans, those plans may be of little use in an actual emergency. The onset of an emergency is not the time to dust off the plan and read it.

The need for emergency management of the medical practice exists at two levels. The first level is management of the medical practice in emergencies, dealing with the practice itself and its medical and nonmedical staff. The second level is characterized by the need for medical personnel to be called on to assist in the broader community emergencies because so many emergencies, whether arising from natural disasters, terrorist attacks, or epidemics, require medical assistance. With this understanding, the importance of emergency management may obviate the need for a practice to decide between two aspects of the cost dilemma.

EMERGENCY MANAGEMENT

As mentioned earlier, at least a basic understanding of the principles and scope of emergency management are helpful to the modern medical practice's management and leadership (Markenson and Reilly 2011). Emergency management encompasses a number of good management practices, such as clear and concise communication and careful planning and training.

Furthermore, although a practice may elect to not be involved in community or regional emergency preparedness and emergency management (EP/EM) efforts, it should be aware of the EP/EM activities and programs where the practice resides. Exhibit 11.1 illustrates the levels of education outreach that typically exist in communities today. Depending on a medical practice's scope, size, and resources, it may be asked to play a significant role in EP/EM.

EXHIBIT 11.1
Education and
Outreach

Preparedness is the shared responsibility of all levels of government, the private and nonprofit sectors, and individual citizens.

Education and outreach are designed to reach out to all partners in preparedness, educate them about their roles, and engage them in the preparedness process.

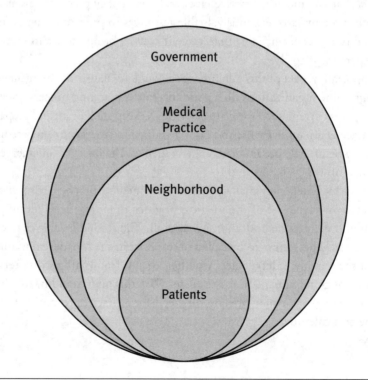

Emergency management is framed by four phases (FEMA 2007):

1. *Mitigation*—those activities a practice undertakes to lessen the severity and impact a potential disaster or emergency may have on its operations.

2. *Preparedness*—those activities a practice undertakes to build capacity and identify resources that may be used should a disaster or emergency occur. In preparedness planning, community integration is key. Community integration is a process of developing relationships with and a mutual commitment to other providers in the community, which can be called on in an emergency to share resources or staff or to accept patients.

3. *Response*—activities that take place at the time of an actual emergency.

4. *Recovery*—a plan to continue or reestablish business operations that involves

    a. disaster recovery, either short or long term;

    b. insurance coverage;

    c. inventory systems;

    d. information systems;

    e. outsourcing of care provision, if necessary;

    f. security, of both facility and documents;

    g. potential to provide assistance to staff; and

    h. public relations and communications with stakeholders.

DEVELOPING AN EMERGENCY PREPAREDNESS PLAN FOR THE PRACTICE

Preparing an emergency plan for the practice is essential for effectively addressing the practice's needs during an emergency or a disaster. The plan must be kept as simple as possible to do the job; it needs to be understandable and usable, not dense with unnecessary detail.

A plan offers a sense of organization, confidence, and awareness for practice members should an emergency arise. Calm demeanor is a key to effectively dealing with emergencies, and a well-designed and -implemented plan helps instill an atmosphere of calm under stressful situations. Recall the story of Captain Chesley "Sully" Sullenberger, the US Air pilot who guided a damaged aircraft to a controlled crash landing on the Hudson River, saving all aboard. He and his crew exhibited no panic, just a calm, well-practiced execution of emergency procedures. Captain Sully had practiced for this potential event on numerous occasions, and his instincts and skill set were honed by those experiences. Medical practices need to be at that same level of readiness to deal with emergencies that arise (Prochnau and Parker 2009).

A necessary first step is to consider the requirements of an emergency preparedness plan from the points of view of all stakeholders affected by the emergency. Often, an emergency preparedness plan is seen as a mandate rather than a living, useful document and is given little additional thought. Practices must avoid this trap and instead put deliberate effort into thinking about who will use the plan, what components will help them in an emergency, and how usable it will be to deploy in the case of a disaster. Many emergency plans are incredibly detailed and overly complex, and they will never be put in effect in an emergency. For example, think about how individuals learn and follow instructions, as with the draw-a-pig exercise in chapter 10. The level of variation demonstrated in that exercise applies to any process or plan, and that variation needs to be accounted for when devising a plan for an emergency.

One recommended method for emergency planning is the all-hazards preparation framework. A medical practice rarely knows with certainty what type of emergency might beset it, even for those practices that undertake a careful analysis of vulnerabilities (vulnerability analyses are discussed in more detail later in the chapter). However, common occurrences characterize any emergency or disaster situation and dictate the need to take the following measures:

◆ Safeguard people

◆ Safeguard property

◆ Ensure communications

◆ Develop alternative operations

◆ Manage the expectations of each member of the practice

Many free educational courses on emergency planning and management are available from the Federal Emergency Management Agency (FEMA) at https://training.fema.gov/.

Exhibit 11.2 illustrates the planning cycle. Note that the plan requires consideration of the nature of the practice and how to equip practice members to respond to emergencies. Training is critical, including exercises for improving proficiency and evaluation and enhancement of the emergency plan. So often, plans are left untested and untouched, and then, of course, they work at a suboptimal level when implemented.

Developing an emergency management plan also requires consideration of the threats and hazards that might be faced by the practice. This process is known as vulnerability analysis (VA). Exhibit 11.3 illustrates the sequence of events needed to complete this portion of the planning process.

Exhibit 11.2
Preparedness
Cycle

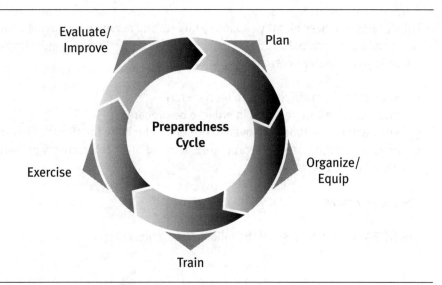

Source: FEMA (2016c).

Of particular importance are the following factors:

◆ *Continuity of the facility*—Is the facility habitable and safe to be used by staff and patients? Are alternative plans in place for having facilities available to the practice to see patients and conduct the work of the practice?

◆ *Continuity of communications*—Are mechanisms in place to communicate with all stakeholders? For example, for your particular practice, should you reach your constituents using social media, e-mail, telephone trees, emergency communications over television or radio broadcast stations, or some combination of these? Should you deploy a special website or front web page that provides a status report on the practice that can be accessed by stakeholders? In large-scale disasters, electronic services may be severely curtailed or overwhelmed, so multiple communication strategies should be considered.

◆ *Essential record-keeping*—What records are essential to see you through this situation, and how are the records safeguarded? Patients being treated under emergencies require documentation of that treatment not only for future care but for liability purposes as well.

◆ *Human resources*—What is your practice doing to safeguard staff? To what extent, if any, are they expected to work in an emergency scenario? Are special

EXHIBIT 11.3
Threat and Hazard
Identification and
Risk Assessment
(THIRA)

THIRA helps practices identify capability targets and resource requirements necessary to address anticipated and unanticipated risks. Specifically, conducting a THIRA can help your practice determine the following:

- What does the practice need to prepare for?
- What resources are required in order to be prepared?
- What actions could be employed to lessen or eliminate the threat or hazard?
- What impacts need to be incorporated onto the practice's recovery preparedness planning?

The THIRA Process

The THIRA process consists of the following four basic steps:

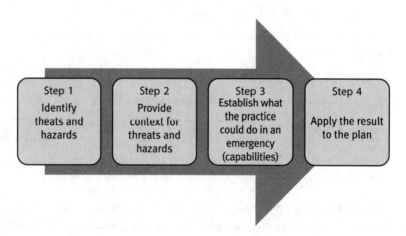

Step 1: The first step is to develop a list of practice-specific threats and hazards based on past experience, forecasting, expert judgement, and available resources.

Step 2: The second step is to add context descriptions to each identified threat and hazard that

- outline the conditions under which a threat or hazard might occur and
- clarify how the timing and location of an incident affect the practice's ability to manage it.

Step 3: The third step is to establish capability targets for each core capability. Capability targets define success and describe what the practice wants to achieve for each core capability. This step looks at

EXHIBIT 11.3
Threat and Hazard
Identification and
Risk Assessment
(THIRA) *(continued)*

- impacts and desired outcomes and how they support development of capability targets,
- guidance on how to develop capability targets, and
- examples of completed capability targets.

Step 4: In step 4, communities apply the results of the THIRA by estimating the resources required to meet capability targets. Communities express resource requirements as a list of resources needed to successfully manage their threats and hazards. It covers the following:

- Capability estimation
- Resource typing, including National Incident Management System–type resources and other standardized resource types
- How to build a completed resource requirement list
- How communities may apply these results to resource allocation decisions and mitigation activities

human resource policies in place regarding pay and other forms of support? If not, should such support be considered? If the practice were unable to operate over an extended period, would any or all staff be laid off, or would they be maintained to help in the recovery phase?

The practice must consider its exercise methodology and how it will bring about the training needed to effectively respond to an emergency. Some of those considerations are shown in exhibit 11.4.

Once the exercise plan is developed, practice managers and leaders must determine how the plan will be implemented. Exercises that the practice can undertake are available in numerous formats. Exhibit 11.5 illustrates some commonly used discussion-based and operationally based exercises for improving response skills as well as the understanding of the emergency plan.

WHO IS AN EMERGENCY MANAGER?

Depending on the size of the practice, the emergency planner for the practice may be the practice manager or administrator or another staff member with an interest in assuming this role. Although designating an emergency planner is important, disaster preparedness should be everyone's job in the practice. Many organizations offer training and information for emergency managers at all levels of expertise, from novice to

EXHIBIT 11.4
Emergency
Preparedness
Exercise
Methodology

The Homeland Security Exercise and Evaluation Program (HSEEP) provides a standardized methodology for planning and conducting individual exercises. The process includes four phases:

- Exercise design and development
- Exercise conduct
- Exercise evaluation
- Improvement planning

Do you have preparations for:

- Determining long-term training and exercise goals and objectives for your practice?
- Creating a multiyear training and exercise plan?
- Identifying members of a planning team?
- Designing and developing training and exercises to achieve your identified goals and objectives?
- Conducting the training and exercises developed by your planning team?
- Evaluating your training and exercises, including development of After Action Reflection?
- Translating lessons learned into measurable steps for improving your practice's response capabilities?
- Assigning responsibility and setting timelines for implementing improvements, and tracking their completion?
- Sharing with others the lessons learned from training and exercising?

Source: Adapted from FEMA (2016c).

expert. Currently, many of these organizations are governmental, as protecting residents has historically been a primary function of government. Internet-based documents, templates, and information are often the most useful because emergency preparedness and management is a rapidly evolving field with new information developed on a continuous basis, rendering other media less useful. The following are useful websites for emergency management resources:

- ◆ Centers for Disease Control and Prevention (CDC)

    — http://emergency.cdc.gov

    — http://emergency.cdc.gov/health-professionals.asp

Exhibit 11.5
Types of
Emergency
Preparedness
Exercises

Exercises fall within two broad categories:

Discussion-Based Exercises

Discussion-based exercises center on participant discussion. They familiarize participants with current plans, policies, agreements, and procedures, or may be used to develop new plans, policies, agreements, and procedures.

Type	Description
Seminar	A seminar is an informal discussion, designed to orient participants to new or updated plans, policies, or procedures (e.g., a seminar to review a new evacuation standard operating procedure).
Workshop	A workshop resembles a seminar, but is employed to build specific products, such as a draft plan or policy (e.g., a training and exercise plan workshop is used to develop a multiyear training and exercise plan).
Tabletop exercise	A tabletop exercise involves key personnel discussing simulated scenarios in an informal setting. Tabletops can be used to assess plans, policies, and procedures.
Game	A game is a simulation of operations that often involves two or more teams, usually in a competitive environment, using rules, data, and procedures designed to depict an actual or assumed real-life situation.

Operations-Based Exercises

Operations-based exercises focus on action-oriented activities such as deployment of resources and personnel and are more complex than discussion-based types. They are used to validate plans, policies, agreements, and procedures; clarify roles and responsibilities; and identify resource gaps in a practice environment.

Type	Description
Drill	A drill is a coordinated, supervised activity usually employed to test a single, specific operation or function within the practice.
Functional exercise	A functional exercise examines and/or validates the coordination, command, and control between the practice and other community partners (e.g., hospital, police, fire department, health department). A functional exercise does not involve any "boots on the ground" (e.g., first responders or emergency officials responding to an incident in real time).
Full-scale exercise	A full-scale exercise is a multiorganizational exercise, involving a "boots on the ground" response (e.g., firefighters, EMS, police, health department, hospital).

Source: Adapted from FEMA (2016c).

— http://emergency.cdc.gov/planning

— http://emergency.cdc.gov/bioterrorism/training.asp

— http://emergency.cdc.gov/bioterrorism

◆ US Department of Homeland Security—http://ready.gov

◆ American Academy of Family Physicians—www.aafp.org/afp/2007/0601/p1679.html

◆ American Red Cross—www.redcross.org/get-help/prepare-for-emergencies/workplaces-and-organizations

One of the most important aspects of emergency preparedness management is keeping preparedness at top of mind in all areas of the practice. Often, medical practices prepare for but then forget about emergency issues, and that learning soon dissipates. The effective emergency manager provides regular updates, training, and information, keeping emergency management on the minds of everyone in the practice.

COMMUNITY EMERGENCY RESPONSE TEAMS

The Community Emergency Response Team (CERT) program educates individuals about disaster preparedness for hazards that may affect their area and trains them in basic disaster response skills, such as fire safety, light search and rescue, team organization, and disaster medical operations. The training is conducted both in the classroom and using exercises. Becoming familiar with the local CERT can be a proactive way to learn about EP/EM, and it also provides a means to connect with the community that may be beneficial in an emergency or disaster situation (FEMA 2016a).

SPECIAL SITUATIONS

In this section, we discuss specific disaster and emergency scenarios that have emerged or become increasingly common in recent years.

TERRORISM

Just in the past decade or so, the likelihood of terrorism affecting medical practices in the United States has shifted from improbable to possible and has emerged as an issue that needs to be addressed. Practices must consider their role in responding to terrorism situations, from a medical care perspective as well as a management function for the practice itself. Much of this response depends on the nature of the practice, whether it is part of a larger organization or an independent practice, where it is located (e.g., urban or rural), and whether the practice is located near other potential targets of terrorist groups.

A Theoretical Example

Your practice is part of a large integrated delivery system (IDS), and you live in a region of the country that has nuclear power plants. More than 2 million residents live in a ten-mile radius of these facilities. Without warning, a nuclear accident occurs due to a suspected terrorist act. Significant amounts of radioactive iodine are released, which requires the population to receive iodine pills to mitigate potential illness. What role does your practice play in this response?

Ideally, this possibility was considered in the health system's VA and in the practice's preparation of the emergency management plan. If the role of the practice has been defined in the context of the larger IDS, the practice's emergency management plan might include helping in the distribution of iodine pills and serving as a repository for this medication.

Although medical practices are traditionally set up to treat patients primarily in a nonemergency situation, the practice should consider what assets it has that can be used in an emergency. Medical supplies, space for treatment, and medical personnel are some examples of what the practice could bring to any disaster or emergency (CDC 2016a).

Bioterrorism

Bioterrorism is one clear emergency situation in which the medical practice can assist the community. According to the Centers for Disease Control and Prevention, bioterrorism potentially involves three primary agent categories, designated as *A*, *B*, and *C* (CDC 2017a).

Category A

These high-priority agents include organisms or toxins that pose the highest risk to the public and national security because of the following traits:

◆ They can be easily spread or transmitted from person to person.

◆ They result in high death rates and have the potential for major public health impact.

◆ They might cause public panic and social disruption.

◆ They require special action for public health preparedness.

Category B

These agents are the second highest priority because they pose the following types of concerns:

◆ They are moderately easy to spread.

◆ They result in moderate illness rates and low death rates.

◆ They require specific enhancements of the CDC's laboratory capacity and enhanced disease monitoring.

Category C

These third highest priority agents include emerging pathogens that could be engineered for mass spread in the future. Their common characteristics include the following:

◆ They are easily available.

◆ They are easily produced and spread.

◆ They have potential for high morbidity and mortality rates and major health impact.

When establishing processes for responding to acts of bioterrorism, the practice manager and leader must consider and plan for all these possibilities.

PANDEMICS

Pandemics are widespread occurrences of infectious diseases affecting large populations or regions (CDC 2017b). What is the role of the medical practice in addressing potential or actual pandemics? Although the answer varies significantly depending on location and type of organization, at a minimum the practice needs to be prepared to deal with significant numbers of patients who are affected by a pandemic flu or other infectious disease. Protection of the staff and other patients is of utmost concern. The American Nurses Association (2008) offers an excellent guide to adapting care standards under pandemic circumstances.

The practice may also have the opportunity to cooperate with local community hospitals and health departments as part of an overall National Incident Management System (Hewitt et al. 2015). Such partnerships bring government and nongovernment organizations and agencies together to manage disasters and emergencies, thereby bringing the whole community together.

Preparing for a Pandemic

One way to address the possibility of a pandemic and how the practice might respond is to conduct a tabletop exercise. The scenario is the development of a flu pandemic in the region served by the practice.

First, the facilitator should provide a space that allows the group to work together on the exercise. If the group is too large, multiple groups may be created. Groups should not exceed seven people. The facilitator also provides flipcharts and markers or other means to record the activities of the groups.

Second, the facilitator gives each group a series of progressive events related to the pandemic, described in stages, and asks the groups to discuss and document how the practice would respond in this situation. They are given a ten-minute time limit for each phase and are instructed to be prepared to share their conclusions with the facilitator and other groups.

◆ Stage I: Reports have been received that the number of cases of a novel strain of flu is on the rise.

◆ Stage II: The practice has begun to see a number of patients with this flu strain.

◆ Stage III: The practice is receiving so many phone calls and visits from patients with this novel strain of flu that the practice is incapable of treating all the patients. This unmanageable volume is exacerbated by the fact that many members of the practice staff are also ill.

Some findings from participating groups might include the following:

◆ Maintain proficiency in addressing a possible pandemic. Do not start cutting corners in safety or quality in an effort to see all the patients who present to the practice. This can be a chaotic time in the practice, so a plan for the surge in patients and how it will be managed is required. Many primary practices get a sense of this issue with outbreaks of the flu.

◆ Take measures to help maintain the health and safety of staff by enacting heightened infection control protocols and enabling use of related equipment. Accidents like needle sticks and exposure to pathogens can more easily occur in a frantic environment than in a normal daily routine, so order and calm need to be maintained, which can only be achieved with preparedness training.

◆   If a known threat exists, establish a protocol for screening, such as asking standard questions about travel, contacts, and location of residence as appropriate.

◆   Remain alert for unusual clusters or unusual patterns of illness, especially when a threat is known or possible. For example, during the Ebola outbreak of 2014, practices began to ask patients with possible Ebola symptoms about their travel history (CDC 2016b).

◆   Establish a diagnosis to determine not only the appropriate prompt treatment for the patient but whether he or she represents an early warning sign of a larger threat.

◆   Alert the proper authorities, such as the local and state health departments. In some cases, the CDC may also be involved.

◆   Assist in the transport of patients as necessary to other facilities, such as a hospital that may be a more appropriate place for the care of the patient.

◆   Assist in the epidemiologic investigation. Government health agencies, such as the CDC and federal and state health departments, rely on the input from providers in the community to help assess the nature and extent of disease outbreaks by reporting the number of cases of the illness under surveillance.

In this simplified example of a tabletop exercise, we see that the progression of a pandemic can quickly become a difficult situation for the practice to handle. What do you do as the manager or leaders of the practice? What plans have been made? What resources can you call on to support your patient volume? Solutions to all these questions and more should be contained in the preparedness plan adopted by the practice, thereby allowing the practice to address an escalating event such as a flu pandemic in a timely and effective way.

CYBERSECURITY THREATS

Security breaches are becoming all too common, and increasingly costly. In 2017, the largest National Health Service trust in the United Kingdom was the victim of a ransomware attack (Donnelly 2017). In 2016, according to a report by Verizon, more than 100,000 incidents of attempted data theft were logged, of which 3,141 were confirmed data breaches where data were stolen. In addition, the motives behind these attempts at data theft were primarily financial or related to espionage.

Cyber criminals have discovered that medical practices and other health-related facilities are rich sources of personal information that can be used for identity theft or, in rare cases, blackmail. These criminals have also learned that medical practices may be easy targets (Kaplan 2016). The medical practice has an obligation to protect patients' private health information as well as the integrity of the practice and its financial well-being.

Consider some of the recent attacks on large and sophisticated organizations in the healthcare field: 94 percent of medical institutions report being the victim of a cyberattack, and 72 percent of providers have reported malicious traffic. A primary reason these incursions are becoming prevalent is that nearly all software applications are now connected to the Internet (Filkins 2014). According to Bloomberg, cyberattacks now cost physician practices and hospitals more than $6 billion per year (Pettypiece 2015).

Common Cyber Risks

Some emerging and longstanding cybersecurity risks include the following:

◆ *Phishing attacks* are typically disguised as e-mails from what appears to be a trusted party asking the receiver to click on a hot link and enter personal information, which then allows the perpetrator access to the accounts or information systems of the practice.

◆ *Trojans and malware* are special software programs (*malware* is malicious software) designed to allow the hacker to access information in systems on the infected computer and the networks to which they are connected.

◆ *Ransomware and advertising scams* are special programs that, if downloaded by the user of the computer system, cause the computer to be infected by one or more viruses. In the case of ransomware, the data in the system become unavailable to the practice until a ransom is paid to the hacker, when a code is provided to unlock the data. Recent cases have shown these attacks to be a real and growing threat (Pot 2016; MGMA Government Affairs 2017).

◆ *Password theft* occurs when an individual simply steals the password of a person who has access to the practice's systems.

◆ *Third-party access breaches* occur through the systems of vendors and other parties that frequently deal with the practice whereby hackers can obtain access and steal data or infect computers with malware.

Responsibilities of the Practice in the Face of a Cyberattack

As with other risk management strategies, the first step is to assess the vulnerability of the practice. Some organizations periodically send staff phishing e-mails as a test of their knowledge and impulse control, for example.

Following that analysis, one of the most important steps the practice can take is to establish clear procedures and policies on the use of all electronic communication devices in the practice. Extensive and comprehensive training of all staff members is necessary on these policies and procedures, including the following:

◆ Proper access of information

◆ Password security

◆ Appropriate management and surveillance of security policies

The practice also needs to have appropriate electronic safeguards in place in the form of firewalls, web and e-mail encryption, and malware protection. An informative introduction to IT security guidelines has been published by the Cybersecurity Working Group of the Healthcare and Public Health Sector, US Department of Homeland Security (2017).

Data breaches often occur despite the best efforts of organizations to prevent them. Depending on the practice's ability to deal with such events, it may consider purchasing cyber insurance, which provides assistance and compensation in the aftermath of damage produced by a cyberattack.

COLLABORATIVE EMERGENCY MANAGEMENT

In any significant emergency or disaster situation, no single entity will likely be able to manage the needs of the entire community. Medical practices, whether freestanding or a part of a large healthcare system, are often called on to assist in these difficult situations. The manager and leaders must acknowledge the practice's expected level of involvement in community emergencies and prepare for the possibility of being asked to assist in a crisis.

EXAMPLES OF COLLABORATION IN EMERGENCY MANAGEMENT

Potential issues that might involve the medical practice in an emergency or disaster situation include a pandemic, such as influenza, as discussed earlier, or contagious diseases, such as the Zika virus, Ebola, or the so-called bird flu (H5N1) virus (CDC 2017b; KFF 2014). A critical point regarding the evolution of new disease threats such as Zika and Ebola is the need to keep clinical personnel updated on the proper methods of surveillance, diagnosis, and treatment. The practice should regularly seek out and incorporate new information about possible disease threats as part of the emergency preparedness plan review and revision process.

The ultimate aim of these considerations is for the medical practice to become an integral part of an overall community response to an emergency. How that effort is organized and who is in charge of it varies from community to community, but the minimum expectation is that the medical practice be involved on some level.

FEMA (2016b) and the CDC assist in developing plans for continuity of operations in times of pandemics or disasters. These resources are logical starting points for medical practices as they prepare their emergency and preparedness plans.

This chapter has provided only a glimpse at some of the important elements of emergency management and preparedness. The practice manager in this new era must continue to seek new information and education and to develop effective plans for the practice and the communities it serves.

DISCUSSION QUESTIONS

1. Outline and discuss the steps in preparing an emergency preparedness plan for the practice.

2. Describe the types of exercises that can be used in the practice to prepare for an emergency.

3. What is the all-hazards approach to emergency planning?

4. Outline and discuss the steps of the preparedness cycle.

5. Identify the important entities in your community for emergency management education and outreach.

REFERENCES

American Nurses Association. 2008. "Adapting Standards of Care Under Extreme Conditions: Guidance for Professionals During Disasters, Pandemics, and Other Extreme Emergencies." Published March. http://nursingworld.org/MainMenuCategories/Workplace Safety/Healthy-Work-Environment/DPR/TheLawEthicsofDisasterResponse/Adapting StandardsofCare.pdf.

Centers for Disease Control and Prevention (CDC). 2017a. "Bioterrorism." Updated May 9. http://emergency.cdc.gov/bioterrorism.

———. 2017b. "Zika Virus." Updated May 4. www.cdc.gov/zika.

———. 2016a. "Preparation & Planning." Updated June 10. https://emergency.cdc.gov/planning.

———. 2016b. "When Caring for Patients Under Investigation (PUIs) or Patients with Confirmed Ebola Virus Disease (EVD)." Reviewed March 22. www.cdc.gov/vhf/ebola/healthcare-us/evaluating-patients/think-ebola.html.

Courier-Journal Staff. 1990. "Feature: A Doctor's Murder." *Courier-Journal*, September 23, 104.

Cybersecurity Working Group, Healthcare and Public Health Sector, US Department of Homeland Security. 2017. "Healthcare and Public Health Cybersecurity Primer: Cybersecurity 101." Accessed May 25. www.phe.gov/Preparedness/planning/cip/Documents/cybersecurity-primer.pdf.

Donnelly, L. 2017. "Largest NHS Trust Hit by Cyber Attack." Published January 17. www.telegraph.co.uk/news/2017/01/13/largest-nhs-trust-hit-cyber-attack.

Federal Emergency Management Agency (FEMA). 2016a. "Community Emergency Response Teams." Updated August 31. www.fema.gov/community-emergency-response-teams.

———. 2016b. "Continuity Planning for Influenza Pandemic." Accessed April 4. www.fema.gov/media-library-data/1410875581685-0729ba3e23e9b0016bbf18efcd6daa59/COOP%20Pandemic%20Influenza.pdf.

———. 2016c. "Preparedness Cycle." Accessed April 4. https://emilms.fema.gov/is910a/EMPFsummary.htm.

———. 2007. "Principles of Emergency Management Supplement." Published September 11. www.fema.gov/media-library-data/20130726-1822-25045-7625/principles_of_emergency_management.pdf.

Filkins, B. 2014. "Health Care Cyberthreat Report: Widespread Compromises Detected, Compliance Nightmare on Horizon." Published February. www.sans.org/reading-room/whitepapers/analyst/health-care-cyberthreat-report-widespread-compromises-detected-compliance-nightmare-horizon-34735.

Gans, D. 2016. "Preparing for a Medical Office Emergency or Disaster." Accessed July 8. www.mgma.com/about/about-mgma-medical-group-management/about-center -for-research/preparing-for-a-medical-office-emergency-or-disaster.

Hewitt, A., S. Wagner, R. Twal, and D. Gourley. 2015. "Closing the Gaps in Public-Private Partnerships and Emergency Management: A Gap Analysis." In *Aligning Community Hospitals with Local Public Health Departments*, edited by M. Hamner, 1–47. Frederick, MD: Lea Tech.

Kaiser Family Foundation (KFF). 2014. "The U.S. Government & Global Emerging Infectious Disease Preparedness and Response." Published December 8. http://kff.org/ global-health-policy/fact-sheet/the-u-s-government-global-emerging-infectious -disease-preparedness-and-response.

Kaplan, J. 2016. "Healthcare Is a Win-Win Target for Hackers." Published June 16. www. beckershospitalreview.com/healthcare-information-technology/doctor-patient -confidentiality-doesn-t-exist-in-a-world-with-ransomware-or-healthcare-is-a-win-win- target-for-hackers.html.

Lyttle, S. 2014. "Hugo 25 Years Later: Rare Charlotte Hurricane Made History." Published September 21. www.charlotteobserver.com/news/local/article9193952.html.

Markenson, M., and D. Reilly. 2011. *Health Care Emergency Management: Principles and Practice*. Sudbury, MA: Jones & Bartlett Learning.

MGMA Government Affairs. 2017. "MGMA Joins HHS Initiative to Protect Practices from Global Cyber Attack." Published May 17. www.mgma.com/government-affairs/ washington-connection/2017/may/mgma-joins-hhs-initiative-to-protect-practices -from-global-cyber-attack.

Pettypiece, S. 2015. "Rising Cyber Attacks Costing Health System $6 Billion Annually." Published May 7. www.bloomberg.com/news/articles/2015-05-07/ rising-cyber-attacks-costing-health-system-6-billion-annually.

Pot, J. 2016. "Ransomware Attackers Refuse to Decrypt Hospital's Files After Being Paid Off." Published May 24. www.digitaltrends.com/computing/ransomware -hospital-hackers-demand-more-money.

Prochnau, W., and L. Parker. 2009. *Miracle on the Hudson: The Survivors of Flight 1549 Tell Their Extraordinary Stories of Courage, Faith, and Determination*. New York: Ballantine.

Ready.gov. 2017. "Medical Reserve Corps." Accessed May 25. www.ready.gov/medical-reserve-corps.

Verizon Communication. 2016. *2016 Data Breach Investigations Report*. Basking, NJ: Verizon.

CHAPTER 12

THE FUTURE AND MEDICAL PRACTICE INNOVATION

Knowing is not enough; we must apply. Willing is not enough;
we must do.

—Johann Wolfgang von Goethe

LEARNING OBJECTIVES

➤ Describe the anticipated changes medicine will experience in the future.

➤ Understand the significance of data analysis and Big Data.

➤ Appreciate the nature and expectations of precision medicine.

➤ Understand the importance of shifting focus from volume-based reimbursement to value-based reimbursement to the medical practice.

➤ Delve into the role of the practice manager in guiding and leading the medical practice of the future.

INTRODUCTION

In the future, as we assume more responsibility for outcomes and as pay-for-volume systems fade away, medical practice revenue will become its cost. That statement might not make any sense until one considers that in a value-based world, reimbursement will be fixed and that whenever a procedure, such as a lab test, is performed, the practice will pay that cost. Currently, that cost is revenue to the practice.

The Gordian knot has long been seen as a metaphor for an unsolvable problem, but it is one that does have a simple solution, if the solver is an innovative thinker. The known cannot be untangled, but it can be cut. We must start to think about what the future should look like for the medical practice; it will be much different than what we see today.

The only way the US healthcare system will achieve a sufficient level of reform is to abandon the philosophy of incrementalism and attack the root cause of the system's failures. This movement will require innovation and a new mind-set, particularly new ways of thinking about the problems of healthcare delivery. This mind-set will feature a significant increase in self-care and collaborative care, and it will require practitioners to provide creative avenues for patients to access services and information. As we discuss in this chapter, behavioral economics will add a new dimension to healthcare by helping medical practices devise methods to help people create changes in their lifestyle and behaviors that have led to significant negative health outcomes. Exhibit 12.1 illustrates the shifts that need to occur for the transition from today's volume-based system to a value-based system to take place.

In the exhibit, the term the *acid river* comes from the team exercise in which a group must build a bridge across an imaginary river of acid (St. John 2017). The goal of the team is to see that all members get across the acid river safely. This task is difficult because materials (resources) for building the bridge are limited; in fact, the bridge must be built by repeatedly removing and replacing segments and experimenting (innovating) to determine what approach will work. It also requires continual monitoring of the team's status and progress. This effort sounds a lot like the task of moving the medical practice

EXHIBIT 12.1

Volume-to-Value
Shifts

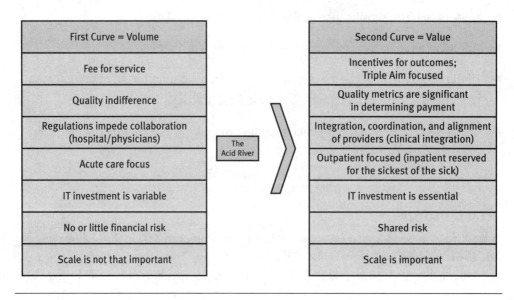

First Curve = Volume	Second Curve = Value
Fee for service	Incentives for outcomes; Triple Aim focused
Quality indifference	Quality metrics are significant in determining payment
Regulations impede collaboration (hospital/physicians)	Integration, coordination, and alignment of providers (clinical integration)
Acute care focus	Outpatient focused (inpatient reserved for the sickest of the sick)
IT investment is variable	IT investment is essential
No or little financial risk	Shared risk
Scale is not that important	Scale is important

The Acid River

from a first-curve, volume-based system to a second-curve, value-based system (see chapter 1 for a discussion of first- and second-curve transformation).

Another fundamental issue faced in the modern medical practice is getting universal adoption of necessary changes. Dr. Everett Rogers (2003) studied and wrote extensively about the types of adopters and stages of adoption. As illustrated in exhibit 12.2, the rate of change in any system is related to the rate of adoption by the different stakeholders. Some will never adopt change, as the graph illustrates, and will not challenge the old paradigm (the way one thinks about how things should be and have been). In fact, those who will never adopt the new ways often hinder adoption by actively working against change (Rogers 2003).

Rogers noted that the vast majority of people wait until they gain more knowledge by observing the early adopters. The late adopters require even more evidence and convincing that the new paradigm is the proper way to go. The implications for practice management are significant: If adoption is spread over too long a period, the practice must operate multiple systems to keep the practice running, thereby increasing cost, adding complexity, and reducing practice effectiveness.

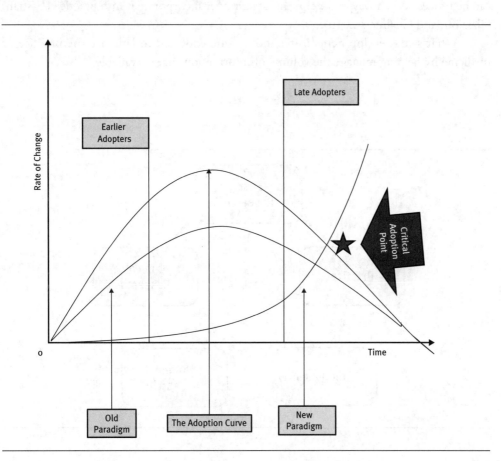

EXHIBIT 12.2
The Second Curve and the Adoption of Innovation

We know change is difficult and adoption takes a long time for administrative and clinical functions—but just how long? Empirical evidence on the adoption rate of clinical innovation has shown that discoveries can take as long as 17 years to be adopted in mainstream medical practice (Morris, Wooding, and Grant 2011). Exhibit 12.3 captures the layers of activity involved in this significant issue.

Clearly, 17 years is much too long in today's rapidly changing world to translate theory to practical application—the window of effectiveness for the discovery may well have passed by the time it is adopted. Thus, a crucial role for practice leaders is to guide the members of the practice to appreciate the new realities of the value-based future. Practice members must be nimble and move quickly to embrace ideas and methods once they are proven to be effective.

Merely encouraging adoption may be inadequate to effect change, however; the lack of will to adjust is just one factor. The sheer amount of new information created regarding the practice of medicine and in healthcare systems and management practices is increasingly difficult to absorb. In 2010, an average of 75 clinical trials and 11 systematic reviews were being published daily, but just a small fraction of this amount of information can be processed in a way that helps the practitioner incorporate it into practice (Bastian, Glasziou, and Chalmers 2010).

That said, developments in technology are expected to enhance the practice of medicine by helping manage the volume of information that is available.

EXHIBIT 12.3

Discovery to Practice

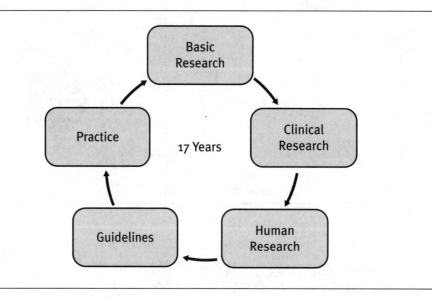

FORCES OF CHANGE

The future direction of healthcare is governed by many forces. They include the current political discussions surrounding healthcare reform as well as the prevailing concerns about access, quality, and cost (discussed in chapter 1). Unprecedented changes are also taking place in private infrastructure and societal values, and they all influence medical practices and practice management.

Many of the compelling forces of change have been discussed elsewhere in the text. Here, as we consider the future delivery of healthcare by the medical practice, we emphasize a few of the most potent drivers faced by medical practices—those that are likely to have the greatest impact on how the US healthcare system and the medical practice function in the future. Later in the chapter, we discuss some implications for medical practices in terms of these forces and other considerations.

DEMOGRAPHIC FORCES

More than 10,000 baby boomers are turning 65 every day, and the aging US population is just one demographic factor shaping the future of healthcare. We all are living longer as well. As people age, they usually need more healthcare services than young individuals, so often the question is not if they will need healthcare, but when, and this issue has significant implications for the amount and types of services practices will need to provide. Another factor is the increasing diversity of US society, which brings the need for a larger scope of services and cultural competence related to delivering healthcare (Livingston and Brown 2017).

ECONOMIC FORCES

In the United States, nearly one in five dollars of the economy is spent on healthcare (KFF 2017). Many observers believe the country cannot afford the cost anymore (Jost 2016). One battle being waged in this area is between the social justice approach and the market approach to healthcare provision. Social justice tends to favor government action and regulatory interventions for the social good, while market proponents favor letting the marketplace dictate outcomes. Whether a true market-based system of healthcare can be sustained in the United States is a continuing debate.

TECHNOLOGICAL FORCES

These forces include the digitization of healthcare, not only medical records but healthcare delivery as well, and any new medical technologies that emerge. In addition, the information available to people through the Internet and other avenues has caused a shift in how patients consume healthcare. They ask more questions than ever before and often know much more about their condition than in the past. Some patients are becoming health literate, but in a confounding turn, health literacy overall seems to be decreasing. Modern medicine and its related technologies offer much hope but also give people a false sense of security. Ultimately, regardless of the advancement of tools and technologies, individuals' behaviors and habits are the primary causes for their health status, not the healthcare system (Resnik 2007), and in that respect, the future is not expected to be much different.

Cost-Effectiveness Research

A fairly new methodology to improve the US healthcare system, known as cost-effectiveness research (CER), is beginning to drive change. This focus of research evaluates the relative performance of different treatments and procedures for similar conditions and determines which approaches are most effective. CER encourages standardization in medicine and discourages overutilization. It accomplishes this aim by tapping large databases from national sources and direct clinical trials to develop evidence-based information on the cost and effectiveness of procedures and treatments. This procedure is always an evidence-based comparison between different treatments (e.g., surgery versus medication) for the same condition or illness. The Agency for Healthcare Research and Quality (AHRQ 2017) conducts significant work in CER, and practice managers should become familiar with these efforts.

Ecological and Other Environmental Factors

With viruses such as Zika emerging and spreading, through globalization, to new areas, additional health concerns are created that require responses from medical practices (Storrs 2016). Practice managers and leaders must see that their practices are equipped with the knowledge and materials needed to address these concerns.

In addition to new diseases, the increasing number of people living in harm's way of natural disasters affects healthcare in a major way. Consider the effects of Hurricane Katrina and Superstorm Sandy on the health of the affected populations as well as on the healthcare delivery system. For example, in the 12 years since Katrina devastated the Gulf Coast, many New Orleans healthcare facilities remain shuttered; however, new facilities have opened with the hope of providing better care and at the same time being more prepared for future emergency events (Rudwitz, Rowland, and Shartzer 2006; Rettner 2013; CNN 2015).

Shifting Values and Beliefs

The values and beliefs of residents continue to be overarching factors that influence the US healthcare system, and these values and beliefs are changing. At one time, questioning the judgment of a physician was unthinkable, but now it is commonplace. People's attitudes about nutrition and alternative therapies have come to the forefront as individuals seek ways to improve self-care, with a greater focus on preventive measures. Lifestyle issues, which have always been major determinants of health, are now influencing the cost of care, becoming widely recognized as quality-of-life indicators. Many of the chronic diseases that plague US society are triggered by lifestyle excesses, such as poor diet and lack of exercise leading to diabetes, obesity, and hypertension.

CULTURAL FACTORS

An increasingly diverse society has created the need for healthcare organizations to employ a culturally competent workforce. According to the US Census Bureau (2015), more than 350 languages are spoken in homes in the United States. To serve the members of all cultural groups at the highest level, medical practices should survey their patient populations to understand the languages and aspects of their cultural background that are important to them in medical office encounters. These surveys and broader community assessments are needed to engage patients in discussions of their needs, wants, and expectations.

POLITICAL FORCES

Political forces at play in the future of healthcare range from educational policies to immigration policies and beyond. However, the most prominent political discussion centers on healthcare reform. Americans remain divided over the Affordable Care Act (ACA), its future, and the role government should play in healthcare delivery (Aaron 2015). In the course of the 2016 presidential election, one major party candidate suggested a complete repeal and replacement of the ACA, while the other major party promised enhancements to the act (Ballotpedia 2016; Motel 2015). As of this writing, the outcome is uncertain, as Congress continues to wrangle along party lines over reform legislation and potential changes to entitlement programs such as Medicare and Medicaid.

For many political stakeholders, the key issue is cost. Getting healthcare costs under control has been a goal for decades, yet costs continue to rise. Another primary issue is universal access. Inequality of both access to and knowledge about healthcare continues despite awareness initiatives aiming to stem it.

GEOGRAPHIC FACTORS

Finally, the distribution of services often hinges on geographic location. Residents of rural areas, regardless of socioeconomic status or level of knowledge about healthcare, face gaps in the availability of many services, an issue that influences the quality of care they receive (Radley and Schoen 2012).

The Lesson of the Affordable Care Act

The current rhetoric and political wrangling over the ACA is reminiscent of the period after Medicare legislation was passed in 1965. Many conversations with physicians and others in the 1970s—years after the program's implementation—yielded questions such as "What are we going to do about Medicare?" The impulse of some was to resist and advocate for revisions to the law. Through the 1980s and 1990s, many practices harbored deep-seated concerns about government involvement in healthcare.

But as we know today, some 50 years later, Medicare is a staple of the healthcare world: Many, if not most, healthcare organizations and practices that care for individuals aged 65 or older receive a significant portion of their revenue from Medicare. With that said, the time Medicare was given to become an accepted and essential part of the healthcare landscape will likely not be afforded the ACA. The fate of the act is very much in question as of this writing. However, the larger context of this long-standing debate and the rancor in the political arena surrounding the ACA, and even thinking back on the aftermath of Medicare's passage, illustrate how important the political environment can be to the medical practice and why leaders and managers must be engaged in understanding and responding to the issues that affect the practice and its patients. Remember that approximately 50 percent of all healthcare dollars come from government entities at all levels, much of that from the federal government. Numerous occasions will likely arise in the future when legislative action affects the practice of medicine and how care is delivered and paid for.

The Promise of Community-Based Primary Care

The practice of medicine historically has been based on the biomedical model (Wade and Halligan 2004). As science has advanced and understanding of disease has improved dramatically, the medical community is beginning to see that much more is involved in health and healthcare than the biomedical science of disease provides. Community-based primary care focuses on the unique needs of the populations providers serve, many of which have been underserved in the past. These practices give special attention to access and the barriers to access, such as transportation, cultural differences, and cost.

We live in a complex society, and many social issues pervade the healthcare system. Violent crime, abuse, addiction, and other social dysfunctions cost the US healthcare system billions of dollars each year. Furthermore, criminal justice, social services, and other elements of the social fabric have a tremendous impact on delivery of services. This tremendous expenditure does not include the substantial impact of crime on the victims beyond their medical care and social harm (Fineline Foundation 2016; McCollister, French, and Fang 2010).

For example, criminal behavior goes beyond inflicting physical injury. One study estimates that healthcare fraud amounts to as much as $272 billion per year (Goldman 2012). Similarly, mental health issues also continue to be a major concern. One in four primary care patients has some diagnosable mental health condition. Primary care practices are beginning to provide innovative solutions by embedding mental health services in the primary care environment (Sampson and Mueller 2017).

FUTURE WORKFORCE CHALLENGES

THE NURSING PROFESSION

The roles of different types of providers in the medical practice are constantly changing. According to a report sponsored by the Robert Wood Johnson Foundation, the scope of nursing will increase to allow nurses to practice to the full extent of their training and licensure (IOM 2011). What will the impact be on the medical practice? One of the key findings of this report is that "nurses should be full partners, with physicians and other health professionals, in redesigning health care in the United States."

Nurses, doctors, and other highly trained healthcare professionals frequently perform jobs that do not require the practitioners' level of education. For example, physicians complete tasks that can be performed by physician assistants and advanced practice nurses, and nurses are doing the work of clerical and other clinical support staff. However, a big shift is in process in which people who have highly specific professional skills are using those skills appropriately. Practice managers need to facilitate this shift by collecting and harnessing better data and information technology skills. We need to make sure practice members work as a team and divide the work on the basis of the scope of practice. For example, nurses can perform certain routine follow-up visits and blood pressure checks, and physician assistants can care for straightforward cases, while the physicians attend to those patients needing more involved care.

Of course, these changes face two significant barriers:

◆ Reluctance on the part of other caregivers to give up clinical responsibilities.

◆ Varied regulations and licensing processes as the result of state-level responsibility. The necessary regulatory changes to allow new modes of practice will progress differently in each state. Practice managers need to be aware of the licensing and regulatory practice limitations on nurses, physician assistants, and nurse practitioners in their practice.

TRAINING IN GERIATRICS

Although primary care needs to be strengthened in general, one particular challenge to the workforce is training in geriatrics. The United States faces a critical shortage of geriatricians currently; by 2025, the number of people over age 65 will double, and approximately 25,000 certified geriatricians will be needed to serve that population. By contrast, in 2014, 7,500 geriatricians were working in the United States (Baruchin 2015).

What are the barriers to attracting geriatricians to the field? Geriatrics is a relatively new specialty and is not particularly glamorous or high paying. In addition, not enough training programs are currently available in geriatrics. According to findings published in the *Journal of the American Medical Association*, only 96 internal medicine or family practice residency graduates entered a geriatric fellowship in 2013 (Brotherton and Etzel 2014).

Practices may be able to increase their ability to care for geriatric patients by utilizing more nurse practitioners and other qualified healthcare professionals who are also receiving advanced training in geriatrics.

GLOBAL THREATS AND INTERNATIONAL COOPERATION

Natural disasters, industrial accidents, and other events occur daily. The nature of global travel contributes to the spread of infectious diseases, posing an additional concern (Pavia 2007). In 2014, the presence of the Ebola virus in the United States, although limited to a handful of infections, caused consternation on the part of health professionals and the public alike. Almost any corner of the world can be reached within 24 hours. As the threat of infectious disease increases, so, too, does the antibiotic resistance of infectious agents, such as tuberculosis, posing enhanced threats to patients. However, antibiotics research lags the ability of infectious agents to become resistant. One reason is that pharmaceutical manufacturers do not garner the same return on investment from antibiotics as they do from other pharmaceuticals, such as those that treat chronic conditions and must be taken for long periods.

The lack of healthcare infrastructure in developing countries has had an influence on global health as well. Often, these resistant strains appear in underdeveloped parts of the world because those regions do not have the medicines available or patients do not take them correctly. Even if infected patients are administered an antibiotic, they may not receive enough to complete the treatment, they may sell part of it, or several people may use one prescription (Reardon 2014). Resistance is increased as a result, and the patient has unwittingly helped the disease agent become less treatable. Patients in the United States are also contributing to the increased resistance by demanding antibiotics when the drugs will do little, if any, good. Practitioners are often reluctant to spend the time to counsel patients on why the antibiotic is unnecessary, due to time pressures and fear of alienating the patient. US patients have been culturally acclimated to expecting a quick pharmaceutical fix for their ailments.

Efforts are under way to address the concerns about antibiotic resistance. The Transatlantic Task Force on Antimicrobial Resistance is focused on developing new antibiotics and other solutions to limit or halt the spread of antibiotic-resistant infections. Additional international health initiatives are being developed as well by the World Health Organization to implement new strategies, policies, and educational efforts to combat the issue of antibiotic resistance (WHO 2017). However, individual country sovereignty poses challenges to their efficacy because the regulations require agreement from leaders and health experts who hold many different cultural beliefs and values and diverse points of view. None of these international bodies can order any government to comply (CDC 2017c).

Why are these issues a concern for practice managers? Two important issues are relevant. First, awareness of global health issues is now a necessity because a practice cannot anticipate when a patient with a disease or infection acquired thousands of miles away may present. As mentioned previously in this text, the practice often serves as the first line of treatment and surveillance for new medical hazards. Second, the practice must continually deliver care at the highest level and most current state of knowledge. To do so requires continuous learning and tuning in to the ever-changing medical landscape.

ADVANCES IN IMAGING AND LABORATORY TESTING

Until the 1960s, exploratory surgery was common; it was the only way available to see inside the body. Today, with multiple imaging technologies, few reasons justify the need for invasive procedures. These procedures include the following:

- Ultrasound

- Magnetic resonance imaging

- Computed tomography

- Medical X-ray (including mammography)

- Fluoroscopy

- Positron emission tomography

- Tactile imaging

- Elastography

- Photoacoustic imaging

- Thermography

- Nuclear medicine

These and a host of other imaging procedures allow virtually every part of the body to be visualized structurally and chemically to make an accurate diagnosis. The number of laboratory tests available to the medical practice is increasing rapidly as well. More than 900 lab tests are commonly performed, which focus on approximately 600 diseases and conditions (Chernecky and Berger 2013). Many of these imaging and laboratory services may soon be provided by the medical practice and serve as a convenience for the patient and the medical staff as well as a source of revenue.

EVIDENCE-BASED HEALTHCARE

Evidence-based healthcare requires the use of research and evidence to determine treatments that produce the best outcomes. This approach to care creates value by limiting variation and the misuse and overuse of procedures, which improves quality and reduces costs. This is another important area of healthcare administration and healthcare research because it offers the promise of effective, high-quality care at reduced cost. AHRQ, the health services and policy research arm of the US Department of Health & Human Services, is leading the way in evidence-based research. A related branch of research, CER, is championed by the Patient-Centered Outcomes Research Institute (PCORI). The formation of PCORI was mandated by the ACA, which is slowly progressing in its mission (GPO 2010). CER activities include the following:

1. Identifying new and emerging clinical interventions

2. Synthesizing the information in more than 40,000 research studies published every year

3. Disseminating the information and tools created to assist the clinician and residents of the United States

4. Identifying the gaps between existing research and clinical practice

STRATEGIES FOR EVIDENCE-BASED CARE

Ongoing emphasis is being placed by government and private payers, as well as patients, on the adoption of evidence-based medical practices. Assisting in this effort are information technologists and high-tech firms developing computer-based models to provide practitioners with ready access to the most current information.

Clearly, a great deal of information is available now. The amount of medical information doubled between 2010 and 2014, with the expectation that it will double every 73 days by 2020 (Densen 2011). Because no human being can know all this information, tools are needed to help bring the latest care to patients.

Keeping guidelines current and then incorporating the economic analysis into evidence-based care creates the cost-effectiveness component. We are beginning to see reimbursement restructured to reward the best achievable outcomes as part of the whole paying-for-value approach.

DATA ANALYTICS AND ARTIFICIAL INTELLIGENCE

It would be difficult to argue that the medical practice does not have a sufficient amount of data to manage and treat its patients. The problem is quite the opposite: Practices have more data than they can manage and use in an unstructured form. Until recently, converting unstructured data into usable and applicable information was extremely difficult. As exhibit 12.4 indicates, unstructured data are almost useless because they are almost impossible to apply to the practice environment. First, the unstructured data must be collected, which helps create information that can be turned into new knowledge about patients and populations served. Only then can this information be put into action.

The ability to convert unstructured data into practicable information is a developing but still nascent science at this time. One leading example of the early progress in this field is IBM's supercomputer Watson. (Watson is one of several supercomputers that provide advanced data analytic solutions. HP, Dell EMC, and other companies are working in this field as well.) Watson mimics human intelligence by quickly iterating nuanced information provided by the user. For example, Watson can read the entirety of existing medical literature in a matter of seconds, an impossible feat for any human being in his or her lifetime; turn the enormous mass of unstructured data into usable information that can respond to questions and problems; and understand nuances in human speech.

How could Watson or another artificial intelligence supercomputer be used in a medical practice? How could it assist providers in treating complex medical conditions? The connection to Watson is made in the cloud. Cloud computing is a means for computer

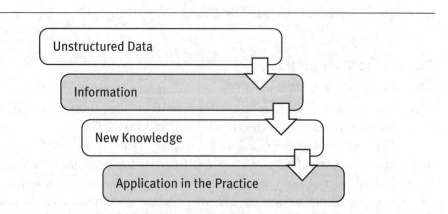

EXHIBIT 12.4
Transformation of Data into Application

users to connect to remote networks of servers that host processing capabilities beyond that of the users' IT capabilities. Following is an outline of Watson's process:

1.   Watson is asked the question.

2.   Watson reviews all medical literature and the clinical information provided.

3.   Watson provides a structured response to the question in the form of possible diagnoses, treatments, and their probability of success.

4.   Watson is given new information and, after a further iteration, provides an additional response.

5.   Watson ultimately provides a complete set of facts on the patient's case.

By using the supercomputer to provide access to all known information regarding the diagnosis of the patient, the provider has an enhanced opportunity to give the best possible response to the clinical issues presented.

Are practices prepared to use new technologies such as Watson? Clearly, the use of this technological platform can benefit patients and assist with the increasing complexity of care and the massive volumes of data being produced. Because artificial intelligence technology is instantaneously updated for new developments and findings in the medical field, the practitioner never needs to be without the latest information.

Exhibit 12.5 illustrates how the provider might interact with a supercomputing technological platform to assist in the treatment of a complex patient.

Although some observers feel artificial intelligence (AI) is the cure for many problems with the US healthcare system (Maney 2017), the use of AI in medical practice is not without controversy. While AI has a place in healthcare delivery, physicians have expressed concern about the lack of human intervention and the erosion of the doctor–patient relationship if care were to become too algorithmic. The concern rests on the importance of the human experience of care, not just the technology (Farr 2017).

POPULATION HEALTH

Why are some people healthy and others not? What determines health, and what is the role of the medical practice in the health of an entire community? These are questions asked by those who study population health (Kindig and Stoddart 2003).

The US healthcare system has long encouraged patient dependency for all medical needs. Medical professionals used a separate language that most patients did not understand, the healthcare system was structured in a complex and confusing way, and at times providers neglected the basics of good health by focusing too much on a particular disease or event and not thinking more about the overall long-term health and well-being of the

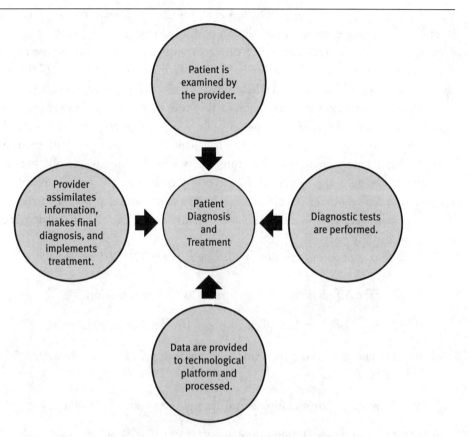

EXHIBIT 12.5
Technology-
Assisted Diagnosis

patient. This last point is likely a by-product of a system that often focused on treatment of disease rather than wellness and prevention. Researchers and practitioners alike now realize that if the goal of the healthcare system is to improve health, every member of the population needs to be engaged and empowered to take steps in ensuring their own health. Simply stated, there will never be enough clinicians or money to provide for all the needs of the population and keep it healthy.

Simply caring for an individual patient in an excellent way is no longer sufficient in the modern practice environment. That individual care is certainly still required, but as made clear by the Triple Aim, the overarching desire is for improved health for the entire population, and achieving that goal requires a different perspective on delivering care.

Population health has been defined a number of ways. It is commonly thought of as the health outcomes and health status of a group of individuals in a community or patient group. Leading expert David Kindig, MD, PhD, defines population health as "the aggregate health outcome of health-adjusted life expectancy (quantity and quality) of a group of individuals in an economic framework that balances the relative marginal returns from the multiple determinants of health" (Kindig 1997).

A key to population health is data, and meaningful, actionable data have until recently been a large missing element of population health management. Performing optimally in population health management is difficult, if not impossible, without the use of powerful data analytical tools as previously discussed. Data facilitate understanding of the nature of the population's health needs and where scarce resources need to be allocated.

Medical practices play an irreplaceable role in population health and its management. Consider the volume of patients a given practice encounters. As emphasized throughout this text, the medical practice is usually the first point of contact for patients with the healthcare system, and therefore it serves as the linchpin in the health of the community, seeing that patients receive necessary treatment and, when appropriate, are referred to other resources. Additionally, physicians and other providers direct virtually all care for patients entering the healthcare system through the emergency department or other points in the hospital.

The data supporting this notion are staggering (CDC 2017a):

◆ Number of physician office visits in 2012: 928.6 million

◆ Number of physician office visits per 100 persons in 2012: 300.8

◆ Percentage of these visits that were made to primary care physicians: 54.6 percent

◆ Number of hospital inpatient discharges per year: 35.1 million

◆ Discharges per 10,000 population: 1,139.6

◆ Average length of hospital stay in days: 4.8

The ratio of hospital admissions to office visits is 26.45 to 1, demonstrating the importance of the relationships developed in the physician practice and in the course of patient care. This statistic is saying that there is 26 times more opportunity to affect the patient's health in the office setting than in the hospital.

According to the Centers for Disease Control and Prevention (CDC 2017a), the average number of visits per person to a medical provider was three per year, so the practice has a much greater opportunity to intervene in basic health issues in the ambulatory setting than the inpatient environment has. In many cases, by the time a patient reaches the inpatient setting, the window for avoiding expensive care or preserving optimal health has closed.

Population health seeks to create a culture that encourages and actively promotes good health. Some of those underlying principles are listed next (reprinted from RWJF 2016):

Culture of Health: Underlying Principles

1. Good health flourishes across geographic, demographic, and social sectors.
2. Attaining the best health possible is valued by our entire society.
3. Individuals and families have the means and the opportunity to make choices.
4. Business, government, individuals, and organizations work together to build healthy communities.
5. No one is excluded.
6. Everyone has access to affordable, quality healthcare.
7. Healthcare is efficient and equitable.
8. The economy is less burdened by excessive and unwarranted healthcare spending.
9. Keeping everyone as healthy as possible guides public and private decision-making.
10. Americans understand that we are all in this together.

Another way to think about the important role medical practices have played in public health (which is closely aligned with population health) is to consider the ten greatest public health achievements of the twentieth century (CDC 1999):

- Vaccination
- Motor vehicle safety
- Safer workplaces
- Control of infectious disease
- Decline in deaths from coronary disease and stroke
- Safer and more healthful foods
- Healthier mothers and babies
- Family planning
- Fluoridation of drinking water
- Recognition of tobacco use as a health hazard

Each of these achievements was either actuated or supported by physicians and other medical practice staff. By providing treatment, knowledge, and surveillance, medical providers have been instrumental in addressing many public health issues and will be integral to implementing new population health strategies in the future.

CHRONIC DISEASE

As demonstrated in chapter 1, the cost and the magnitude of chronic disease in the United States is astonishing. One issue of concern in practice management is how to effectively deal with patients experiencing chronic disease. Changing reimbursement schemes and increasing expectations of the physician practice to provide enhanced patient experiences and high-quality care at lowered cost have placed responsibility squarely on practices to manage chronic disease effectively. A common belief among observers has traditionally been that the healthcare system has a limited ability to influence the health behaviors that lead to disease; therefore, linking payment to demonstrating improvements in these behaviors seems unfair. In addition, payment and time devoted to the care and prevention of chronic disease has long been limited because the healthcare system has been focused on treatment instead of preventive care. In truth, we have a sick care system, not a healthcare system.

However, that perception is changing, albeit slowly right now. One of the most important concepts in managing chronic disease is patient activation, which indicates a person's ability to manage their health and healthcare. Ways to increase patient activation include providing patients with the knowledge, skills, and confidence to be engaged in their care. Patients who score low in activation are much less likely to take an active role in their healthcare and do not seek care as advised or as appropriate, especially with regard to chronic disease.

As reimbursement focuses more on value-based outcomes programs that in part encourage healthy behaviors, medical practices will need to effectively activate patients in their care, thereby improving health results.

UPSTREAMING

What the healthcare industry has begun to recognize is that population health strategies cannot be executed without the integration of medical providers, either through a clinical integration approach or by bringing providers into the organization in an employment model (Hegwer 2016). Upstreaming provides a refreshed view of overall health-related issues. Upstreaming is a public health concept that can best be described as looking at the root causes of health problems and concerns and directing resources to address those problems. An often-told story may help to further explain the concept:

> One day, two individuals were walking along the riverbank when they looked out and saw a child struggling in the water. They quickly jumped in to rescue the child, and although the water was swift, through the heroic efforts of the two rescuers, they were able to safely bring the child to shore.

The child went happily along his way, and the two individuals proceeded on their walk. Again, they looked out in the water and saw another child struggling and on the verge of drowning in the rapidly moving current. In heroic fashion, the two again rescued the child. No sooner had they made it to shore when they saw another child in the same predicament. One of the rescuers began to walk upstream in a rapid pace, while his friend looked dismayed and said, "Where are you going? More children need to be saved." To that the rescuer replied, "I'm going to see who's throwing these children in the water."

Our view of medical practice has always been that the practice is responsible only for treating acute illness and injury. As our understanding of health and health-related issues has increased, we now know that treatment is not enough if we are to bring the healthcare system into a new era. Although practices will always need to provide lifesaving and quality-of-life enhancing treatments to their patients, they will also need to "take an upstream view" of health-related issues. This point can be illustrated with another story about upstreaming and the practice environment:

A young uninsured man presented to the practice on a regular basis with his diabetes continually out of control. Each time, the physician ascertained the problem and prescribed treatment for the patient, which required hospitalization. Following each treatment, the man's condition stabilized and he resumed his normal life. However, the treatment was expensive for the healthcare system to provide, and it had to write off the cost as either bad debt or charity care because the patient was uninsured.

Eventually, after this sequence of events had occurred over and over again, the physician began to wonder why, considering this patient's disease could be controlled with medication, diet, and exercise. The next time the patient presented to the practice, the physician spent some time talking with him. The physician asked, "Why is it that every six weeks you're in the office, needing to have your diabetes brought under control?" The young man replied, "Well, Doc, I am a laborer and often have to work out of town. Because I have no health insurance, I only receive 30 days of medication from the medical assistance program here in the city. Unfortunately, I run out of medicine about two weeks before I'm able to return home. After two weeks with no medicine, my sugar is too high." The physician replied, "Well, no wonder. We can see about getting you an additional allotment of medication that will last you until you return home between jobs." After that solution was implemented, the young man was not seen under those circumstances again.

This is upstreaming.

By simply treating what presented to the office, the real cause of the problem was not evident. The patient had to be asked—be engaged in a dialogue—to bring the source of the problem to light. The average physician spends less than 12 seconds listening to a patient before he or she interrupts and begins to speak (Rhoades et al. 2001). This study is more than 15 years old, but with so much else in healthcare changing, this finding has not. The rigidly timed 15-minute office visit erodes physician and patient relationships and has been driven by the need to produce volume rather than value (Rabin 2014). Dialogue, which must include listening to patients, is a very powerful tool—one that must be used in the medical practice.

Other ways that upstreaming can be supported by medical practices include paying attention to public policy updates and supporting policies that reflect the well-being of the practice's patients. They need to care about the condition of sidewalks, street lighting, and safe places for children to play. They also should think about the availability of nutritious food at reasonable prices, such as provided through urban gardens, and encourage policymakers to make decisions for the community that promote health and healthful behavior.

Providers must abandon the "don't ask, don't tell" policies that practices have often followed, reluctant to delve deeply into social and other concerns that patients may have beyond their medical complaints. The provider often feels helpless to address them. To combat that sense of helplessness, practices can develop a list of resources available in the community to assist patients with needs that extend beyond the practice's limits (Manchanda 2014).

Payment reform will also encourage collaboration and cooperation in addressing problems that lead to negative health outcomes. As has been stated often in this text, the volume-based reimbursement system has led to less-than-optimal health outcomes because "we don't get what we don't reimburse." Busy practitioners have difficulty in the current system balancing the financial needs of the practice and the needs of the patient. In the 2012 documentary *Escape Fire*, Donald Berwick, MD, states that every person in the healthcare system is doing exactly what he or she should be doing on the basis of his or her needs and incentives. Until the system encourages cooperation and a greater focus on upstreaming, practices will continue to struggle to meet the increasing demands of the chronically ill as well as the spiraling cost of care (Heineman and Froemke 2012). The time has come to stop blaming and start working together to bring about an enhanced reality for the US healthcare system and the patients served.

UNDERSERVED AREAS AND COMMUNITY HEALTH CENTERS

Many practitioners would like to serve rural and other underserved communities but have difficulty doing so because of the economic situation inherent to many such communities. For example, 20 percent of the population lives in rural communities, while only 9 percent of medical practices serve those areas. In addition, rural communities often have older populations, and as we know, older populations require more medical care than younger populations do.

Community health centers are a form of medical practice that may receive federal and state funding to provide primary care to underserved areas. They typically are unable to operate entirely on their own because the economic base is lacking to support them. They are found in both urban and rural areas. Though the people served by them may have insurance, as in many rural areas, the population base is not large enough to support a thriving practice and these community services need to be supported for them to exist. A community needs medical services even if the population is too small to support a practice.

Practices in these environments should consider seeking governmental support to maintain and expand their practice when the local population is not able to do so. The Health Resources and Services Administration (HRSA) of the US Department of Health & Human Services is one resource for these existing practices and for those interested in starting practices in underserved areas (HRSA 2012). Many of the programs that apply to rural areas also apply to underserved areas in urban communities, such as the Health Professional Shortage Area program (HRSA 2016).

An example of how practices can become involved in their underserved communities was demonstrated by the Sanger Clinic a few years ago. As part of a Reach 2010 coalition project sponsored by the CDC (2017b), the clinic engaged with 45 neighborhoods and 25 other agencies for the purpose of improving the cardiovascular health of the community. The practice built coalitions, provided education, and increased awareness of related health-care issues. In the process, it promoted goodwill and reduced the reluctance of patients to seek help while positioning itself as an active member of the community. As shown in exhibit 12.6, in the initiative's early phase, more than 5,000 people received information and follow-up treatment, and an outreach clinic treated more than 40 people with serious, potentially life-threatening issues. "Why are you here, and what do you bring to the table?" was the practice's motto in this exemplary community movement (Wagner 2003).

GENOMICS AND PRECISION MEDICINE

Another rapidly developing game changer in technology is occurring in the field of genetic mapping and testing. Coupling genetic testing with advanced analytics has ushered in a whole new dimension of medical practice. Genomics provides the medical practitioner with the promise of providing precision medicine to each patient instead of treating patients based on more general criteria (Collins and Varmus 2015).

The first sequencing of the human genome took more than 15 years and cost over $3 billion to complete. On subsequent sequencing rounds, the cost began to come down. The dramatic cost reduction has been due to the development of automated technologies for sequencing and improved techniques. Today, private-sector companies can conduct a human gene sequence in a matter of days or hours at a cost of less than $1,000 (Illumina 2016; *Nature* 2010). Exhibit 12.7 shows the incredible reduction in the cost of sequencing a genome.

EXHIBIT 12.6

The Role of
Physician Group
Practices in
the Healthy
Communities
Movement

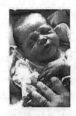
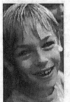
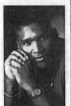
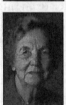
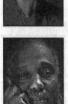

Healthy Families, Healthy Communities

A collaborative effort of more than 45 neighborhoods and 25 agencies to help improve the physical and mental health of underserved communities.

General Strategy

- Increase awareness of health care issues
- Increase community leadership and goodwill
- Position the medical group as a active and contributing member of the community

Benefits

Efforts such as *Healthy Families, Healthy Communities* cannot be measured entirely by financial statements or traditional measures of success. We must also consider the intrinsic value to ourselves and the communities we serve, including:

- Better, stronger, healthier communities
- Personal and professional fulfillment by medical staff
- Placing medical staff communities as leaders and builders for the future

Serving The Entire Community

With 50 staff physicians specializing in cardiovascular medicine and thoracic and cardiovascular surgery, we combined our individual efforts into community success. An Outreach Clinics was established at a local health center, we participated in sponsorship of health fairs, Heart Walks, a speakers bureau and the distribution of Heart/Health Assessment literature in underserved communities.

Results

To date, approximately 5,000 people have been provided information, initial and/or follow-up treatment through this collaborative effort. The Outreach Clinic has treated 41 seriously ill patients thus far. These people would not have had traditional access to a health care system, or would have done so only on an emergency basis.

Your Turn

"Why are you here, and what do you bring to the table?"
If you have questions, or would like
information on starting a program in
your community, contact:

Dr. Stephen Wagner. Ph.D., FACMPE
Administrator
Sanger Clinic
1001 Blythe Blvd.
Suite 300
Charlotte, NC 28203
(704) 373-0212 • Fax (704) 372-1488

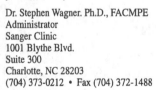

Not Just Meeting Health Care Needs, Exceeding Them.

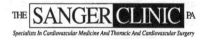

Source: Sanger Clinic (2017).

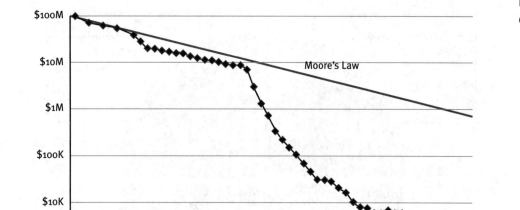

EXHIBIT 12.7
Cost per Genome

Source: National Human Genome Research Institute (2016).

From this breakthrough research, one can now envision the day patients enter the medical practice and present the clinician a thumb drive with their genome on it and say, "Treat me." Implicit in this statement is treat *me*, meaning, specifically me, not some average person between the ages of 18 and 64 who weighs between 100 and 250 pounds. The significant variation among people likely has an important role in the efficacy of treatment (Tsimberidou, Eggermont, and Schilsky 2014). How will medical practices meet that coming reality? Are they even thinking about it? Will medical practices' response depend on the emergence of a generation of physicians that embraces genomics before it becomes reality? All these questions remain unanswered for now, but we can be certain that practices will see technology and the knowledge base related to genomics and precision medicine advance rapidly in the coming years.

Exhibit 12.8 illustrates a model for how one might conceive of precision medicine working in the medical practice. The patient and his or her genetic profile interacts with the provider and the data analytics platform through a connection to the cloud. A specific diagnosis is determined, and all treatment options known at the time are assessed for that patient. As databases containing specific genetic interactions with medications and treatments grow, the ability to pinpoint those treatments will likely increase.

A cohort initiative, which follows a specific group of people of all ages, genders, and backgrounds, called the Precision Medicine Initiative Cohort Program is currently under way by the National Institutes of Health (2016). About 1 million people are involved in the research and will share biological samples of genetic data, dietary behaviors, and lifestyle

EXHIBIT 12.8
Precision Medicine

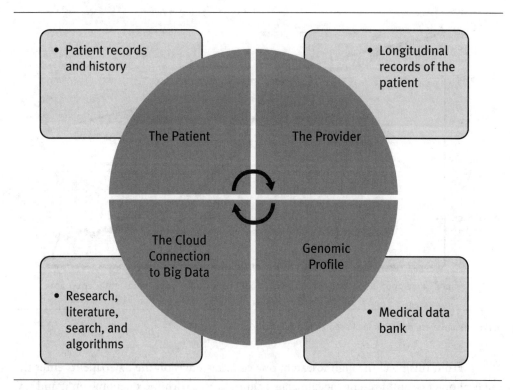

patterns. This information will be linked to their electronic health record to determine how resulting actionable data can be brought to the clinical practice for care delivery. Exhibit 12.9 illustrates the important features of the Precision Medicine Initiative Cohort Program. The medical practice and its management and leaders need to be cognizant of developments in this emerging field, as this and similar studies will likely yield new practice protocols.

THE INTERNET AND SELF-EFFICACY

In the past 50 years, we have seen a dramatic change as society has moved from the Industrial Age to an age of information, and many of the predictions and the ideas presented in Alvin Toffler's 1984 book *The Third Wave* have come to pass.

The Internet has had, and will continue to have, a dramatic impact on the delivery of healthcare. It has democratized healthcare information such that it is widely available to virtually everyone in the society who has access to the Internet, which has led to the ability of the patient and caregivers to be more fully informed and engaged in healthcare decisions. In the past, most consumers of healthcare were almost completely reliant on the provider for this information.

In the 2016 book by the same title, Steve Case discusses the impact the Internet will have on many aspects of our lives, one of those being healthcare. The first wave of the

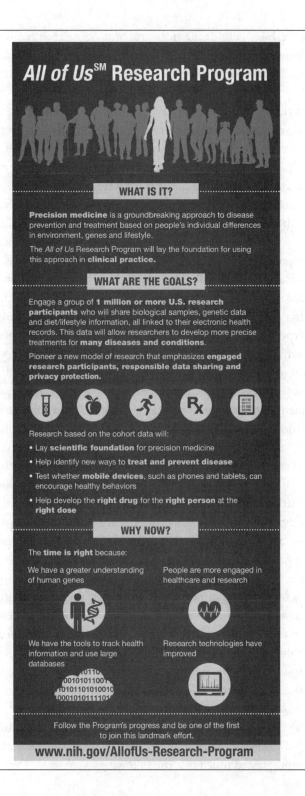

EXHIBIT 12.9
National Institutes
of Health's All of Us
Research Program

Internet was the establishment of the infrastructure. Some may recall the days of dial-up modems, slow connections, no spam, and few e-mails. Of course, those days are gone, and we now see the Internet as heavily integrated into our lives. The second wave is the increasing application of the Internet to the world, which is seen in how we purchase products, how we find our way to locations using interactive maps and navigation apps, the way we obtain information, how we interact with one another, and many other aspects of our daily lives.

However, healthcare is only beginning to adapt to the information age. In the future, the Internet may have the most profound impact on healthcare delivery of any transformation seen to date. This is represented in the third wave, where industries are revolutionized by incorporating and using the Internet in ways not previously seen (Case 2016).

Although the availability of information offers many benefits, it also creates challenges. Healthcare delivery is a complex activity, and often, information found on the Internet is either unreliable or difficult for a nonclinician to interpret, which can lead to misunderstandings and distrust. Enlightened providers help their patients seek information about their conditions by directing them to appropriate sites that offer helpful information about their health needs. They also encourage patients to discuss the information they find and assist in interpreting what it means. Given the time constraints of the volume-driven practice world we have discussed, finding the time to guide patients in this way is difficult. But that situation will need to change because, in the end, a better-informed patient can be a better partner in her care, which will then lead to better outcomes.

Practice management professionals are coming to realize that the healthcare provider cannot bear the entire burden for healthcare outcomes. When discussing many of the new payment models that tie outcomes to reimbursement, providers often express concern that they have no control over patient behavior, which is frequently the primary cause of negative results. Therefore, self-efficacy has become an important issue in practice management. The practice needs to find effective and efficient ways to help patients manage their conditions, especially those of the chronic nature. The more the patient understands and believes in her ability to influence her medical outcome through her efforts, the more likely she is to be successful.

One effective way to support patients in this effort is to use online engagement tools. These tools offer several important features that improve patient engagement and ultimately patient outcomes. The features are often targeted to a specific patient group. Patients volunteer to participate in studies that help delineate the different groups, which increases the likelihood of the successful utilization of the tools.

For example, a study by Solomon, Wagner, and Goes (2012) found that the use of online tools increased patient activation. In this study, patients were given information either online or in a more traditional written form. The information provided to the online group included modules driven by algorithms that met the patient at the educational level appropriate for his or her knowledge regarding the condition. For example, the online diabetes program progressed much like the following:

The patient logs in to the educational program presented to him on diabetes. The patient enters the interactive module and receives this prompt: "Hi, my name is Linda. I understand you have diabetes."

On the basis of the patient's response (for purposes here, that response is affirmative), the module continues: "So, how much do you know about your diabetes?"

The patient selects an option from a menu ranging from very little to significant amounts of knowledge. On the basis of that selection, the interaction continues. If the patient selects an intermediate level of knowledge, the module responds: "That's good; so you know a quite a bit about your condition. Would you like to know more about the A1c level and what it means to your diabetes care?"

If the patient responds "yes," Linda explains in some detail about the A1c level and its importance in the treatment of diabetes.

Online modules of this type have been shown, in this study and others, to be more engaging and to increase the level of activation by the patients who use them. In the Solomon, Wagner, and Goes (2012) research, the traditional written format approach to providing patient educational materials had significantly less impact on engagement. Regular reminders also helped patients follow through with the necessary steps to optimize their care (Lorig et al. 2008; Solomon, Wagner, and Goes 2012).

The number of medical apps and web locations available for smartphones is now well in excess of 1 million. As of July 2013, nearly 900,000 medical applications were offered in Apple's iTunes, and nearly 800,000 were available in Google's Play Store, with Microsoft offering more than 100,000 applications (Aungst 2013). And the number continues to grow, offering an unprecedented amount of new information and tracking and monitoring capabilities, and providing tremendous empowerment to patients to care for themselves. The implications for medical practice are similarly unprecedented, as, for example, physicians can now prescribe medical apps for their patients to assist them in managing their care.

PATIENTS' INTERACTIONS WITH HEALTHCARE PROVIDERS

The Internet allows seemingly unlimited ways for patients to interact with healthcare providers, monitor health status, obtain healthcare information, and exercise increasing control over healthcare consumption. Some of the infrastructure building for provider interactions, however, is being driven by nontraditional providers, or nonproviders, and innovators in other areas of industry. In a report produced by the Silicon Valley Bank (2015), research found that initial public offerings increased dramatically in the healthcare space between 2013 and 2014. Examples of such companies and activities are the following:

◆ Biological pharmaceutical (biopharma) companies' engagement in preclinical and phase I stages of development of new medications increased by 320 percent.

- ◆ Biopharma companies participating in phase 2 and 3 and commercial stages of development increased by 210 percent.

- ◆ Device companies producing new imaging equipment, monitors, and medication delivery systems increased by 500 percent.

- ◆ Companies focused on providing diagnostic services and developing medical diagnostic tools increased by 230 percent.

Silicon Valley is taking a very big interest in life sciences (e.g., CBS News 2016), and all this investment and activity in healthcare will have an impact on the modern medical practice by increasing consumer expectations and demands and by providing numerous alternatives to the traditional office.

NONTRADITIONAL PROVIDERS

The impact of nontraditional providers on the traditional medical practice might best be illustrated with a story.

One day, Steve woke up and did not feel so well—probably nothing serious, but he thought he could use some medical attention. He placed a call to his regular doctor inquiring about the availability of an appointment. "I'm in the neighborhood and I'm not feeling so well today," Steve said. "Would you have time to see me?" The receptionist replied, "I am very sorry, Steve, but we have no appointments until the day after tomorrow." Steve responded, "Wow, I'll either be much worse or better by then. By the way, how much will it cost to see the doctor? I have a high-deductible health plan (HDHP) and have to pay the cost myself for the first few thousand dollars." The receptionist replied, "I'm not really sure what it will cost. It depends, but our typical office visit is approximately $150." Feeling that he really needed some symptomatic relief, Steve headed to his local pharmacy thinking that the pharmacists might be able to recommend something for his symptoms. On arriving, he was surprised to see an urgent care clinic, and further surprised that he could see a provider right away and the cost for the visit would be $80. Steve saw the clinician at the urgent care center and as a courtesy canceled his appointment with his doctor scheduled two days later.

The moral of the story is twofold. The modern medical practice will need to be more responsive to the needs of patients and their desire for immediate service or forgo offering this type of service. In the past, practices have scheduled their resources on their own terms and on the basis of their own needs, not on the demands of patients. In addition, the advent of the HDHP as the dominant form of insurance in the United States is making patients economically sensitive, more like consumers of other goods and services, where price matters.

The tremendous growth in nontraditional provider offerings has come about because these new entrants in the healthcare space see the opportunity in providing more convenient or cost-effective services to the patient by incorporating retail concepts into the delivery of healthcare. Currently, about 3,000 retail clinics are operating in the United States. The largest players are Walgreens, Walmart, and CVS. Virtually all large health systems have developed services in the urgent care format (Gensler 2016). The nontraditional provider limits the services it offers, defines those services carefully, and focuses on convenience to attract customers. As a result, retail clinics are serving ever-increasing numbers of people. One study estimates a 50 percent growth in the number of retail clinics between 2013 and 2018 (Gensler 2016). Modern medical practices must keep this competitive model in mind and seek ways to improve access and convenience. Some recommended steps toward this end include the following:

◆ Extending hours, which may require the addition of providers such as nurse practitioners and physician assistants

◆ Offering clinics for specific services such as sports physicals

◆ Offering virtual care services

◆ Providing clinic hours on weekends and holidays during specified times for established patients

SITE-BASED CORPORATE MEDICAL SERVICES

Corporations often join forces with medical practices to provide on-site medical services to their employees. The organization provides a facility that is staffed by members of the medical practice. Services provided by on-site clinics include some or all of the following:

◆ Employee physicals

◆ Screening programs for early detection of disease

◆ Episodic care for minor illness and injuries

◆ Short and long-term disability follow-up

◆ Chronic disease management

◆ Health education

Site-based clinics offer a number of advantages for the employees as well as the organization. They may be less costly than employees seeking care on their own, and they certainly allow for reductions in the amount of time employees are away from the workplace, enhancing productivity. Employees appreciate the opportunity to seek medical services without missing work and losing income. Many employers allow the employee to seek medical services on-site without docking their pay.

CONCIERGE PRACTICES

Although not a new concept, concierge practice has gained popularity in recent years. The basic aspects of this form of practice involve a monthly or annual fee paid directly to the practice in exchange for a heightened level of service. Such enhanced service may take the following forms:

◆ On-demand phone and virtual consultations

◆ E-mail privileges with the provider

◆ Quick access for on-site services (most concierge practices do not have waiting rooms)

◆ A closely developed relationship with the provider

What makes this level of attention possible is that concierge practices accept a limited number of patients. A typical primary care practice may have as many as 2,500 to 4,000 patients, whereas a concierge practice might have only 400 to 600. These practices usually do not take or bill insurance. However, some insist on the patient having private insurance for services not provided in the concierge practice agreement. Only the services defined in the agreement with the practice are covered under the fees charged.

Although at one time these practices were considered the domain of the wealthy in society, this paradigm is beginning to change. Frustration with the current healthcare system has led more patients to opt for the concierge practice, and more providers are finding satisfaction in practicing this way. As one can imagine, this satisfaction is due to lowered operational complexity, reduced cost, and the reduced patient load, allowing concierge providers to deliver more thorough services and spend more time with their patients than typical providers can. Most providers who have switched to a concierge format do not experience a reduction in income even though they see significantly fewer patients (Leonard 2012).

WEARABLES AND INTERNET-BASED MEDICAL SERVICES

"Many people will wear devices that let them connect to the Internet and will give them feedback on their activities, health and fitness. They will also monitor others (their children or employees, for instance) who are also wearing sensors, or moving in and out of places that have sensors" (Anderson and Rainie 2014). Whereas in the past patients visited the medical practice to be monitored, the Internet and sophisticated devices now allow for that monitoring to be done continuously and without going to the office. Monitoring for heart arrhythmias is an example of this type of monitoring.

TELEHEALTH AND TELEMEDICINE

Telehealth and *telemedicine* are often used synonymously; however, the two terms refer to different activities: *Telehealth* refers to a variety of educational, public health–related, and other services that can be offered in a digital format. *Telemedicine* refers specifically to providing a medical service in a digital format (Sood et al. 2007). *E-health* is another term that is frequently used. For our purposes, the common term *telehealth* is used to refer to all three.

Telehealth offers a number of potential benefits to the medical practice:

- It provides healthcare access for people in remote or rural environments or those who are unable to travel easily.

- It provides a tool for managing long-term chronic illnesses without the need for expensive and time-consuming office visits.

- It can help minimize hospitalizations by addressing nonemergent problems quickly.

- It increases the number of patients who can be seen or treated in a given time.

- It provides a new, innovative servicing practice that is in demand by patients.

- It helps prevent the spread of infectious diseases by allowing patients to be evaluated remotely.

VIRTUAL CARE

In 1962, Hanna-Barbera produced the cartoon show *The Jetsons*. In episode 10, the cartoon showed what is probably the first example of a virtual physician visit, where the son, Elroy, sees the doctor over a video screen. Little did viewers know at that time that the episode was predicting what would become a reality decades later.

Virtual care visits are expected to capture $13.7 billion of healthcare outlays by 2018 and are becoming an increasingly common service provided by medical practices (Wang 2014). If the modern medical practice is not proficient at providing telemedicine services, it could become a significant competitive disadvantage for the practice. The barriers of technology and payment for virtual services have largely been overcome, as both insurers and patients are increasingly comfortable paying for this new utility (Herman 2016). HDHPs make the use of virtual services attractive as well because they are typically less expensive than office visits for the patient.

SOCIAL MEDIA

Social media are having an impact on medical practices that is likely to grow in the coming years. Practices can use social media to perform the following functions:

◆ Communicate with patients. Social media can provide one or more effective tools for reminding patients about needed medical services or reminding them of necessary healthcare compliance issues. A presence on the web can establish the practice as an authority and expert in patient care and provide a social media channel (sometimes called a portal), which allows easy communication for both the patients and the practice; 80 percent of adults use online searches when considering medical treatment (Fox 2011).

◆ Communicate with colleagues by text, direct message, chat, and e-mail. Some practices have internal websites to facilitate interactions and information sharing, such as schedule changes or emergency closings, among providers and other members of the practice.

◆ Communicate with the public, such as to convey up-to-the-minute wait times, health-related events, disasters or other disruptions to the office operations, location changes, new providers and services, and so on.

Social media can also lend positive or negative exposure to the practice. A patient having an unsatisfactory experience with the practice can quickly tweet or post an unfavorable review of the practice online, which can have an influence on existing and potential patients.

Practices considering the use of social media should carefully craft policies and procedures that maintain professionalism and privacy for patients and help practice members understand just how cautious they need to be about what information is shared. Practice managers must be sure that members of the practice are versed in the proper use of this medium (Hayon, Goldsmith, and Garito 2014).

ALTERNATIVE AND COMPLEMENTARY MEDICINE

Alternative medicine refers to medical practices that are not commonly used in Western societies. *Complementary medicine* refers to the combination and concomitant use of alternative and traditional medical practices. We consider both together as the term *alternative and complementary medicine* (CAM). Because few people in the United States forgo conventional treatment altogether, the term *integrative medicine* is often used (Mayo Clinic 2014).

The most common forms of CAM are reported by the National Center for Complementary and Integrative Health (2016) to be the following:

- Natural products, such as herbs and supplements

- Deep breathing

- Yoga, tai chi, and qi gong

- Chiropractic and osteopathic manipulation

- Meditation

- Massage

- Special diets

- Homeopathy

- Progressive relaxation

- Guided imagery

In 2012, $57.7 billion of out-of-pocket costs were spent on CAM practitioners, products, education, and other materials. A substantial portion of that cost was used for more than 300 million visits to CAM providers each year (CMS 2014).

Some medical practices are beginning to incorporate CAM services into traditional medical offerings. However, many are cautious about doing so as, to date, relatively few rigorous research studies have been conducted on CAM practices, although these have been around for thousands of years. Some observers suggest this absence relates more to a knowledge gap than an indictment of CAM, although efficacy and safety must always be a prime concern for the patient (NIH 2013).

BEHAVIORAL ECONOMICS AND CHANGING PATIENT BEHAVIOR

One of the greatest challenges facing healthcare today is getting patients to understand and comply with medical advice. Virtually everyone knows they should not smoke or engage in risky behavior, make good choices about eating, get exercise, and get regular medical checkups. In a study published in 2016, researchers found that a substantial number of cancer cases might be prevented by behavior modification (Song and Giovannucci 2016).

Why don't we do it? Behavioral economics studies show promise in offering solutions to help patients make good decisions and to change negative behaviors. Unlike traditional economics, behavioral economics incorporates psychological insights and neurobiology and takes into consideration that people are not always rational but rather make emotionally based decisions (Thaler 2015).

Medical practitioners and their patients alike fall into decision traps such as the following that prevent them from making good decisions (Plous 1993):

◆ *Overconfidence bias*—Holding unrealistically positive views about oneself and one's performance

◆ *Immediate gratification bias*—Choosing alternatives that offer immediate rewards and that avoid immediate costs; also known as discounting future value

◆ ***Heuristics***—Using rules of thumb to simplify decision making

◆ *Anchoring effect*—Fixating on initial information and ignoring subsequent information

◆ *Selective perception*—Selecting, organizing, and interpreting events on the basis of the decision maker's biased perceptions

◆ *Confirmation bias*—Seeking information that reaffirms past choices and discounts contradictory information

◆ *Framing bias*—Selecting and highlighting certain aspects of a situation while ignoring other aspects

◆ *Availability bias*—Losing decision-making objectivity by focusing on the most recent events

◆ *Representation bias*—Drawing analogies and seeing identical situations when none exist

◆ *Randomness bias*—Creating unfounded meaning out of random events

◆ *Sunk cost errors*—Forgetting that current actions cannot influence past events and relate only to future consequences

◆ *Self-serving bias*—Taking quick credit for successes and blaming outside factors for failures

Heuristics
Mental shortcuts that provide the decision maker with a predetermined conclusion about a situation based on past experiences.

◆   *Hindsight bias*—Mistakenly believing that an event could have been predicted once the actual outcome is known

The medical practice should incorporate many of these behavioral economic ideas into patient care to produce improved outcomes (Thaler and Sunstein 2009). In doing so, it needs to consider several factors of a behavioral economics approach related to patient compliance issues. Society is bombarded constantly by messages from fast-food companies, drink manufacturers, and many other marketing efforts that encourage people to engage in activities that may be detrimental to their health. The healing and treatment efforts undertaken by practitioners are often ineffective against advertisements that are seductive and highly engaging. The behavioral economics factor provides an emotional hook to the activity being encouraged, and flashy advertisements are effective at sharpening that hook. Compare the brochures on display at medical practices—the ones with all the facts and figures—to an ad that features attractive people enjoying a 1,000-calorie sandwich with a 500-calorie drink. Particularly insidious is the fact that the people shown indulging in high-calorie, high-sugar, or high-fat fare are not obese but instead thin, lean, and attractive with a lot of energy: the picture of health. Medical practices must determine a way to combat that imagery by making good choices appealing.

Research shows that a number of behavioral techniques, such as providing incentives, can be effective in helping change patient behavior (Rice 2013). The first is the patient contract. Creating a contract between the provider and the patient to comply with certain instructions on diet or another healthcare issue has been found to be effective for ensuring compliance. The act of signing a contract improves compliance, even though no real consequence results other than the fact that the patient has violated the contract if he or she digresses. This approach has a strong cultural basis that makes it effective.

An example of a contractual intervention is the Ulysses contract. Ulysses, the main character of the Odyssey series, wanted to hear the siren song but knew that it would mean sure death to him and his crew. To avoid this fate, he asked his crew to lash him to the mast of his ship so that he could not be tempted to leave the ship. The crew filled their ears with wax to prevent them hearing the song, and no matter how much Ulysses asked, he was not released from his tethers (Homer 2015).

The point of the Ulysses contract in the patient health context is to make the activity impossible (or at least difficult) to do. An example is to ask one household member to lock snacks in a cabinet and deny access to the person needing to refrain from eating them. Another example is to lock a driver's cell phone in the trunk of the car to prevent texting and driving (Ariely 2009).

Another tool is anti-charity giving. This technique involves the patient or the practice depositing a small amount of money into an account that is earmarked to be given to a charity. The patient selects two charities. One is a charity the patient likes and prefers giving to, and the other is a charity the patient dislikes and would never give to. The patient and provider agree that if the patient follows the instructions regarding a health intervention for a specified period (e.g., discontinue smoking for three months), the money will be donated to the charity chosen by the patient. If the patient fails to comply, the money is given to the charity the patient does not like. This simple technique has been shown to be effective in motivating new behavior (Ariely 2014).

These two ideas may help patients overcome one of the most difficult psychological decision traps, discounting future rewards. All of us have said, "I'll only do this one more time, and then I'll never do it again," only to break the promise and repeat the undesired action. Humans value current rewards more highly and disproportionately than future rewards, making health behaviors particularly difficult to influence. This adjustment also requires behavior change—for example, removing the temptation by not buying the foods that are unhealthful—because willpower lasts only so long. People are likely to engage in unwanted behavior if the temptation remains.

As we move to a new era that rewards outcomes, practices have a greater need to engage patients to comply and improve their health behaviors; these and other behavioral economic techniques may be useful in that effort. Companies are developing techniques and tools based in behavioral economics to engage patients, and several resources are available that practices can share with patients. For example, the American Heart Association (2017) provides information through its website, www.heart.org, and offers ideas on helping patients and families change their eating behaviors through videos that feature good decision making when eating out and selecting foods.

As we have seen in this text, healthcare in general and the medical practice in particular are undergoing dramatic changes. The rate of change is likely to increase, and practice leaders and managers will need to incorporate new ideas and strategies to effectively meet the needs and expectations of the future. Practices that remain stuck in the old paradigms of delivering care may find themselves facing a future fraught with difficulties. Armed with new information and new strategies, practice managers and leaders can actively lead positive change in a new era of medical practice. We must take the initiative to create positive change in our communities and not simply follow what others decide is right.

DISCUSSION QUESTIONS

1. Describe the difference between first-curve and second-curve elements for medical practices.

2. What are some barriers to spreading innovation in the medical practice?

3. List examples in your community of physician practice outreach efforts to connect and serve the community beyond the office.

4. Discuss the importance of genomics to the future of medical practice.

5. Discuss the importance of precision medicine to the future of medical practice.

6. Describe some ways payment for medical services will likely change in the future.

7. How do you think the role of the medical practice manager will change in the future?

8. How would you describe the future of practice management?

REFERENCES

Aaron, H. J. 2015. "Five Years Old, Going on Ten: The Future of the Affordable Care Act." Published March 27. www.brookings.edu/blog/health360/2015/03/27/five -years-old-going-on-ten-the-future-of-the-affordable-care-act.

Agency for Healthcare Research and Quality (AHRQ). 2017. "Healthcare Cost and Utilization Project (HCUP)." Reviewed May. www.ahrq.gov/research/data/hcup/index.html.

American Heart Association. 2017. "5 Easy Ways to Find Healthier Options at the Grocery Store." Updated January 10. https://healthyforgood.heart.org/Eat-smart/Articles /5-Easy-Ways-to-Find-Healthier-Options-at-the-Grocery-Store.

Anderson, J., and L. Rainie. 2014. "The Internet of Things Will Thrive by 2025." Published May 14. www.pewinternet.org/2014/05/14/internet-of-things.

Ariely, D. 2014. "A Beginner's Guide to Irrational Behavior." Course presented at Duke University.

———. 2009. *Predictably Irrational: The Hidden Forces That Shape Our Decisions*. New York: HarperCollins.

Aungst, T. 2013. "Apple App Store Still Leads Android in Total Number of Medical Apps." Published July 12. www.imedicalapps.com/2013/07/apple-android-medical-app.

Ballotpedia. 2016. "2016 Presidential Candidates on Healthcare." Accessed August 9. https://ballotpedia.org/2016_presidential_candidates_on_healthcare.

Baruchin, A. 2015. *More Seniors, Fewer Geriatricians: Shifting Demographics Pose Challenges for Medical Education*. Washington, DC: Association of American Medical Colleges.

Bastian, H., P. Glasziou, and L. Chalmers. 2010. "Seventy-Five Trials and Eleven Systematic Reviews a Day: How Will We Ever Keep Up?" Published September 21. http://journals. plos.org/plosmedicine/article?id=10.1371/journal.pmed.1000326.

Brotherton, S. E., and S. I. Etzel. 2014. "Graduate Medical Education, 2013–2014." *Journal of the American Medical Association* 312 (22): 2427–45.

Case, S. 2016. *The Third Wave: An Entrepreneur's Vision of the Future*. New York: Simon & Schuster.

CBS News. 2016. "Billionaire Sean Parker Donates $250 Million to Cancer Research." Published April 13. www.cbsnews.com/videos/billionaire-sean-parker-donates-250-million -to-cancer-research.

Centers for Disease Control and Prevention (CDC). 2017a. "Ambulatory Care Use and Physician Office Visits." Updated March 31. www.cdc.gov/nchs/fastats/physician-visits.htm.

———. 2017b. "Division of Community Health (DCH): Making Healthy Living Easier." Updated June 13. www.cdc.gov/nccdphp/dch/index.htm.

———. 2017c. "Transatlantic Taskforce on Antimicrobial Resistance (TATFAR)." Updated June 24. www.cdc.gov/drugresistance/tatfar.

———. 1999. "Ten Great Public Health Achievements—United States, 1900–1999." Published April 2. www.cdc.gov/mmwr/preview/mmwrhtml/00056796.htm.

Centers for Medicare & Medicaid Services (CMS). 2014. "National Health and Expenditure Data." Updated May 5. www.cms.gov/Research-Statistics-Data-and-systems/ Statistics-Trends-and-reports/NationalHealthExpendData.

Chernecky, C., and B. Berger. 2013. *Laboratory Tests and Diagnostic Procedures*, 6th ed. Philadelphia, PA: Saunders.

CNN. 2015. "Charity Hospital: 10 Years Later." Accessed June 2, 2017. www.cnn.com/videos /us/2015/08/29/hurricane-katrina-anniversary-new-orleans-charity-hospital-gupta- dnt-ac.cnn/video/playlists/hurricane-katrina-10-years-later.

Collins, F. S., and H. Varmus. 2015. "A New Initiative on Precision Medicine." *New England Journal of Medicine* 372: 793–95.

Densen, P. 2011. "Challenges and Opportunities Facing Medical Education." *Transactions of the American Clinical and Climatological Association* 122: 48–58.

Farr, C. 2017. "Silicon Valley Is Trumpeting A.I. as the Cure for the Medical Industry, but Doctors Are Skeptical." Published May 27. www.cnbc.com/2017/05/27/ai-medicine-doctors-skeptical.html.

Fineline Foundation. 2016. "Cost of Violent Crimes." Accessed July 12. www.fineline foundation.org/cost-of-violent-crimes.

Fox, S. 2011. "The Social Life of Health Information, 2011." Published May 12. www.pew internet.org/2011/05/12/the-social-life-of-health-information-2011.

Gensler. 2016. "Retail Health, Retail Medicine and the New Healthcare Experience." Accessed July 14. www.gensler.com/research-insight/in-focus/retail-health -retail-medicine-the-new-healthcare-experience.

Goldman, T. R. 2012. "Eliminating Fraud and Abuse." Published July 31. www.healthaffairs. org/healthpolicybriefs/brief.php?brief_id=72.

Government Publishing Office (GPO). 2010. "Public Law 111-148—Mar. 23, 2010." Published March 23. www.gpo.gov/fdsys/pkg/PLAW-111publ148/pdf/PLAW-111publ148.pdf.

Hanna-Barbera Productions. 1962. "Uniblab." *The Jetsons*. Broadcast November 25. Story by B. E. Blitzer, teleplay by T. Benedict.

Hayon, K., T. Goldsmith, and L. Garito. 2014. *A Guide to Social Media for Physician Practices*. Boston: Massachusetts Medical Society.

Health Resources and Services Administration (HRSA). 2016. "Health Professional Shortage Areas (HPSAs)." Reviewed October. https://bhw.hrsa.gov/shortage-designation/hpsas.

———. 2012. "Rural Guide to Federal Health Professions Funding." Published May. www. hrsa.gov/ruralhealth/pdf/ruralhealthprofessionsguidance.pdf.

Hegwer, L. R. 2016. "6 Business Imperatives for Population Health Management." *Healthcare Executive* 31 (4): 16–20.

Heineman, M., and S. Froemke (directors). 2012. *Escape Fire: The Fight to Rescue American Healthcare*. Documentary film. Aisle C Productions and Our Time Projects.

Herman, B. 2016. "Virtual Reality: More Insurers Are Embracing Telehealth." Published February 20. www.modernhealthcare.com/article/20160220/MAGAZINE/302209980.

Homer. 2015. *The Odyssey*. Translated by S. Butler. Seattle, WA: CreateSpace.

Illumina. 2016. "Sequencing Kits for Every Lab." Accessed February 4. www.illumina.com/content/illumina-marketing/amr/en_US/products/sequencing-kits.html.

Institute of Medicine (IOM). 2011. *The Future of Nursing: Leading Change, Advancing Health*. Washington, DC: National Academies Press.

Jost, T. 2016. "Affordability: The Most Urgent Health Reform Issue for Ordinary Americans." Published February 29. http://healthaffairs.org/blog/2016/02/29/affordability-the-most-urgent-health-reform-issue-for-ordinary-americans.

Kaiser Family Foundation (KFF). 2017. "New Dashboard Provides Key Data on the U.S. Health System." Published May 24. http://kff.org/health-costs/press-release/new-dashboard-provides-key-data-on-u-s-health-system-quality-spending-access-outcomes.

Kindig, D. 1997. *Purchasing Population Health: Paying for Results*. Ann Arbor, MI: University of Michigan Press.

Kindig, D., and G. Stoddart. 2003. "What Is Population Health?" *American Journal of Public Health* 93 (3): 380–83.

Leonard, D. 2012. "Is Concierge Medicine the Future of Health Care?" Published November 29. www.bloomberg.com/news/articles/2012-11-29/is-concierge-medicine-the-future-of-health-care.

Livingston, G., and A. Brown. 2017. "Intermarriage in the U.S. 50 Years After Loving v. Virginia." Published May 18. www.pewsocialtrends.org/2017/05/18/intermarriage-in-the-u-s-50-years-after-loving-v-virginia.

Lorig, K. R., P. L. Ritter, D. D. Laurent, and K. Plant. 2008. "The Internet-Based Arthritis Self-Management Program: A One-Year Randomized Trial for Patients with Arthritis or Fibromyalgia." *Arthritis Care & Research* 59 (7): 1009–17.

Manchanda, R. 2014. "What Makes Us Sick? Look Upstream." Filmed August. www.ted.com/talks/rishi_manchanda_what_makes_us_get_sick_look_upstream.

Maney, K. 2017. "How Artificial Intelligence Will Cure America's Sick Health Care System." Published May 24. www.newsweek.com/2017/06/02/ai-cure-america-sick-health-care-system-614583.html.

Mayo Clinic. 2014. "Complementary and Alternative Medicine." Published January 24. www.mayoclinic.org/tests-procedures/complementary-alternative-medicine/basics/definition/prc-20021745.

McCollister, K. E., M. T. French, and H. Fang. 2010. "The Cost of Crime to Society: New Crime-Specific Estimates for Policy and Program Evaluation." *Drug and Alcohol Dependence* 108 (1–2): 98–109.

Morris, Z. S., S. Wooding, and J. Grant. 2011. "The Answer Is 17 Years, What Is the Question: Understanding Time Lags in Translational Research." *Journal of the Royal Society of Medicine* 104 (12): 510–20.

Motel, S. 2015. "Opinions on Obamacare Remain Divided Along Party Lines as Supreme Court Hears New Challenge." Published March 4. www.pewresearch.org/fact-tank/2015/03/04/opinions-on-obamacare-remain-divided-along-party-lines-as-supreme-court-hears-new-challenge.

National Center for Complementary and Integrative Health. 2016. "Complementary, Alternative, or Integrative Health: What's in a Name?" Modified June 28. https://nccih.nih.gov/health/integrative-health.

National Human Genome Research Institute. 2016. "The Cost of Sequencing the Human Genome." Accessed February 4. www.genome.gov/sequencingcosts.

National Institutes of Health. 2016. "Precision Medicine Initiative Cohort Program." Accessed July 14. www.nih.gov/precision-medicine-initiative-cohort-program.

———. 2013. "Complementary and Alternative Medicine." Updated March 29. https://report.nih.gov/NIHfactsheets/ViewFactSheet.aspx?csid=85.

Nature. 2010. "Human Genome at Ten: The Sequence Explosion." *Nature* 464: 670–71.

Pavia, A. T. 2007. "Germs on a Plane: Aircraft, International Travel, and the Global Spread of Disease." *Journal of Infectious Diseases* 195 (5): 621–22.

Plous, S. 1993. *The Psychology of Judgement and Decision Making*. New York: McGraw-Hill.

Rabin, R. C. 2014. "15-Minute Visit Takes a Toll on the Doctor-Patient Relationship." Published April 21. http://khn.org/news/15-minute-doctor-visits.

Radley, D. C., and C. Schoen. 2012. "Geographic Variation in Access to Care—the Relationship with Quality." *New England Journal of Medicine* 367: 3–6.

Reardon, S. 2014. "Antibiotic Resistance Sweeping Developing World." *Nature* 509 (7499): 141–42.

Resnik, D. B. 2007. "Responsibility for Health: Personal, Social, and Environmental." *Journal of Medical Ethics* 33 (8): 444–45.

Rettner, R. 2013. "Hurricane Sandy's Toll on Health." Published October 28. www.livescience. com/40754-hurricane-sandy-health-impact.html.

Rhoades, D., K. McFarland, W. Johnson, and A. Finch. 2001. "Speaking and Interrupting During Primary Care Office Visits." *Family Medicine* 33 (7): 528–32.

Rice, T. 2013. "The Behavioral Economics of Health and Healthcare." *Annual Review of Public Health* 34: 431–47.

Robert Wood Johnson Foundation (RWJF). 2016. "Building a Culture of Health." Accessed March 31. www.rwjf.org/en/how-we-work/building-a-culture-of-health.html.

Rogers, E. M. 2003. *Diffusion of Innovations*, 5th ed. New York: Free Press.

Rudwitz, R., D. Rowland, and A. Shartzer. 2006. "Healthcare in New Orleans Before and After Hurricane Katrina." *Health Affairs* 25 (5): w393–w406.

Sampson, D., and M. Mueller. 2017. "Integrating Behavioral Health into Rural Primary Care Clinics Utilizing a Telehealth Model." In *Career Paths in Telemental Health*, edited by M. Maheu, K. Drude, and S. Wright, 277–83. New York: Springer.

Sanger Clinic. 2017. "Healthy Families, Healthy Communities." Charlotte, NC: Sanger Clinic.

Silicon Valley Bank. 2015. "Trends in Healthcare Investments and Exits 2015." Santa Clara, CA: Silicon Valley Bank.

Solomon, M., S. Wagner, and J. Goes. 2012. "Effects of a Web-Based Intervention for Adults with Chronic Conditions on Patient Activation: Online Randomized Controlled Trial." *Journal of Medical Internet Research* 14 (1): 1–13.

Song, M., and E. Giovannucci. 2016. "Preventable Incidence and Mortality of Carcinoma Associated with Lifestyle Factors Among White Adults in the United States." Published September. http://oncology.jamanetwork.com/article.aspx?articleid=2522371.

Sood, S., V. Mbarika, S. Jugoo, R. Dookhy, C. Doarn, N. Prakash, and R. Merrell. 2007. "What Is Telemedicine? A Collection of 104 Peer-Reviewed Perspectives and Theoretical Underpinnings." *Telemedicine and e-Health* 13 (5): 573–90.

St. John, C. 2017. "Acid River Activity." Accessed May 26. www.leadershipchallenge.com/resource/acid-river-activity.aspx.

Storrs, C. 2016. "As Zika Reaches US Shores, States and Cities Struggle to Respond." *Health Affairs* 35 (7): 1156–59.

Thaler, R. 2015. *Misbehaving: The Making of Behavioral Economics.* New York: W. W. Norton.

Thaler, R., and C. Sunstein. 2009. *Nudge: Improving Decisions About Health, Wealth, and Happiness.* New York: Penguin.

Toffler, A. 1984. *The Third Wave.* New York: Bantam.

Tsimberidou, A., A. Eggermont, and R. Schilsky. 2014. "Precision Cancer Medicine: The Future Is Now, Only Better." *American Society of Clinical Oncology Education Book* 34: 61–69.

US Census Bureau. 2015. "Census Bureau Reports at Least 350 Languages Spoken in U.S. Homes." Published November 3. www.census.gov/newsroom/press-releases/2015/cb15-185.html.

Wade, D. T., and P. W. Halligan. 2004. "Do Biomedical Models of Illness Make for Good Healthcare Systems?" *British Medical Journal* 329: 1398–401.

Wagner, S. L. 2003. "Defining the ACMPE Fellow." *College View* (Fall): 27–30.

Wang, H. 2014. "Virtual Healthcare Will Revolutionize the Industry, if We Let It." Published April 3. www.forbes.com/sites/ciocentral/2014/04/03/virtual-health-care-visits-will-revolutionize-the-industry-if-we-let-it/2/#1ec2a8ef3c35.

World Health Organization (WHO). 2017. "Antibiotic Resistance." Published May. www.who.int/antimicrobial-resistance/en.

APPENDIX

The following are lists of recommended resources applicable to practice management. Of course, any of hundreds more organizations may be of interest to the practice manager, so explore and find the organizations and sites that serve you best.

JOURNALS AND MAGAZINES

American Journal of Health Behavior
American Journal of Health Promotion
American Journal of Health Studies
American Journal of Preventive Medicine
American Journal of Public Health
Australian and New Zealand Journal of Public Health
Frontiers of Health Services Management
Health Affairs
Health Care Management Review
Health Care Supervisor
Health Education and Behavior
Health Education Research
Health Policy
Health Promotion International
Health Psychology
Health Services Management Research

Health Values
Healthcare Executive
Hospital & Health Services Administration (see *Journal of Healthcare Management*)
Journal of Behavioral Medicine
Journal of Disaster Studies, Policy and Management
Journal of Emergency Management
Journal of Family and Community Health
Journal of Healthcare Management
Journal of Homeland Security and Emergency Management
Journal of Public Health Management and Practice
Journal of School Health
Journal of the American Medical Association
MGMA Connection
Milbank Quarterly
Modern Healthcare
New England Journal of Medicine
Public Health Reports
Social Science & Medicine

PROFESSIONAL ASSOCIATIONS AND ORGANIZATIONS

American Association of Homes and Services for the Aging (www.aahsa.org)
American Association of Integrated Healthcare Delivery Systems (www.aaihds.org)
American Association for Physician Leadership (www.physicianleaders.org)
American College of Healthcare Executives (www.ache.org)
American College of Physician Executives (www.acpe.org)
American Health Care Association (www.ahca.org)
American Health Information Management Association (www.ahima.org)
American Managed Behavioral Healthcare Association (www.ambha.org)
American Medical Association (www.ama-assn.org)
American Medical Group Association (www.amga.org)
American Organization of Nurse Executives (www.aone.org)
American Public Health Association (www.apha.org)
American Society for Healthcare Human Resources Administrators (www.ashhra.org)
American Society for Healthcare Risk Management (www.ashrm.org)
Association for Health Services Research (www.ahsr.org)
Association of University Programs in Healthcare Administration (www.aupha.org)
Blue Cross and Blue Shield Association (www.bluecares.com)
Center for Healthcare Ethics (www.chce.org)
Commission on Accreditation of Rehabilitation Facilities (www.carf.org)
Council of Teaching Hospitals and Health Systems (www.aamc.org/coth)

Healthcare Financial Management Association (www.hfma.org)

Healthcare Information and Management Systems Society (www.himss.org)

Health Insurance Association of America (www.hiaa.org)

The Joint Commission (www.jointcommission.org)

Medical Group Management Association and American College of Medical Practice
      Executives (www.mgma.com)

National Association for Home Care (www.nahc.org)

National Association of Managed Care Physicians (www.accme.org)

National Hospice Organization (www.nho.org)

Robert Wood Johnson Foundation (www.rwjf.org)

Society for Healthcare Strategy and Market Development (www.shsmd.org)

DATA SETS AND DATABASES

Dartmouth Atlas of Health Care (www.dartmouthatlas.org)

Healio (www.healio.com)

HealthSTAR (http://igm.nlm.nih.gov)

Medline (www.nlm.nih.gov)

Medlink National Directory (www.biostats.com)

National Institutes of Health (www.nih.gov)

National Library of Medicine (www.nlm.nih.gov)

US Department of Health & Human Services (www.hhs.gov)

FOUNDATIONS AND OTHER NOT-FOR-PROFIT ORGANIZATIONS

Center for Health Care Strategies (www.chcs.org)

Center for Studying Health System Change (www.hschange.com)

Commonwealth Fund (www.cmwf.org)

Foundation for Informed Medical Decision Making (www.dartmouth.edu/dms/cecs/fimdm)

Healthgrades (www.healthgrades.com)

Institute of Medicine (www.nas.edu/iom)

Leapfrog Group (www.leapfroggroup.org)

Medical Outcomes Trust (www.outcomes-trust.org)

GOVERNMENT AGENCIES

Agency for Healthcare Research and Quality (www.ahrq.gov)

Centers for Medicare & Medicaid Services (www.cms.gov)

US Department of Veterans Affairs (www.va.gov)

Health Resources and Services Administration (www.hrsa.gov)

National Institute for Health and Care Excellence (www.nice.org.uk)

GLOSSARY

Additional useful terms may be found at the MGMA Knowledge Center of the Medical Group Management Association (www.mgma.com/Libraries/Assets/Practice%20 Resources/Tools/Glossary-of-terms-used-in-medical-practice-management.pdf).

Account. A record of financial transactions; usually refers to a specific category or type, such as travel expense account or purchase account.

Accountant. A person who is trained to prepare and maintain financial records.

Accounting. A system for keeping score in business, using dollars.

Accounting period. The time over which profits are calculated. Normal accounting periods are months, quarters, and years (fiscal or calendar).

Accounts payable. Amounts owed by the practice for the goods or services it has purchased from outside suppliers.

Accounts receivable. Amounts owed to the practice by its customers.

Accrual accounting system. An accounting system that records revenues and expenses at the time the transaction occurs, not at the time cash changes hands.

Ambulatory care. Healthcare services provided to patients on an outpatient basis, rather than by admission to a hospital or another healthcare facility.

Analytical. Decision-making style in which the decision maker gives careful consideration to the uniqueness of situations. This style is typically used when tolerance for ambiguity is high and decision makers are rational in their thinking.

Ancillary services. Range of services provided to support the work of a primary physician, classified into three categories: diagnostic, therapeutic, and custodial.

Asset. Item of value owned by a business. May be a physical property, such as a building; a physical object, such as a stock certificate; or a right, such as the right to use a patented process.

Attitude. Mental state indicating level of readiness.

Audit. A careful review of financial records to verify their accuracy.

Bad debt. Amount owed to a practice that will not be paid.

Balance sheet. A statement of the financial position of a practice at a specific time, often at the close of business on the last day of the month, quarter, or year.

Behavior. How an individual acts, especially toward others.

Breakeven point. The amount of revenue from sales that equals the amount of expense. Often expressed as the number of units that must be sold to produce revenues equal to expenses. Sales above the breakeven point produce a profit; sales below produce a loss.

Capital. Resources, usually cash available to invest or use for operations.

Capitation. Payment to the provider as a fixed amount for each patient he or she agrees to treat, regardless of whether or not those patients seek care. Payment is typically based on a set number of dollars per member per month.

Cash accounting system. Method of accounting by which income is recognized as it is received and expenses are recognized when they are paid.

Cash flow. The amount of cash generated by business operations, which usually differs from profits. Calculated as operating revenue minus operating cost.

Certificate of need (CON). Approval issued by a governmental body to an individual or organization proposing to construct or modify a health facility or to offer a new or different service.

Certification. A voluntary system of standards that practitioners meet to demonstrate accomplishment or ability in their profession. Certification standards are generally set by nongovernmental agencies or associations.

Chart of accounts. A listing of all the accounts or categories into which business transactions are classified and recorded. Each account is assigned a number, and transactions are coded by this number for computer analysis and manipulation.

Chronic illness. Diseases characterized by one or more of the following criteria: They are permanent; leave residual disability; are caused by nonreversible pathological alteration; require special training of the patient for rehabilitation; or require a long period of supervision, observation, or care.

Credit. An accounting entry on the right or bottom of a balance sheet usually reflecting an increase in liabilities or capital or a reduction in assets.

Current asset. An asset that is expected to be turned into cash within a year, including cash, marketable securities, accounts receivable, and inventory.

Dashboard. Similar to a car's dashboard, provides a medical practice integrated and consistently presented operational data for decision making.

Depreciation. An expense that is intended to reflect the loss in value of a fixed asset.

Environmental factors. Forces that influence the business but are external to the business itself, such as public policy, regulations, and economic conditions.

Equity. The owners' share of a business.

Expenditure. Occurs when an item is acquired for a business, an asset is purchased, salaries are paid, and so on.

Expense. An expenditure that is chargeable against revenue during an accounting period, resulting in the reduction of an asset.

Fixed cost. A cost that does not change as sales volume changes (in the short run). Fixed costs normally include such items as rent, depreciation, interest, and any salaries unaffected by ups and downs in sales.

Goal. A specific target that an individual or a company tries to achieve.

Governance. A system of policies and procedures designed to facilitate oversight of the management of the enterprise. Serves as the foundation of how the practice will behave, compete, and document its actions.

Health Insurance Portability and Accountability Act (HIPAA). Legislation covering many aspects of patient privacy and the sharing of private health information.

Heuristics. Mental shortcuts that provide the decision maker with a predetermined conclusion about a situation based on past experiences.

Interest. A charge assessed for the use of money.

Inventory. The supply or stock of goods and products that a practice has for sale.

Liability. An amount owed by a practice to an individual or entity.

Licensure. A mandatory system of state-imposed standards that practitioners must meet to practice a given profession.

Medicare Advantage. Program established by the Balanced Budget Act of 1997 whereby an eligible individual may elect to receive Medicare benefits through a managed care organization. Formerly called Medicare+Choice and still informally known as Medicare Part C.

Medigap. A supplemental health insurance policy sold by private insurance companies that is designed to pay for healthcare costs and services not paid for by Medicare or any private health insurance benefits.

Organizational change. A process by which the organization evolves to help it adapt to a new set of environmental and competitive factors.

Organizational dynamics. The script for the organization's human capital, or the ways in which individuals and processes interact in the company.

Paradigm shift. A change in the way a practice views its business.

Pay for performance (P4P). Mechanism whereby providers are reimbursed on the basis of their level of success in meeting specific performance measures.

Point-of-service (POS) plan. A health insurance plan in which members do not have to choose how to receive services until they need them. The most common use of the term applies to a plan that enrolls each member in both an HMO (or HMO-like) system and an indemnity plan. These plans provide different benefits, depending on whether the member chooses to use plan providers or go outside the plan for services.

Post. To enter a business transaction into a journal, a ledger, or another financial record.

Preferred provider organization (PPO). A health insurance plan with an established provider network ("preferred providers") that covers maximum benefits when members visit a preferred provider.

Present value. A concept that compares the value of money available in the future with the value of money in hand today. Used to analyze investment opportunities that have a future payoff. For example, $78.35 invested today in a 5 percent savings account will grow to $100 in five years. Thus, the present value of $100 received in five years is $78.35.

Profit. The amount left over when expenses are subtracted from revenues. Also referred to as *income*, *net income*, or *earnings*.

Resource-based relative value scale (RBRVS). Means by which to determine the rate at which Medicare reimburses physicians on a fee-for-service basis. Calculated using the costs of physician labor, practice overhead, materials, and liability insurance, with the resulting amounts adjusted for geographical differences.

Retained earnings. Profits not distributed to shareholders as dividends; the accumulation of a practice's profits less any dividends paid out. Retained earnings are not spendable cash.

Return on investment. A measure of the effectiveness and efficiency with which managers use the resources available to them, expressed as a percentage.

Revenue. The amounts received by or due to a practice for goods or services it provides to customers. Receipts are cash revenues; revenues may also be represented by accounts receivable.

Risk. The possibility of loss, inherent in all business activities. High risk requires high return. All business decisions must consider the amount of risk involved.

Stakeholder. An individual or a group that has a vested interest in the practice.

Stock. A certificate (may be electronic or another type of record) that indicates ownership of a portion of a corporation; a share of stock.

Strategy. The science of business planning whereby an organization plans its approach to achieving its goals.

SWOT. A strategic planning technique that systematically looks at a company's strengths, weaknesses, opportunities, and threats.

Telemedicine. Involves the use of electronic communication and information technologies to provide or support clinical care at a distance.

Transformational leadership. A form of leadership intended to create change in individuals and the medical practice by encouraging valuable and positive change in followers and promoting growth in both followers and leaders.

Utilization review. An organized procedure carried out through committees to review admissions, duration of stay, and professional services furnished and to evaluate the medical necessity of those services and promote their most efficient use.

Values. The beliefs and guidelines an individual uses to make choices when confronted with a situation.

Variable cost. A cost that changes as sales or production change. If a business is producing nothing and selling nothing, the variable cost should be zero.

INDEX

Note: Italicized page locators refer to figures or tables in exhibits.

Cultural competence: diversity and, 337

Culture: aligning with positive behavior, 51–52; defined, 50; of health, underlying principles in, 349; organization and, 50–52, *51*

Current assets: defined, 198

Current Procedural Terminology (CPT), 30, 176

CVS: health clinics in, 361

Cyber breaches, 93–94

Cyber criminals, 95, 326

Cyber insurance, 328

Cybersecurity threats, 326–28; common cyber risks, 327; practice responsibilities in face of cyberattack, 327–28

Cycle of practice development, *126*

Damages: malpractice insurance caps and, 118

Dartmouth Atlas, 8, 379

Dashboards, 78, 204

Data: breaches of, 93–94, 95, 328; cloud service and loss of, 91; lack of utility of, 305; population health and, 348; population health management and, 81, 85; process improvement projects, 296; transformation of, into application, 345, *345*

Data analytics: artificial intelligence and, 345–46; quality improvement and, 305

Data breach protection insurance, 117

Data management: effective medical practice operations and, 77; important functions of, 77–78

Data warehouse, 77

Days of receivables outstanding, *206*

Debt obligations: corporations and, 44

Decision support: data management and, 77

Deductibles, 156, 157. *See also* Coinsurance; Copayments; Health insurance premiums; High-deductible health plans (HDHPs); average, four plan categories for healthcare exchanges, 159, *160*; CDHPs and, 30

Defects: Lean and, 293

Deming, W. Edwards, 2, 285, 290

Deming Institute: resource for improvement, 236

Demographic forces of change, 337

Denial: alcoholic or addicted physicians and, 264

Denial stage: in change process, 233

Denied claims: financial metrics and, 203–4

Depreciation, 196

Depression stage: in change process, 233

Determinants of health, 21, *22, 29*

Diabetes, 20, 21

Diagnosis: technology-assisted, 346, *347*

Dialogue: importance of, in medical practice, 352

Dictating (or direct) leadership style, 252

Digital photography: example of paradigm shift, 27

Digitization of healthcare, 25–26, 337–38

Direct costs, 189

Direct mail: as example of high-involvement advertising media, 147

Disaster preparedness: CERT program and, 322

Disaster scenarios, special situations, 322–28; bioterrorism, 323–24; cybersecurity threats, 326–28; pandemics, 324–26; terrorism, 322–23

DiSC, 241, 259

Discounted fee-for-service, 155

Discounting future value, 366

Discrimination: interview questions and basis for, 222

Discussion-based emergency preparedness exercises, *321*

Disease burden: changing, 19–20

Disease management, 169

Disruptive behaviors: addressing, 263; spectrum of, *264*

Diversity, 25; cultural competence and, 337; dimensions of, 242; inclusion and, 241–42; leadership and issues with, 269–71; in thinking, openness to, 271; workforce, 26

DMAIC methodology: Six Sigma and, 303–4

Doctors of osteopathy (DOs), 13

"Don't ask, don't tell" policies: abandoning, as part of upstreaming, 352

DOs. *See* Doctors of osteopathy

Double taxation: avoiding, 201

"Draw-a-pig" exercise: emergency preparedness planning and, 316; red bead experiment and, 292–93; variation, QI, and stages in, 291–92, *292*

Drucker, Peter, 39, 50, 151, 215, 260

Dual eligibility, 172

Dyad leadership agreement: development template for, *258*

Dyad leadership model: in practice management, 256–60

ABOUT THE AUTHOR

Stephen L. Wagner, PhD, FACHE, FACMPE, FACEM, FACHT, has been active in the field of healthcare as an executive, a teacher, and a researcher for more than four decades. He recently retired from a long career as a medical practice administrator, including many years as the senior administrator of the Sanger Clinic, where he was instrumental in the creation of the Sanger Heart and Vascular Institute.

Dr. Wagner is now an executive in residence and assistant professor in the School of Health and Medical Sciences at Seton Hall University. In addition, his work as an expert on the US healthcare system and its transformation focuses on managing the difficult process of changing the healthcare organization to meet the challenges of the future.

He earned his master's degree in healthcare fiscal management from the Wisconsin School of Business at the University of Wisconsin–Madison and his doctorate in healthcare public policy analysis from the University of Louisville College of Business.